Solutions for Complex Upper Extremity Trauma

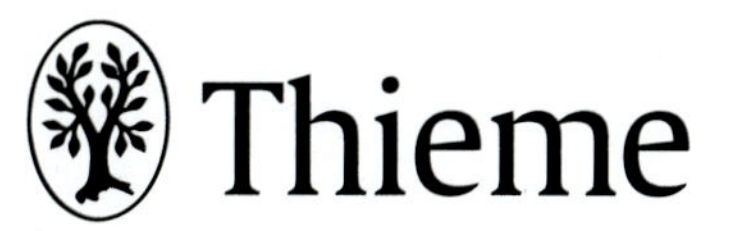

Solutions for Complex Upper Extremity Trauma

Edited by

David M. Dines, MD
Professor of Orthopedic Surgery
Albert Einstein College of Medicine
Senior Attending Physician
Sports Medicine and Shoulder Service
The Hospital for Special Surgery
New York, New York

Dean G. Lorich, MD
Assistant Professor of Orthopedic Surgery
Weill College of Medicine of Cornell University
The Hospital for Special Surgery
New York, New York

David L. Helfet, MD
Professor of Orthopedic Surgery
Weill College of Medicine of Cornell University
The Hospital for Special Surgery
New York, New York

Thieme
New York · Stuttgart

Thieme Medical Publishers, Inc.
333 Seventh Ave.
New York, NY 10001

Editor: Esther Gumpert
Managing Editor: J. Owen Zurhellen IV
Vice President, Production and Electronic Publishing: Anne T. Vinnicombe
Production Editor: Heidi Pongratz, Maryland Composition
Vice President, International Marketing: Cornelia Schulze
Chief Financial Officer: Peter van Woerden
President: Brian D. Scanlan
Compositor: Thomson Digital
Printer: Everbest

Library of Congress Cataloging-in-Publication Data
Solutions for complex upper extremity trauma / [edited by] David M. Dines, Dean G. Lorich, David L. Helfet.
p. ; cm.
Includes bibliographical references and index.
ISBN 978-1-58890-504-8 1. Arm—Wounds and injuries. 2. Arm—Surgery. 3. Orthopedic surgery. I. Dines, David M. II. Lorich, Dean G. III. Helfet, David.
[DNLM: 1. Arm Injuries—diagnosis. 2. Arm Injuries—surgery. 3. Bones of Upper Extremity—injuries. 4. Orthopedic Procedures—methods. WE 805 S689 2008]
RD557.S64 2008
617.5'74044—dc22
2007038563

Important note: Medical knowledge is ever-changing. As new research and clinical experience broaden our knowledge, changes in treatment and drug therapy may be required. The authors and editors of the material herein have consulted sources believed to be reliable in their efforts to provide information that is complete and in accord with the standards accepted at the time of publication. However, in view of the possibility of human error by the authors, editors, or publisher of the work herein or changes in medical knowledge, neither the authors, editors, nor publisher, nor any other party who has been involved in the preparation of this work, warrants that the information contained herein is in every respect accurate or complete, and they are not responsible for any errors or omissions or for the results obtained from use of such information. Readers are encouraged to confirm the information contained herein with other sources. For example, readers are advised to check the product information sheet included in the package of each drug they plan to administer to be certain that the information contained in this publication is accurate and that changes have not been made in the recommended dose or in the contraindications for administration. This recommendation is of particular importance in connection with new or infrequently used drugs.

Some of the product names, patents, and registered designs referred to in this book are in fact registered trademarks or proprietary names even though specific reference to this fact is not always made in the text. Therefore, the appearance of a name without designation as proprietary is not to be construed as a representation by the publisher that it is in the public domain.

Printed in China

5 4 3 2 1

ISBN: 978-1-58890-504-8

Dedication

To our respective families, spouses, children, and parents, whose love and support make this book and all other aspects of our professional careers possible.

To our mentors, teachers, and colleagues, who have inspired us to be the best surgeons and educators that we could be, allowing us to share our knowledge with others.

To our students, residents, and fellows, who by their thirst for learning have stimulated us to be better orthopedic surgeons and educators.

To our patients, who may benefit from the current knowledge that we have imparted in this text and who always inspire us and challenge us to find better ways to treat their maladies.

Contents

Foreword

The intended goal of this book is to provide a practical and useful compendium of indications and techniques for managing the full array of upper extremity trauma from the shoulder to the forearm. The three editors have certainly achieved their stated objective.

A textbook covering this particular topic is long overdue. In my opinion, the management of upper extremity trauma has lagged behind that of lower extremity for obvious reasons. The fractures involving the elbow and the shoulder can be extremely complex and seem to have an equal, if not sometimes greater, functional impact than comparable fractures of the lower extremity. These injuries have typically been managed in a trauma setting and, due to the relatively lower frequency of such injuries, expertise in their management has not been comparable to that of the lower extremity. The editors of this important text, David Dines, Dean Lorich, and David Helfet, are to be commended; first for identifying a void in the literature, and second for their willingness to fill this void with a comprehensive textbook. The three editors and the contributors are experienced as traumatologists and upper extremity surgeons. This in itself brings great credibility to this effort. The subject of complex upper extremity trauma is thoroughly addressed in the 18 chapters of this volume. In addition to the topic selection, of particular importance is the breadth of experience brought to bear on this important question by the editors and contributors. This book features an international perspective on this topic with numerous contributions from Europe and Canada as well as from the United States. The organization of the book is most logical, beginning with the clavicle and ending at the forearm. As is the appropriate trend today, the three editors place a particular emphasis on surgical technique and have complimented the description of an operation with useful photographs to facilitate the understanding of the surgical strategy being described. The chapters are written in a uniform fashion, and thus there is a clear strength of editorial presence and focus, making the entire text easy to read and easy to navigate.

Toward this end, the layout of the text is very logical, describing first the acute injury and its management, then following with a second chapter discussing its complications and reconstructive options. This format certainly facilitates the use of this text to identify topics in a fast and efficient manner. The editors and contributors have achieved a nice balance between a concise yet comprehensive bibliography. Thus, the references are relevant and useful and speak to the topic at hand. Similarly, the illustrations and art are carefully chosen to compliment the text message.

In summary, Drs. Dines, Lorich, and Helfet have, in my judgment, very successfully carried out the intended purposes of providing a comprehensive yet focused text on the current status of management of upper extremity trauma. This textbook is an important contribution to the orthopedic literature and would be essential for those individuals who have a direct responsibility to manage upper extremity injuries.

Bernard F. Morrey, MD

Preface

With the ever-increasing population, the incidence of traumatic injuries has likewise continued to increase. With people of all ages, including the elderly, participating in more sports and other activities, the number of complicated and complex injuries to the upper extremity has increased dramatically in recent years. The orthopedic traumatologists of all experience levels are now faced with the difficult tasks of recognition and treatment of more complex and complicated fracture patterns in patients of all ages who are interested in continuing their active life styles.

Over the last decade, many improvements in diagnostic modalities have allowed the orthopedic surgeon to recognize more complex injury patterns after trauma to the upper extremity. This recognition in conjunction with significant technological advances in exposure, instrumentation, standard and minimally invasive fracture fixation devices, and external fixation and range of motion apparatus has significantly improved the results in treatment.

With these concepts in mind, we felt the need to produce a book that addresses these contemporary issues in trauma to the upper extremity from the shoulder girdle to the forearm. We have asked some of the premier upper extremity trauma experts from around the world to share their most up-to-date principles in dealing with the diagnosis, treatment, and postoperative rehabilitation in both the acute and the complicated chronic situations. Since we are all aware of the ever-burgeoning changes in technology, we have asked these authors to emphasize the "basic principles of care" which remain at the heart of excellent outcomes. The chapters are organized in such a way to allow the reader easy access to those specific issues which they face in clinical practice while allowing a more comprehensive view for reference at other times. The book is technique-oriented with many figures and intraoperative photographs for easy review of specific case situations.

Our purpose in writing this book is to present to the orthopedic surgeon/traumatologist of all levels, from the generalist taking emergency call to the orthopedic traumatology specialist, state-of-the-art techniques to treat these complex injuries in a way that will improve outcomes for all affected patients.

David M. Dines, MD
Dean G. Lorich, MD
David L. Helfet, MD

Acknowledgments

We gratefully acknowledge the contributions of artist Peggy Firth for her outstanding drawings, Esther Gumpert and J. Owen Zurhellen at Thieme for their editorial assistance, and all the contributing authors for their outstanding efforts, which helped to bring this project to fruition.

David M. Dines, MD

Dean G. Lorich, MD

David L. Helfet, MD

Contributors

Joseph A. Abboud, MD
Clinical Assistant Professor of Orthopedic Surgery
University of Pennsylvania
Philadelphia, Pennsylvania

Kenneth J. Accousti, MD
Fredericksburg Orthopaedic Associates PC
Fredericksburg, Virginia

Frank A. Cordasco, MD, MS
Associate Professor of Orthopedic Surgery
Weill College of Medicine of Cornell University
The Hospital for Special Surgery
New York, New York

Edward V. Craig, MD
Professor of Clinical Orthopedic Surgery
Weill College of Medicine of Cornell University
Attending Surgeon
The Hospital for Special Surgery
New York, New York

David M. Dines, MD
Professor of Orthopedic Surgery
Albert Einstein College of Medicine
Senior Attending Physician
Sports Medicine and Shoulder Service
The Hospital for Special Surgery
New York, New York

Joshua S. Dines, MD
Department of Orthopedic Surgery
Sports Medicine and Shoulder Service
The Hospital for Special Surgery
New York, New York

Diego L. Fernandez, MD
Professor of Orthopedic Surgery
Lindenhof Hospital and University of Bern
Bern, Switzerland

Evan L. Flatow, MD
Department of Orthopedic Surgery
Mount Sinai Medical Center
New York, New York

Michael J. Gardner, MD
Fellow of Orthopedic Trauma
Department of Orthopedic Surgery
Harborview Medical Center
Seattle, Washington

Andreas M. Hartmann, MD
Department of Traumatology and Sports Injury
Paracelsus University Hospital of Salzburg
Salzburg, Austria

David L. Helfet, MD
Professor of Orthopedic Surgery
Weill College of Medicine of Cornell University
The Hospital for Special Surgery
New York, New York

Paul S. Issack, MD, PhD
The Hospital for Special Surgery
New York, New York

Jesse B. Jupiter, MD
Hansjorg Wyss/AO Professor of Orthopedic Surgery
Harvard Medical School
Director of Hand and Upper Limb Surgery
Massachusetts General Hospital
Boston, Massachusetts

Bryan T. Kelly, MD
Assistant Professor of Orthopedic Surgery
Weill College of Medicine of Cornell University
Assistant Attending Orthopedic Surgeon
The Hospital for Special Surgery
New York, New York

Peter Kloen, MD, PhD
Director of Orthoaedic Trauma
Department of Orthopedic Surgery
Academic Medical Center
Amsterdam, The Netherlands

Margaret H. Lauerman, BS
The Hospital for Special Surgery
New York, New York

Dean G. Lorich, MD
Assistant Professor of Orthopedic Surgery
Weill College of Medicine of Cornell University
The Hospital for Special Surgery
New York, New York

René K. Marti, MD, PhD
Professor of Orthopedics
Academic Medical Center
Amsterdam, The Netherlands

Michael D. McKee, MD, FRCS(C)
Associate Professor of Surgery
Division of Orthopedic Surgery
University of Toronto
St. Michael's Hospital
Toronto, Ontario, Canada

Ladislav Nagy, MD
Assistant Professor of Hand
and Peripheral Nerve Surgery
University Hospital Balgrist
Zurich, Switzerland

Matthew L. Ramsey, MD
Associate Professor of Orthopedic Surgery
University of Pennsylvania
Presbyterian Medical Center
Philadelphia, Pennsylvania

Herbert Resch, MD
Professor of Traumatology and Sports Injury
Paracelsus University Hospital of Salzburg
Salzburg, Austria

David C. Ring, MD, PhD
Assistant Professor of Orthopedic Surgery
Harvard Medical School
Orthopedic Hand and Upper Extremity Service
Massachusetts General Hospital
Boston, Massachusetts

Jonas R. Rudzki, MD
Washington Orthopedics and Sports Medicine
Washington, DC

Peter C. Strohm, MD
Department of Orthopedics and Traumatology
Albert-Ludwigs University Freiburg
Freiburg, Germany

Norbert P. Südkamp, MD
Professor of Medicine
Department of Orthopedics and Traumatology
Albert-Ludwigs University Freiburg
Freiburg, Germany

Christian J. H. Veillette, MD, MSc, FRCSC
Assistant Professor of Orthopedic Surgery
University of Toronto
Toronto, Ontario, Canada

Russell F. Warren, MD
Department of Orthopedic Surgery
The Hospital for Special Surgery
New York, New York

Christian van der Werken, PhD
Professor of Surgery
Division of Surgical Specialties
University Medical Center Utrecht
Utrecht, The Netherlands

1 Operative Treatment of Fractures of the Clavice

Andreas M. Hartmann and Herbert Resch

> We are proud that our brains are more developed than the animals: we might also boast of our clavicles. It seems to me that the clavicle is one of man's greatest skeletal inheritances, for he depends to a greater extent than most animals, except the apes and monkeys, on the use of his hands and arms.
>
> E. A. Codman, 1934

The incidence of clavicle fractures accounts for ~50 per 100,000 inhabitants per year; only 4% of all fractures involve the clavicle. The management of this fracture, however, has recently evolved because new evidence has demonstrated the importance of the proper healing of the clavicle. With the newfound importance of fitness as a principle of life and the resulting increase in sports activities, clavicle fractures are occurring more frequently in the general population, predominantly in young people. Today, fast, successful treatment without sequelae is a matter of economic importance and a topic of discussion in public affairs.

Anatomy and Embryology of the Clavicle

The clavicle is an S-shaped tubular bone with a medial anterior and a posterior lateral convexity. The length varies proportionally to the size of the individual, whereas the male clavicle usually is longer in the middle. The diameter at the medial metaphysic measures 18 mm, at the lateral 15 mm, and at the diaphysis ~7 mm. The narrowest diameter is measured at the meeting point of the two half circles of the S-shaped clavicle, the most frequent location of clavicle fractures. The medial clavicle shows a tubular form; however, laterally it becomes more and more flat on the cranial and caudal face to provide a congruent articulation with the corresponding acromion. It provides attachments for the deltoid, trapezius, sternocleidomastoid, pectoral, and subclavius muscles, which are responsible for the typical displacement seen in midshaft fractures. As the clavicle lies subcutaneously throughout its length and contours the upper trunk with its connection to the upper extremity, the fracture deformity also becomes an aesthetic problem.

The clavicle is the only tubular bone with a mesenchymal ossification, which starts in the embryo and ends in the third decade (mean age: men, 26 years; women, 25 years). The medial epiphyseal end is responsible for 80% of the clavicle's growth. Because of the late closure of the epiphyseal growth zone, growth plate separations must be considered in children or younger patients experiencing pain or tenderness proximally or distally over the clavicle.

Function of the Clavicle

The clavicle is the only link connecting the trunk with the arm. With the above-mentioned muscles, it contributes, together with the thoracoscapular and glenohumeral joints, to the movement of the upper extremity. As a distance holder and strut, it represents an unavoidable link for overhead work, stabilizing the glenohumeral joint, especially in the sagittal plane, and providing a stable, efficient center of rotation for the shoulder joint.[1] In the case of trauma, the middle third of the clavicle has to withstand the greatest bending and torsional forces. The clavicle also protects the underlying neurovascular structures. With the surrounding muscles, especially the sternocleidomastoid muscle, the clavicle has an important function in respiratory function; hence, the treatment of injury to the clavicle must be considered in situations where there is a concomitant injury to the rib cage.

Classification

Based on anatomic peculiarities and typical fracture conditions, the clavicle is divided into three thirds as classified by Allman **(Fig. 1–1)**.[2] The medial or proximal part is small and extends from the sternoclavicular joint to the lateral attachment of the costoclavicular ligament. The midportion is the biggest and reaches to the medial beginning of the conoid part of the coracoclavicular (CC) ligament. Fractures lateral to the conoid are therefore described as distal clavicle fractures. For each third, a separate structure classification exists, whereas the one for the medial fractures described by Craig[3] lacks the

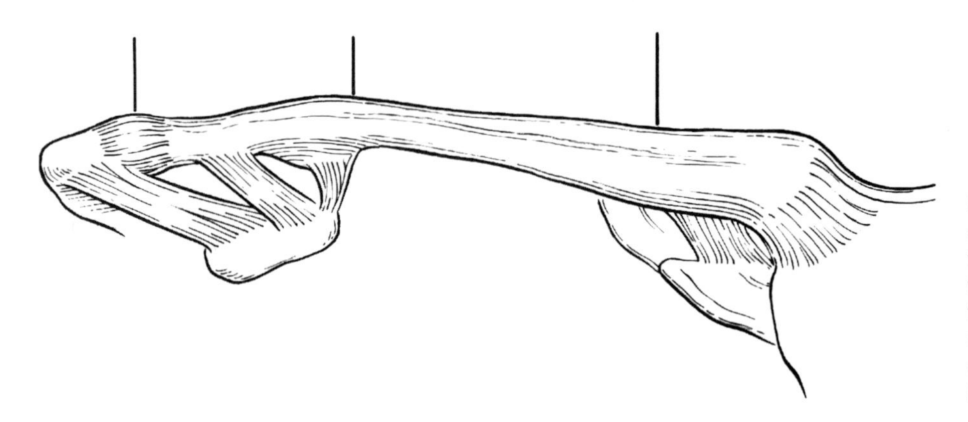

Figure 1–1 Classification of midshaft clavicle fractures as per Allman.[2] **(A)** proximal fractures from the sternoclavicular joint to the costoclavicular ligaments, **(B)** midshaft fractures from the costoclavicular ligaments to the coracoclavicular ligaments, and **(C)** distal fractures from coracoclavicular ligaments to the acromioclavicular joint.

benefit of general classification itself. Medial fractures are rare, and the scarcity of data makes evidence-based conclusions about treatment difficult. We do not use this classification in our clinic; however, we recognize its significance when involved in a comparative investigation. The Academy of Orthopedics/American Association for the Study of Internal Fixation (AO/ASIF) classification is widely used for fractures of the middle third and has been found helpful in therapy decisions. Type A is described as a simple transverse fracture, type B is a wedge fracture, and type C is a comminuted fracture with no contact with the main fragments.

For the lateral third of clavicle fractures, Neer's classification[4] remains the gold standard. Adaptations by Rockwood[5] or Breitner and Jager,[6] offer no additional benefit particularly in treatment decisions. Neer's type I **(Fig. 1–2)** is a stable fracture located laterally from the nondisabled CC ligaments. In Neer's type II **(Fig. 1–3)**, the fracture lies between the conoid and trapezoid components of the CC ligaments. The medial part, the conoid ligament, is ruptured, but the distal one, the trapezoid, remains intact. Infrequently, both ligaments are ruptured and combined with a distal clavicle fracture. If we have intact ligaments with a proximal fracture we classify it with the midshaft fractures. Occasionally, distinction is difficult if radiographic displacement of the proximal fragment gives no hint of ligament damage. Neer's type III **(Fig. 1–4)** describes a fracture extending into the acromioclavicular (AC) joint. The division in stable and unstable fractures is helpful for dictating further treatment.

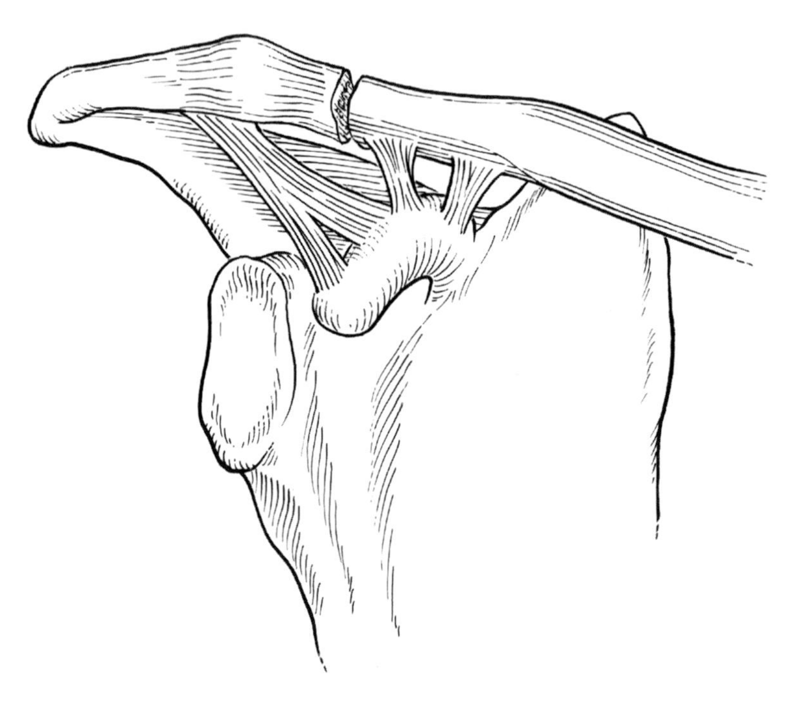

Figure 1–2 Classification of distal clavicle fractures: type I. Fractures distal to the coracoclavicular ligaments, which remain intact.

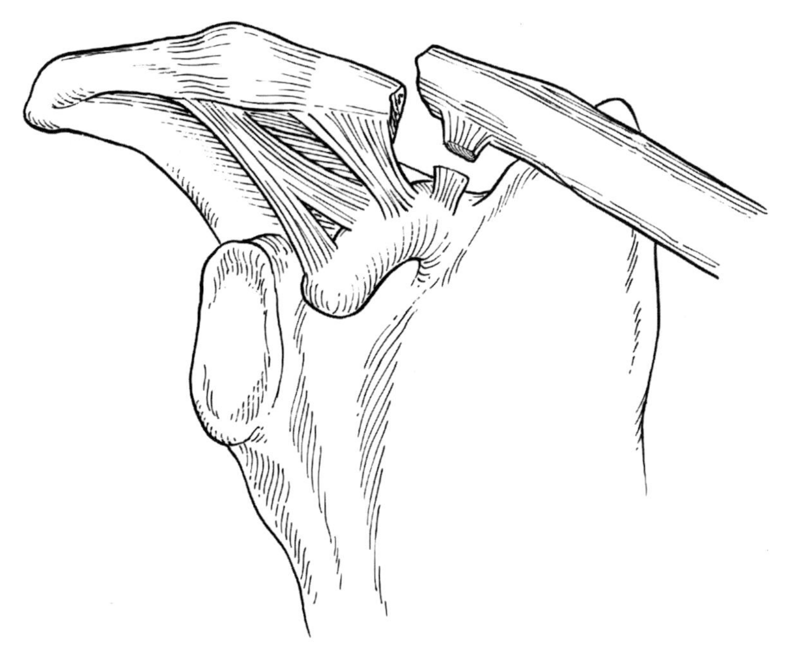

Figure 1–3 Classification of distal clavicle fractures: type II. Fractures in between the coracoclavicular ligaments with rupture of the conoid ligament.

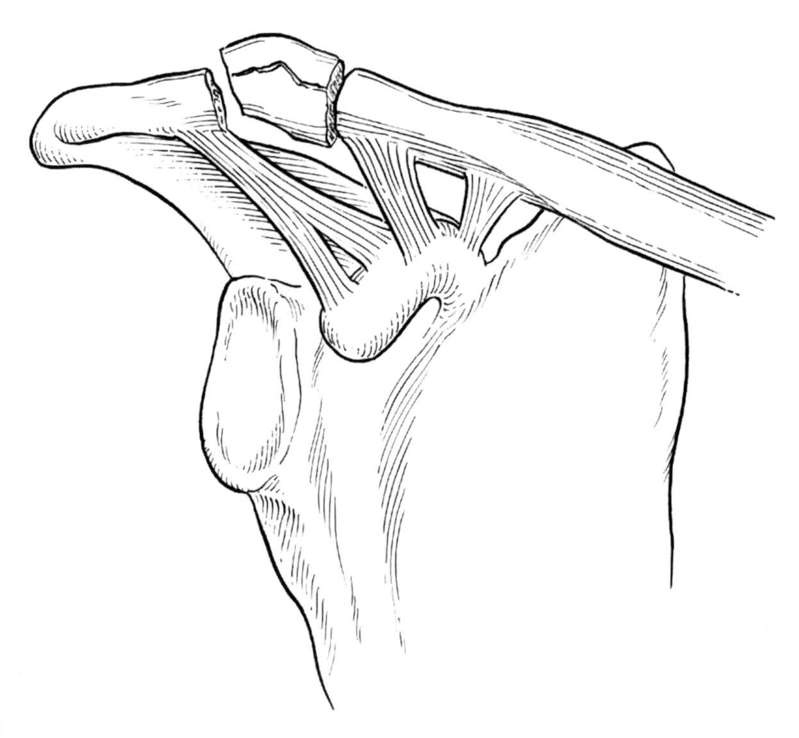

Figure 1–4 Classification of distal clavicle fractures: type III. Fractures distal to the coracoclavicular ligaments (like type I) with extension into the acromioclavicular joint.

Epidemiology

The frequency of clavicle fractures due to trauma is 2.6 to 4%.[7,8] Although this is a small percentage, with increasing recreational activities clavicle fractures are occurring more frequently, 52 in 1952 compared to 64 per 100,000 in 1987.[9] In the only prospective trial, Nowak et al[8] found in the years 1989 to 1990 a frequency of 50/100,000 inhabitants (males 71/100,000, females 30/100,000). Clavicle fractures represent 35 to 44% of all fractures of the shoulder girdle.[7,10] They are more common in males under 30 years of age. Because of the strong fixation of the ends of the clavicle by surrounding ligaments the thinner middle part, 80% are located in the midthird. Among these, 48% are displaced and 19% comminuted[7]; 10 to 18% of these fractures are distal, and 2 to 10% of fractures are of the medial third of the clavicle.[11] Fractures of the medial third show a mean age of 51 years, of the midthird 21 years, and of the distal third 47 years. Patients over 75 years in age show an increasing frequency of medial or distal third clavicle fractures.[9] Regarding the fracture displacement, age distribution, nondisplaced fractures have a mean age of 11 years, minimally displaced fractures have a mean age of 27 years, and comminuted fractures have a mean age of 43 years.

Patient Assessment

During clinical examination, the complaints and posture of the patient, local signs of swelling, bruising, and deformity may make the diagnosis evident. The diagnosis is confirmed by an anteroposterior (AP) and 45% cranially and caudally angled radiograph of the injuries located in the middle third of the clavicle. Evaluation should be performed on the vertebral column, proximal humerus, shoulder girdle, and upper thorax and lung, particularly in multiply injured patients. Ignorance of these concomitant injuries can lead to inappropriate treatments. Lateral fractures additionally need axillary radiographs centered on the AC joint. To distinguish stability of lateral fractures, it is sometimes necessary to perform a radiograph with a 5-kg weight pulling on the arm. In these cases, we highly recommend local anesthesia on the affected side.

Secondary to the multiple overlying structures of the upper thorax, a fracture of the medial clavicle is often difficult to visualize on plain x-ray. A computed tomography (CT) scan is recommended in cases with obvious signs of injury. Ultrasound can be helpful in children and newborns. Careful neurologic and vascular examinations should be performed in all patients with clavicular injuries. Concomitant injuries such as pneumo- and hemothorax or neurovascular damage have been reported, but are uncommon.

Fracture Mechanism

In 87% of clavicle fractures, the cause is a fall on the shoulder – either a direct blunt trauma or a fall on the outstretched arm. These injuries are often common in contact sports and cycling, motorcycling, skiing, and riding.

Treatment

Nonsurgical Treatment

The results of operative treatment are always compared with the results of a conservative therapy treatment. Lester in 1929 described the use of plaster spicas, splinting devices, bandages, or simple slings (more than 200 methods) in the treatment of midclavicular fractures. Some clinicians favor reduction, putting a knee between both shoulder blades, others a redressing figure-eight bandage. In a 1987 prospective randomized study, Andersen[12] demonstrated identical functional and cosmetic results, comparing a figure-eight bandage and a simple sling. The initial displacement remained unchanged in each group, whereas the simple sling caused less discomfort and perhaps fewer complications. The widely accepted treatment is a simple immobilizer from a few days up to 3 weeks to reduce pain. Elevation over 90 degrees and strengthening should begin after clinical consolidation of the fracture is evident. After 8 to 12 weeks and radiographic healing, shoulder strengthening work and contact sports may be considered. Nondisplaced and minimally displaced fractures will heal with symptomatic treatment and little concern regarding either cosmesis or function.

Nordqvist et al[13] found among 225 conservatively treated midclavicle fractures, 185 (82%) asymptomatic, 39 (17%) with moderate pain, and 1 (0.4%) with significant pain. In this retrospective study with a mean follow-up of 17 years (12 to 22 years), 68% were displaced and comminuted fractures. This study showed a 24% malunion and a 3% nonunion rate; however, the majority of these patients with radiographic abnormalities had good outcome in this long-term investigation.

In contrast, Hill et al[14] reviewed 52 midclavicle, completely displaced fractures with a mean follow-up of 38 months, and found 15% nonunions and 31% unsatisfactory results. No patient had significant impairment of range of motion; however, 13 (25%) patients had mild to moderate pain, 15 (29%) had some evidence of brachial plexus irritation, and 28 (56%) had cosmetic complaints.

In 2005, Nowak et al[15] evaluated prospectively an evaluation of 222 patients with clavicle fractures. They showed 42% of patients treated nonoperatively continued to have significant sequelae 6-months postinjury. The nonunion rate was only 7%; therefore, other symptoms were responsible for their complaints. Displacement of more than one bone width was the strongest radiographic risk factor for symptoms and sequelae. A comminuted fracture and older patients were associated with increased risk of symptoms persisting at 6 months.

Regarding sequelae after clavicle fractures, it is important to focus not only on nonunion, which may have no clinical symptoms, but to concentrate more on malunion, which can be responsible for pain, neurovascular symptoms, cosmetic complaints, and functional deficits.

Surgical Treatment

Because of the results related above, the decision for operative treatment results in extremely controversial discussions. Without a doubt, therapy for children is in the domain of nonoperative treatment. In children, even displaced fractures are treated with a short immobilization in a sling or a figure-eight bandage.

In adults, only absolute indications for surgical treatment include open fractures, fractures with neurovascular damage, refracture, or floating shoulders with midclavicular and Neer's type II fractures of the distal clavicle. More controversial indications for operative treatment include displacement, comminution or shortening, multiply injured patients, and patients with injuries of the lower extremity and the need for the use of crutches. These questions concern predominantly midclavicular fractures; surgical indications for the proximal and distal clavicle are more evident.

Fractures of the Proximal Third of the Clavicle

Secondary to the low incidence (2% of clavicle fractures), recommendations for treatment of the sternal and clavicle fractures are based on case reports or small series reported in the literature. We find that these fractures, which seldom are significantly displaced, can be treated conservatively in a sling for a few weeks. As patients with this fracture are middle-aged on average, one must be careful not to overlook fractures in younger patients where epiphyseal fusion may not have yet taken place. Because the medial epiphyses typically remain open into the third decade of life, it is important to recognize that apparent sternoclavicular dislocations in some young adults may actually be epiphyseal separation injuries.[16,17] Epiphyseal fracture can be difficult to recognize on a CT scan. In rare cases such as an open fracture, operative stabilization may be indicated. Plating should be chosen because pin migration after tension band wiring is a concern with potentially devastating complications. Pin displacements into the aorta and a pin coughed up in the lung have been reported in the literature. Some authors recommend conservative treatment in general because of good therapy options with resection of the sternal end of the clavicle, if the deformity is symptomatic later.

Fractures of the Middle Third of the Clavicle

The most frequent fracture is the midthird fracture. The middle third of the clavicle actually represents nearly half of the length of the clavicle from the costoclavicular to the CC ligaments. All former studies unanimously called for conservative treatment of all clavicle fractures; however, recently there is some doubt as to the best treatment choice. The sentence "Most clavicle fractures are treated conservatively and heal uneventfully with good outcome" is not true. On behalf of the Evidence-Based Orthopaedic Trauma Working Group, Zlowodzki et al[18] published a systematic review of 2,144 midshaft clavicle fractures reported from 1975 to 2005. The operative treatment took place in 47% of all cases. This is about the same percentage we would estimate in our patients. Therefore, there appears to be a large gap between surgeons or clinics who treat all clavicle fractures conservatively and others who operate on most of these injuries. Widely accepted indications for operative treatment are open fracture, the one with associated neurovascular damage, the refracture and floating shoulder, i.e., the clavicle fracture combined with a scapular neck fracture. The latter indication is called into question by Edwards et al,[19] presenting excellent results with conservative treatment. After a mean follow-up of 28 months, 20 patients treated with short (3 to 14 days) immobilization were examined and showed a Constant score of 96 points.[20] Others have shown excellent data after operative treatment[15] and poor outcomes with conservative treatment.[14] Many have proposed operative treatment for displaced, comminuted fractures and patients who are multiply injured or have fractures of the lower limb with the need for crutch use.

In the literature of the past 30 years, Zlowodzki et al[18] in a meta-analysis of clavicle fractures found only three randomized controlled trials (RCTs), three additional cohort studies with control group, and two prospective observational studies, comparing operative versus nonoperative treatment. The majority of all identified studies were retrospective (18/23), had no control group (15/21), and did not use any randomization if there was a control group (3/6).

In a RCT (evidence-based medicine [EBM-] level 2 therapy) Smith et al[21] compared nonoperative treatment with plating in two groups of 50 patients with 100% displaced midshaft fractures. The nonunion rate was 24% in the nonoperative group and 0% with plating. In the nonoperative group, 30% (6% for operative group) developed neurological and 44% cosmetic complaints. However, in the plating group, 30% of patients requested hardware removal upon fracture healing.

Judd et al[22] found in their RCT (EBM-level 2 therapy) with 29 patients with displaced clavicle fractures treated with intramedullary plating. They showed 3.4% nonunion rate with two refractures (6.9%). In their nonoperative group, 28 patients showed 0% nonunion and 3.4% refractures.

Zlowodzki et al's study[18] found a 5.9% overall nonunion rate for nonoperative treatment, and a 15.1% nonunion rate in the subset with displaced fractures. Risk fractures for nonunion after conservative therapy were displacement, comminution, female gender, and advanced age. Risk reduction for nonunion could possibly be achieved by operative treatment.

A larger multicenter study has provided results for meaningful interpretation in this population of patients with fractures of the midshaft of the clavicle. Descriptions such as "some neurologic complaints" and "complaints about the cosmetic appearance of their shoulder" are unclear. The results from published studies become uncomparable. In the end, the physician's therapy advice has to value possible sequelae presented like nonunion, pain, loss of strength, or cosmetic complaints. The view of most orthopedic surgeons that displaced midshaft fractures can generally be treated nonoperatively with few functional deficits may be an incorrect perception. The views tend to be based on studies of radiographic surgeon-based outcomes. McKee et al[23] recently has evaluated patient-based outcomes and objective muscle strength testing in 30 patients treated nonoperatively for displaced midshaft clavicle fractures. Strength and endurance of the injured shoulder was compared with the noninjured extremity and was found to be slightly diminished in all motions on the affected side. The mean Constant score was 71 points and the mean DASH score[24] was 24.6, indicating substantial residual disability.[40] Further, McKee et al[23] using the same type of critical evaluation of shoulder function and patient-oriented outcome, evaluated 132 patients with displaced and midshaft fractures in a randomized, prospective multicenter study comparing nonoperative treatment to plate fixation of these injuries. They found Constant shoulder scores and DASH scores were significantly improved in the operative fixation group at all time points evaluated. This study showed a significantly increased time to radiographic union in the operative groups: 16.4 weeks in the operative group compared with 28.4 weeks in the nonoperative group. Two of the 67 patients treated with plate fixation went on to nonunion compared with 9 of 65 patients in the nonoperative group. Further, symptomatic malunion developed in 9 patients in the nonoperative group and none in the operative group.

Nowak et al[25] presented in their prospective study the 9- to 10-year follow-up of patients with nonoperatively treated clavicle fractures: 46% of the patients complained of sequelae, 9% at rest, 39% pain during work, and 27% cosmetic defects. Predictors for sequelae, pain, and cosmetic complaints were the displacement and comminution, whereas shortening only affected cosmetic complaints. Patients with risk factors such as fractures with displacement, especially if there is no bony contact and/or fracture comminution, should be considered for more active treatment options. Treatment and follow-up of clavicular fractures should therefore not only be focused on nonunions, but on the risk of nonunion with increasing age, female gender, displacement of the fracture, and the presence of comminution.[17]

For operative treatment three methods are available. Stabilization with external fixator is infrequently indicated for widely open fractures with comminution, or after hardware removal in the case of deep infection. On the other hand, plating and intramedullary pinning can be used for all other situations.

Plating

Many surgeons prefer to use plating techniques. The one-third tubular plate appears to be too thin to withstand the three-dimensional forces addressing the clavicle. Reconstruction, dynamic compression (DC-), limited-contact dynamic compression (LCDC-), or preformed plates also with locking screws are suitable. Plating **(Figs. 1–5** and **1–6)** can provide a satisfactory outcome, but can have complication rates up to 23%,[26,27] the major ones being deep infection, plate breakage, nonunion, plate loosening leading to malunion, and refracture after plate removal. We believe many of these complications are technique related: they can be avoided with more meticulous handling of the soft tissues and the soft tissue attachments to the bony fragments. However, the risks for a second operation to remove the hardware and cosmetic complaints

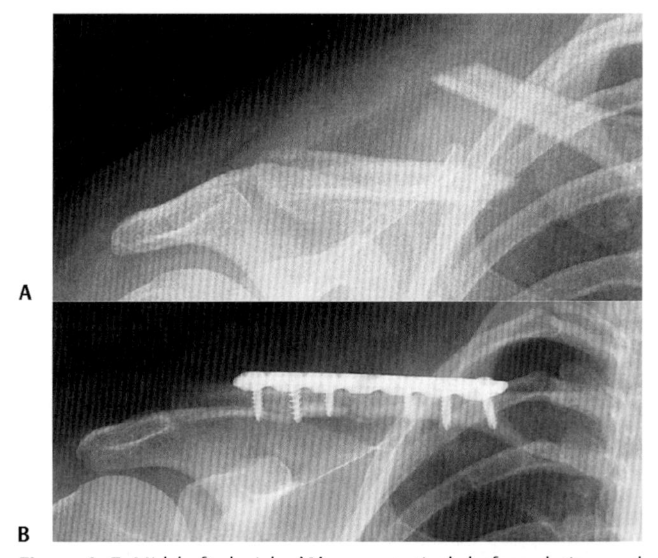

Figure 1–5 Midshaft clavicle: **(A)** preoperatively before plating, and **(B)** 3 weeks postoperatively.

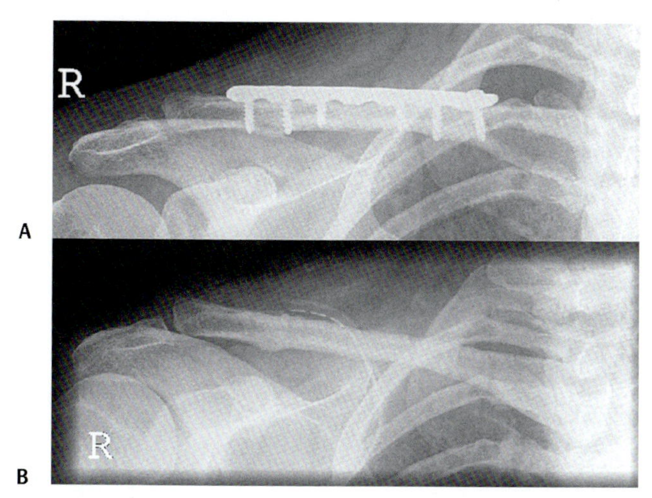

Figure 1–6 Midshaft clavicle: **(A)** 6 months after plating, and **(B)** after hardware removal (1 year).

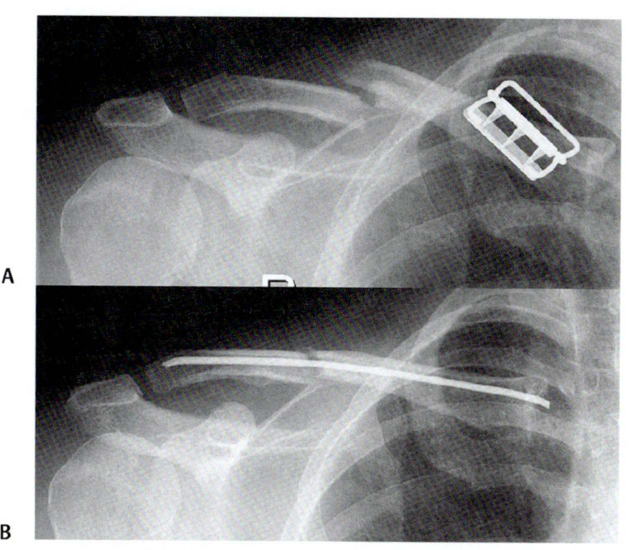

Figure 1–7 Midshaft clavicle: **(A)** preoperatively before antegrade nailing, and **(B)** 4 weeks postoperatively.

are important factors influencing treatment options. In the case of clavicular nonunion, plating seems to continue to be the treatment of choice. The position of the plate superior may biomechanically be able to support axial loading better than the anteroinferior side.[28] However, Lim et al[29] found 34 patients had significantly better Visual Analogue Scale scores in patients undergoing anteroinferior plating.

Intramedullary Pinning

Kirschner wires (K-wires) and threaded pins have been used, with different techniques of insertion and with attempts to prevent migration of these wires. However, reports of significant problems arising from pin migration and significant complication rates have been reported. Secondary to these complications, Grassi et al[30] concluded in their competitive cohort study that nonoperative treatment appears more advantageous than open intramedullary fixation for the management of most midclavicular fractures. In contrast, there are some studies suggesting advantages outweigh the disadvantages with intramedullary pinning.[18,30,33] The risk of catastrophic pin migration can be minimized by the use of different materials, like elastic titanium wires,[34,35] threaded pins or screws,[32,36] or other operative techniques.[33] There are two methods for intramedullary fixation from medial to lateral or vice-versa. First described by Lengua et al[37] in France in 1987, 25 fractures were treated with K-wire from medial to lateral with good results. They did a closed reduction in all 25 cases and found no nonunions. The wire was bent at the site of insertion to prevent migration. In one case the pin perforated the skin and was removed. In 2003, Jubel et al[31,35] presented their technique “elastic stable intra-medullary nailing” with a titanium nail inserted from medial **(Figs. 1–7** and **1–8)**. A closed reduction of the fracture was successful in 50% of 65 fractures.

Fifty-eight patients showed a Constant score of 96 in 6 months after pin removal performed approximately 7 months after operation. Jubel et al's[31, 35] indication for stabilization included not only fractures with a displacement over 2 cm, with neurovascular damage or floating shoulders, but also multiply injured patients for better nursing care and patients with injuries of lower extremity with a need for crutch use. Complications in this series included 1 nonunion, 4 skin problems making a shortening of the nail necessary, 4 shortening of the fracture 1.5 cm, and 2 hypertrophic scars. The advantage of insertion from the medial is the possible closed reduction with minimized risk of iatrogenic injury to the subclavicular structures.

On the contrary, the procedure performed from distal to proximal is indispensably bound to an open reduction. Some devices like the Knowles, Hagie, or Rockwood pins can bring compression of the fracture gap and have good

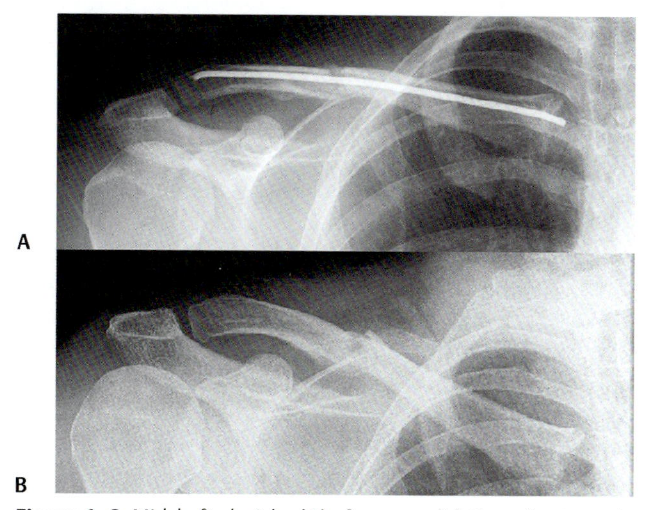

Figure 1–8 Midshaft clavicle: **(A)** after consolidation of antegrade nailing, and **(B)** after hardware removal (9 weeks).

results and healing; however, they have been associated with significant complications with the locking nut in 23% of cases (AE Kenneth, oral presentation, American Academy of Orthopaedic Surgeon Annual Conference, February 2005, Washington, DC). To avoid this, Chen et al[36] use a simple cannulated screw and have had good results in short-term follow-up. Ngarmukos et al[33] presented an intramedullary stabilization with two K-wires grasping two cortices in each main fragment. Three pins had to be removed before bone healing; however, they found a high percentage of nonunions (10%) in this study of 110 clavicle fractures.

Regarding the nailing techniques, the nonunion rates among all therapy options are the lowest (1.6 to 1.8%) yet reported.[15,18] Closed reduction and nailing from a medial starting side should theoretically be more dangerous; however, the only reported complication with plexus palsy is reported with an open procedure.[38] Jubel et al[35] published the largest series with 65 fractures. They reported no iatrogenic injuries in their series, in which a closed fracture reduction was performed in 48% of fractures. The patients reported significantly less pain and an increase in abduction ability on postoperative day 3, compared with examination 1 day preceding surgery. There were problems with the end of the pin in 5%, making shortening necessary. Nail displacement was not seen, nor was infection noted. In one patient (1.7%) with a comminuted fracture, a secondary shortening of 1.5 cm appeared. All authors using retrograde nailing reported problems with the pin end at the dorsal side of the clavicle in some cases, making a second operation because of skin perforation necessary.

In our own unpublished series, we have evaluated 30 midshaft clavicle fractures treated with pin fixation with minimal follow up of 12 months. Half of the patients were multiply injured: 16 simple, oblique fractures, 10 with two and 1 with four fragments were seen. We experienced complications including one infection, one pin shortening, and three migrations making early removal necessary. We had one malunion, one delayed union, and the other 28 of the 30 united uneventfully.

Comparing intramedullary pinning with nonoperative treatment, there is undoubtedly a large advantage compared with nonunion for nailing among all midclavicular fractures (1.6 versus 5.9%) and displaced fractures (2 versus 15%).[18] Shortening or malunion is rare in operative treatment, whereas malunion occurs in 29% with conservative treatment.[13] Nordqvist et al[13] reported with conservative treatment significantly more frequent fair or poor results among malunions and nonunions compared with healed radiologically aligned fractures. Shortening, they suggest, is common after initially displaced fractures, but has no clinical significance.[39] Matis et al[40] found a significantly higher nonunion rate among fractures with shortening over 2 cm.

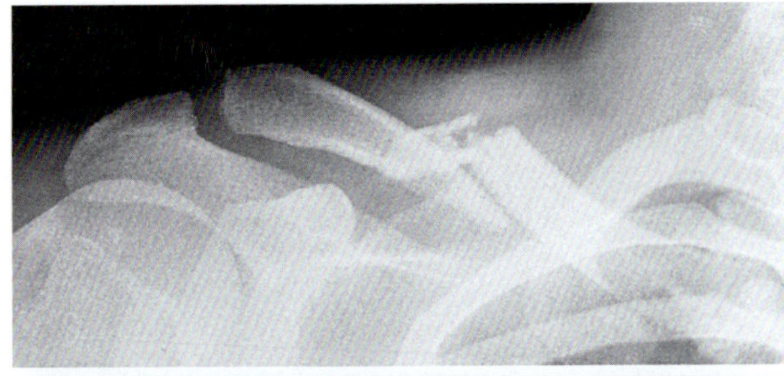

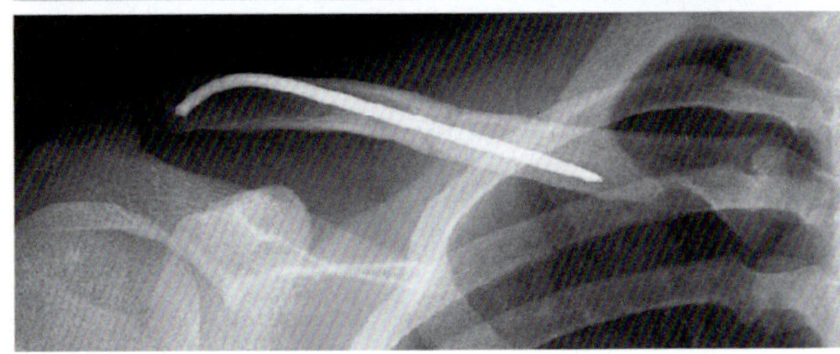

Figure 1–9 Midshaft clavicle: **(A)** preoperatively before retrograde nailing, and **(B)** 10 days postoperatively.

Preferred Technique

We recommend operative treatment in young active patients with midshaft clavicle fractures in which the shaft width is displaced and comminuted. Also, fractures with shortening of more than 2 cm or lengthening with a wide gap are treated operatively. The intramedullary retrograde pinning **(Figs. 1–9** and **1–10)** with open reduction is the preferred method in our clinic. We believe an open reduction of the fracture with the use of elastic titanium nails is the safest means to perform the procedure **(Fig. 1–11)**. General anesthesia combined with interscalene block is performed, the patient is set in a beach-chair position, the arm is prepped and draped free. A 2-cm-long oblique skin incision over the fracture gap is performed and the fracture exposed, taking great care to protect soft

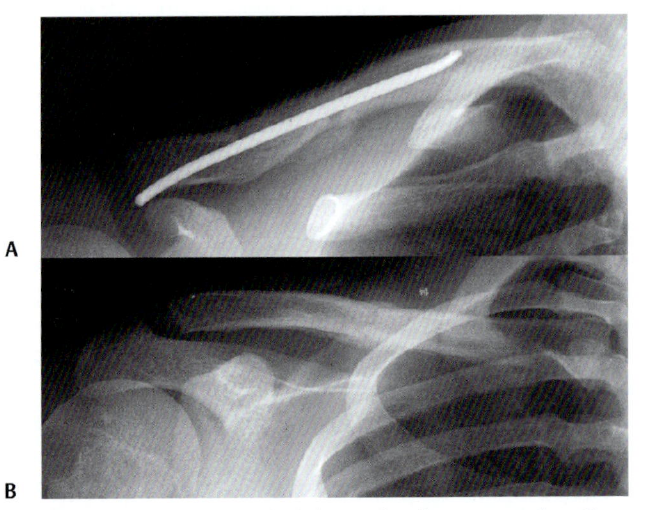

Figure 1–10 Midshaft clavicle: **(A)** 4 weeks after retrograde nailing, and **(B)** after hardware removal (10 weeks).

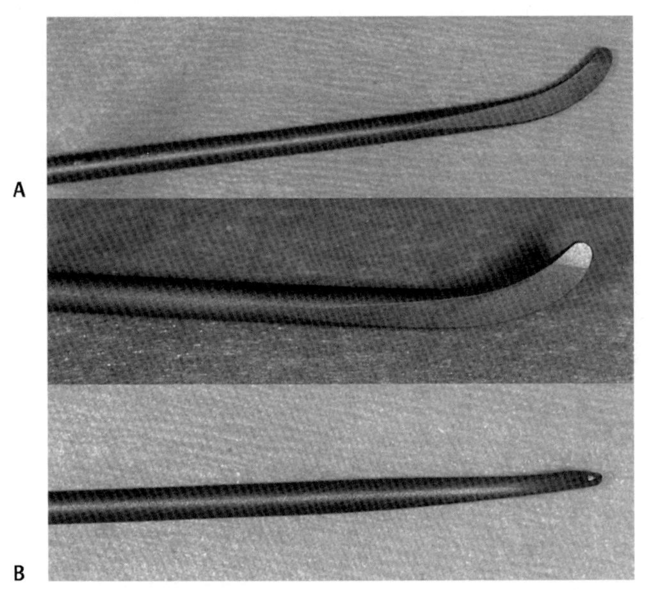

Figure 1–11 Three views of an elastic intramedullary titanium nail.

tissue bridges to bone. The ends are grasped and reamed in both directions with a 3.2-mm drill. In the distal fragment the dorsal cortex must be perforated. In most cases, a 3-mm thick pin is used, seldom a 2.5- or 3.5-mm is utilized. The terminal end is bent slightly to ensure easier passage through the intramedullary canal. The nail is also shortened to facilitate retrograde passage into the medial fragment. The pin is clamped in a T-handle, introduced into the distal main fragment, and driven through the dorsal cortex of the distal third of the clavicle. After a small skin incision, the T-handle is changed to the other end of the pin. The nail is now driven retrograde into the proximal medial fragment. The elasticity and bent nail make it easier to anchor the nail in the proximal end without perforating the cortex. Fragments with tissue connections should be fixed by sutures. The end of the dorsal side is bent up to 90 degrees and the head embedded in the surrounding soft tissues. After the operation, the patient is placed in a sling for 2 to 3 weeks, just to reduce pain. Elevation over 90 degrees is not allowed until clinical consolidation of the fracture appears.

Fractures of the Distal Third of the Clavicle

In the 1970s, Neer published his classification of distal clavicle fractures. He noted the importance of concomitant rupture of the two CC ligaments. Type I injuries **(Fig. 1–2)** described as a distal fracture without damage of these ligaments are classified as stable fractures. The overall accepted treatment is nonoperative. A sling is used until there is pain relief. Elevation over 90 degrees should be avoided until clinical consolidation; contact sports should be avoided until there is overt bone healing.

In type II **(Fig. 1–3)**, one or both ligaments are ruptured. In this case, the large lever arm created by the sternocleidomastoid muscle significantly displaces the fracture. Secondary to this displacement and the unopposed muscular forces, an unstable situation is created with poor healing preconditions. Neer and others reported a nonunion rate of 30%[41]. Due to these data operative stabilization is recommended.

In contrast, Robinson and Cairns[42] published in 2004 a series of 120 conservatively treated displaced distal clavicle fractures and found 21% nonunions without clinical disadvantage. The Constant score was 93 points. Only 14% required secondary surgery. There were no significant differences in the short-form 36 score between the patients with healed fractures, compared with those with nonunions or those who had been operated on secondarily.

Type III fractures **(Fig. 1–4)** are treated like type I because the CC ligaments are intact. In this group, the option of excising the lateral end of the clavicle is possible should symptoms continue. In these cases, nonoperative management of these fractures is recommended; therefore only type II fractures remain to be considered for surgical options. For operative treatment of type II fractures, extraarticular wires with tension band or mini-fragment T-plates (AO/ASIF) are used if the distal fragment is big enough, or a hook plate if it is small or comminuted. Transarticular fixation of the AC joint should be avoided because of a high amount of migration and skin problems, including infection.[43]

A hook plate can be too short; if fractures lie more proximal, then plating should be considered. Mini-fragment plates are sufficient if they are chosen large enough to catch at least six cortices of each main fragment. For patients with bad bone quality a tension band wire is the best therapy option. Of critical importance is to avoid compromising the AC joint, as symptoms can persist even after hardware removal. Additionally the immobilization time may not exceed 6 weeks with transarticular pins, which is more often too short for ligament healing. On the other hand, extraarticular positioned pins can be removed even 3 months later. If the distal fragment is too small or comminuted, the injury should be treated like an AC joint dislocation with a bone fragment. This can be excised later.

A disadvantage of plating is the need for hardware removal, with its potential complications of clavicle refracture.[44] Secondary to the proximity of the AC joint, the tension band wires also should be removed after bone healing.

In the era of minimally invasive surgery, a few authors have also described diverse attempts in the use of mini-incision techniques. In a series of 12 patients, Levy et al[45] showed a tension band with a PDS suture performed with four stab incisions and a closed reposition or a mini-open technique. All fractures healed in an anatomic position

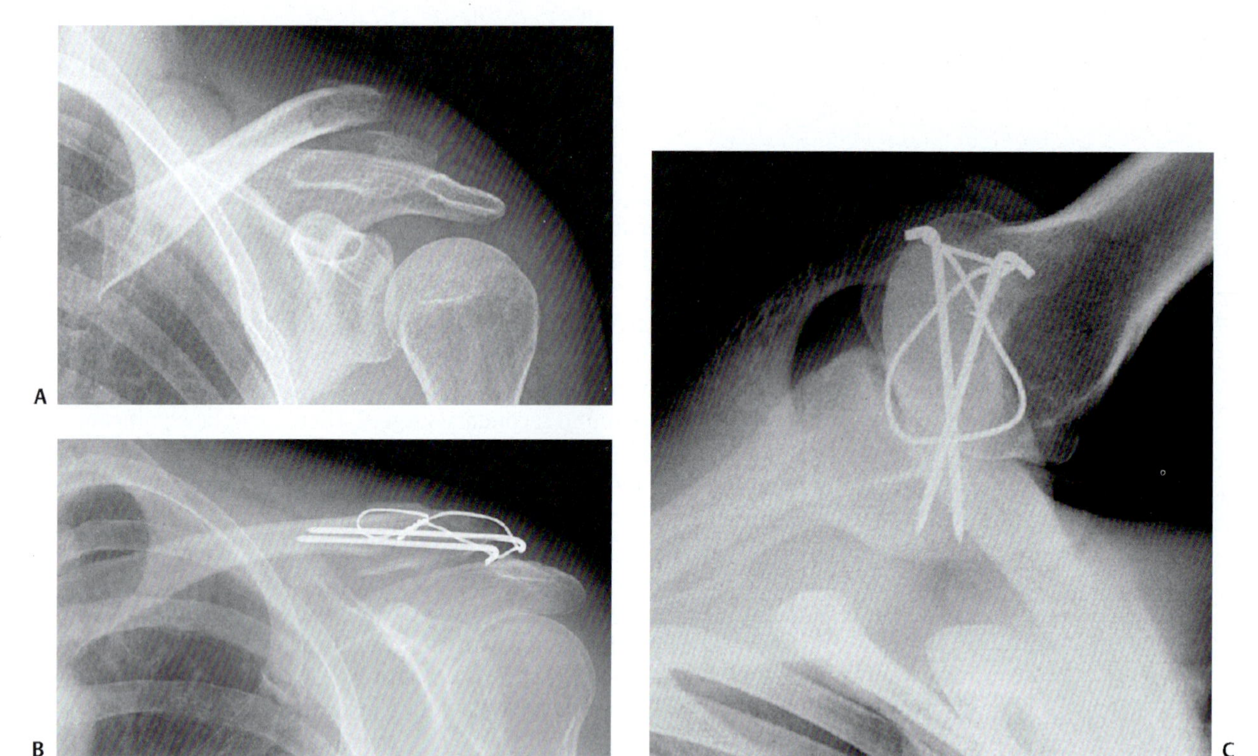

Figure 1–12 Distal clavicle: **(A)** preoperatively before applying a tension-band wire, and **(B,C)** postoperatively.

after 12 weeks with the Constant Score of 97 points. At final follow-up, none of the patients had any symptoms and all returned to full activity. Using Bezer et al's[46] method, the CC ligaments are restored by a suture anchor fixation and the fracture by a single transarticular wire. In this case series with 10 patients, there was one pin migration and an infection caused by a K-wire. The mean Constant score at 24 months was 96.6 points. Larger studies should be undertaken to justify the value of these new methods. A comparison between tension band wire and hook plate was performed by Flinkkila et al[47] They found a Constant score of 84 points in the K-wire group and 90 points in the hook plate. K-wires were mostly transarticular and had more complications. The mean follow-up was 6 years in the K-wire group, 2 years in the other group.

Preferred Technique

Minimally invasive techniques in the treatment of distal clavicle fractures are few in number and typically small in nature. They need to be critically evaluated prior to their routine usage in these cases. In our estimation, tension band wires and the hook plate are equal implants. Fracture location and comminution dictate the treatment methods: a more distal or comminuted fracture is fixed with a hook plate, and the more proximal fracture without comminution is more amenable to a tension band wire **(Fig. 1–12)**. Pins are placed extraarticularly.

Postoperative Care

In conservative treatment, it is advantageous to use a simple sling or figure-eight bandage, which is maintained until pain relief. Maintenance of fracture reduction after attempted closed reduction has not been validated in the literature. The sling works as a pain reducer and should be worn up to 3 weeks until soft tissue consolidation minimizes fracture movement. Full elevation and overhead activity can be performed after 6 weeks. Push-ups and contact sports are allowed only after radiographic and clinical bone healing has occurred, usually at 10 to 12 weeks.

After surgical intervention, a sling is needed for comfort until operative pain disappears. Range of motion is limited to 90 degrees of abduction for 2 weeks for younger patients, and for 4 weeks for older patients. Shoulder-demanding activities are not allowed before radiographic evidence of bone consolidation has occurred. Intramedullary pins can be removed at 3 months, and plates at 6 months after the operation.

Conclusion

Fractures of the proximal third of the clavicle are rare and are treated conservatively in the most cases. For the most patients with midshaft clavicle fracture, conservative treatment will bring good functional results, but operative therapy is an option in young active patients. In some studies far dislocated fractures give better results with an operative treatment. In this group, intramedullary pinning, when performed by closed reduction, shows lesser scars while the outcome is equal to plating. Regarding the literature, a general recommendation for conservative or operative treatment cannot be made; an individual therapy has to be performed. Dislocated fractures of the distal third of the clavicle can be fixed with a nontransacromially passed figure-eight band if located in the far lateral and with a hook plate, if the fracture involves the coracoclavicular ligaments.

References

1. Inman VT, Saunders JB, Abbott LC. Observations of the function of the shoulder joint – Verne T. Inman, MD, PhD (1905–1980), J.B. dec M. Saunders (1903–1991), and Leroy C. Abbott, MD (1890–1965). Clin Orthop Relat Res 1996;330:3–12
2. Allman FL. Fractures and ligamentous injuries of the clavicle and its articulation. J Bone Joint Surg Am 1967;49: 774–784
3. Craig EV. Fractures of the clavicle. In: Rockwood CA Jr, Matsen FA III, eds. The Shoulder. Philadelphia: W.B. Saunders, 1990:367–412
4. Neer CS. Fractures of the distal third of the clavicle. Clin Orthop 1968;58:43–50
5. Robinson CM. Fractures of the clavicle in the adult. Epidemiology and classification. J Bone Joint Surg Br 1998; 80:476–484
6. Jager M, Breitner S. Therapy related classification of lateral clavicular fracture. Unfallheilkunde 1984;87(11):467–473
7. Postacchini F, Gumina S, De Santis P, Albo F. Epidemiology of clavicle fractures. J Shoulder Elbow Surg 2002;11(5): 452–456
8. Nowak J, Mallmin H, Larsson S. The aetiology and epidemiology of clavicular fractures – a prospective study during a two-year period in Uppsala, Sweden. Injury 2000;31(5):353–358
9. Nordqvist A, Petersson C. The incidence of fractures of the clavicle. Clin Orthop Relat Res 1994;300:127–132
10. Graves ML, Geissler WB, Freeland AE. Midshaft clavicular fractures: the role of operative treatment. Orthopedics 2005;28(8):761–764
11. Robinson CM. Fractures of the clavicle in the adult – epidemiology and classification. J Bone Joint Surg Br 1998; 80(3):476–484
12. Andersen K, Jensen PO, Lauritzen J. Treatment of clavicular fractures. Figure-of-eight bandage versus a simple sling. Acta Orthop Scand 1987;58:71–74
13. Nordqvist A, Petersson CJ, Redlund-Johnell I. Mid-clavicle fractures in adults: end result study after conservative treatment. J Orthop Trauma 1998;12(8):572–576
14. Hill JM, McGuire MH, Crosby LA. Closed treatment of displaced middle-third fractures of the clavicle gives poor results. J Bone Joint Surg Br 1997;79(4):537–539
15. Nowak J, Holgersson M, Larsson S. Sequelae from clavicular fractures are common – a prospective study of 222 patients. Acta Orthop 2005;76(4):496–502
16. Cope R. Dislocations of the sternoclavicular joint. Skeletal Radiol 1993;22(4):233–238
17. Lewonowski K, Bassett GS. Complete posterior sternoclavicular epiphyseal separation – a case-report and review of the literature. Clin Orthop Relat Res 1992;281: 84–88
18. Zlowodzki M, Zelle BA, Cole PA, Jeray K, McKee MD. Treatment of acute midshaft clavicle fractures: systematic review of 2144 fractures – on behalf of the Evidence-Based Orthopaedic Trauma Working Group. J Orthop Trauma 2005;19(7):504–507
19. Edwards SG, Whittle AP, Wood GW. Nonoperative treatment of ipsilateral fractures of the scapula and clavicle. J Bone Joint Surg Am 2000;82(6):774–780
20. Constant CR, Murley AHG. A clinical method of functional assessment of the shoulder. Clin Orth 1987;214:160–164
21. Smith CA, Rudd J, Crosby LA. Results of operative versus non-operative treatment for 100% displaced mid-shaft clavicle fractures: a prospective randomized trial. Paper presented at: Proceedings of the 68th Annual Meeting of the American Academy of Orthopaedic Surgeons, 2001
22. Judd DB, Bottoni CR, Pallis MP, et al. Intramedullary fixation versus nonoperative treatment for mid-shaft clavicle fractures. Paper presented at: Proceedings of the 72nd Annual Meeting of the American Academy of Orthopaedic Surgeons, 2005
23. McKee MD, Pedersen EM, Jones C, et al. Deficits following nonoperative treatment of displaced midshaft clavicle fractures. J Bone Joint Surg Am 2006;88(1):35–40
24. Hudak PL, Amadio PC, Bombardier C. Development of an upper extremity outcome measure: the DASH (disabilities of the arm, shoulder and hand) [corrected]. The Upper Extremity Collaborative Group (UECG). Am J Ind Med 1996;29(6):602–608
25. Nowak J, Holgersson M, Larsson S. Can we predict long-term sequelae after fractures of the clavicle based on initial findings? A prospective study with nine to ten years of follow-up. J Shoulder Elbow Surg 2004;13(5):479–486
26. Bostman O, Manninen M, Pihlajamaki H. Complications of plate fixation of fresh displaced midclavicular fractures. J Trauma 1997;43(5):778–783
27. Shen WJ, Liu TJ, Shen YS. Plate fixation of fresh displaced midshaft clavicle fractures. Injury 1999;30(7):497–500
28. Iannotti MR, Crosby LA, Stafford P, Grayson G, Goulet R. Effects of plate location and selection on the stability of midshaft clavicle osteotomies: a biomechanical study. J Shoulder Elbow Surg 2002;11(5):457–462
29. Lim M, Kang J, Kim K, et al. Anterior inferior reconstruction plates for the treatment of acute midshaft clavicle fractures. Paper presented at: Proceedings of the 20th Annual Meeting of the Orthopaedic Trauma Association, 2003
30. Grassi FA, Tajana MS, D'Angelo F. Management of midclavicular fractures: comparison between nonoperative treatment and open intramedullary fixation in 80 patients. J Trauma 2001;50(6):1096–1100

31. Jubel A, Andermahr J, Schiffer G, Tsironis K, Rehm KE. Elastic stable intramedullary nailing of midclavicular fractures with a titanium nail. Clin Orthop Relat Res 2003;408:279–285
32. Chu CM, Wang SJ, Lin LC. Fixation of mid-third clavicular fractures with Knowles pins – 78 patients followed for 2–7 years. Acta Orthop Scand 2002;73(2):134–139
33. Ngarmukos C, Parkpian V, Patradul A. Fixation of fractures of the midshaft of the clavicle with Kirschner wires – results in 108 patients. J Bone Joint Surg Br 1998;80(1): 106–108
34. Jubel A, Andermahr J, Prokop A, Lee JI, Schiffer G, Rehm KE. Treatment of midclavicular fractures in adults. Early results after rucksack bandage or elastic stable intramedullary nailing. Unfallchirurg 2005;108(9):707–714
35. Jubel A, Andermahr J, Schiffer G, Rehm KE. The technique of elastic-stable intramedullary nailing of midclavicular fractures. Unfallchirurg 2002;105(6):511–516
36. Chen PY, Lin CC, Wang CC, Tsai CL. Closed reduction with intramedullary fixation for midclavicular fractures. Orthopedics 2004;27(5):459–462
37. Lengua F, Nuss JM, Lechner R, Baruthio J, Veillon F. The treatment of fractures of the clavicle by closed medio-lateral pinning. Rev Chir Orthop Reparatrice Appar Mot 1987;73(5):377–380
38. Ring D, Holovacs T. Brachial plexus palsy after intramedullary fixation of a clavicular fracture – a report of three cases. J Bone Joint Surg Am 2005;87(8):1834–1837
39. Nordqvist A, Redlund-Johnell I, von Scheele A, et al. Shortening of clavicle after fracture. Acta Orthop Scand 1997;68(4):349–351
40. Matis N, Kwasny O, Gaebler C, Vecsei V. Effects of clavicle shortening after clavicle fracture. Hefte Unfallchirurg 1999;275:314–315
41. Neer CS. Fracture of the distal clavicle with detachment of the coracoclavicular ligaments in adults. J Trauma 1963;3:99–110
42. Robinson CM, Cairns DA. Primary nonoperative treatment of displaced lateral fractures of the clavicle. J Bone Joint Surg Am 2004;86(4):778–782
43. Hughes PJ, Bolton-Maggs B. Fractures of the clavicle in adults. Curr Orthop 2002;16:133–138
44. Nadarajah R, Mahaluxmivala J, Amin A, Goodier DW. Clavicular hook-plate: complications of retaining the implant. Injury 2005;36(5):681–683
45. Levy O. Simple, minimally invasive surgical technique for treatment of type 2 fractures of the distal clavicle. J Shoulder Elbow Surg 2003;12(1):24–28
46. Bezer M, Aydin N, Guven O. The treatment of distal clavicle fractures with coracoclavicular ligament disruption. J Orthop Trauma 2005;19(8):524–528
47. Flinkkila T, Ristiniemi J, Hyvonen P, Hamalainen M. Surgical treatment of unstable fractures of the distal clavicle – a comparative study of Kirschner wire and clavicular hook plate fixation. Acta Orthop Scand 2002;73(1): 50–53

2 Nonunions of the Clavicle

René K. Marti and Peter Kloen

Clavicle fractures are common, comprising ~44% of all shoulder injuries and ~3% of all fractures. Most fractures of the clavicle involve the midshaft (69 to 81%). Fortunately, surgery is rarely indicated for these fractures because nonoperative treatment will lead to a good result in the vast majority of patients. Established indications for operative fixation of clavicle fractures include open fractures, pathological fractures, segmental fractures, fractures that compromise neurovascular structures, impending skin penetration by fracture ends, and significant displacement. There is no clear guideline, however, as to what amount of displacement can be accepted. Other reasons to operate on these fractures include (1) the presence of a so-called floating shoulder, or (2) if the procedure would promote early mobilization in a polytrauma patient. Finally, acute operative treatment can be called for in the throwing athlete to allow for earlier recovery and for cosmesis.[1–3]

A recent systematic review of 2144 midshaft clavicle fractures showed that nonoperative treatment of 1145 fractures resulted in a nonunion rate of 5.9%. When limited to 159 displaced fractures, the nonunion rate of nonoperative treatment increased to 15.1%.[2]

Etiological factors suggested to predispose to a nonunion include open fracture, initial displacement, comminution, refracture, inadequate immobilization, and initial open operative treatment.[1] Given these statistics the surgeon will be more likely to operate on a clavicle nonunion than on an acute clavicle fracture. Various tactics have been described for treating these nonunions utilizing either internal (plates and screws or intramedullary devices) and external fixation.[2,3]

Fractures on either end of the clavicle are much less common, but require surgical intervention relatively more often. Medial clavicle fractures can (partly) obstruct the esophagus and upper airway when the displacement is posterior, and most of these will need reduction and stabilization.[4] Although a large Scandinavian study reported good results after nonoperative treatment of lateral clavicle fractures, there is an ongoing debate whether lateral clavicle (intra- and extraarticular) fractures need fixation.[5] Although nonunion of the medial and (mostly) lateral clavicle are not uncommon, literature on how to treat these is sparse.

Classification

Fractures of the clavicle are often classified based on location according to Allman[6] into middle third (type I), outer third (II), and medial third (III). The nonunion type of the clavicle is most often classified according to Weber and Çech[7] into atrophic, oligotrophic, and hypertrophic. In their classic treatise on nonunions, they describe clavicle nonunions with shortening, those with a defect and shortening, and distal clavicle nonunions. Distal or lateral clavicle fractures and nonunions have also been classified according to Neer on the basis of their relation with the coracoclavicular (CC) ligaments (types I and II) and whether or not the fracture extends into the acromioclavicular (AC) joint (type III).[8] Medial clavicle fractures and resulting nonunions are often a growth plate fracture-dislocation (Salter–Harris I or II) when seen in patients younger than 25 years of age when the growth plate of the medial end of the clavicle finally closes.

Patient Assessment

History

Patients' complaints typically range from a mild aching during overhead activities to a severe and disabling resting pain with impaired function and rapid fatigability of the shoulder girdle and upper limb. Backpacks or other devices with shoulder straps often cause discomfort. In ~30% of patients symptoms of brachialgia are present.[9,10] Brachialgia is defined as a paresthesia or any numbness in the arm with or without associated muscle weakness. Usually, this involves the medial aspect of the arm.

Physical Examination

With the subcutaneous position of the clavicle, patients with midshaft clavicle nonunion do not generally require extensive diagnostic evaluation. The defect is often easy to palpate and motion and/or crepitus (usually painful) are obvious. The medial fragment is usually more prominent because of the downward pull on the lateral fragment. Often there are altered shoulder mechanics secondary to

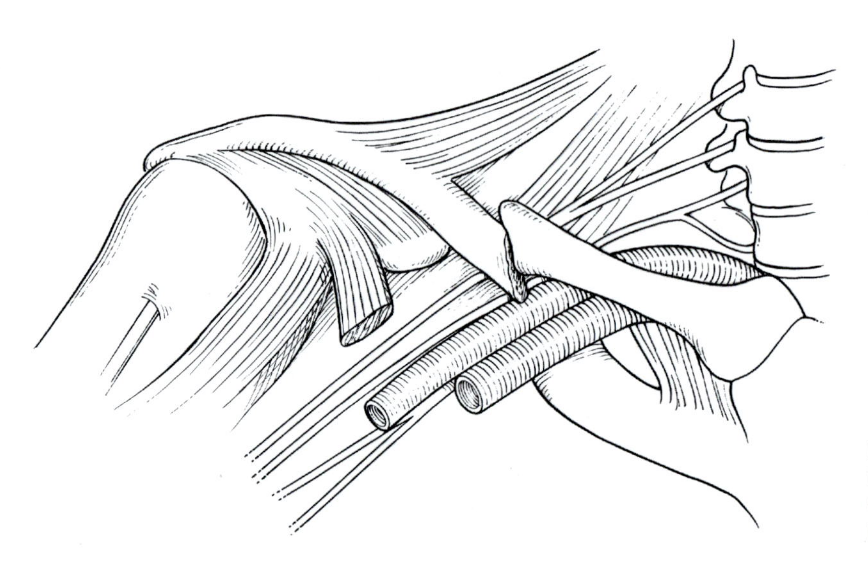

Figure 2–1 Brachialgia is relatively common in patients with a (most often) hypertrophic midshaft clavicle nonunion. The medial cord of the brachial plexus is impinged upon by the nonunion.

pain or malposition, resulting in a characteristic "drooping" or "ptosis" of the shoulder.[10] More difficult is the diagnosis of a medial or lateral clavicle nonunion, as these injuries can often mimic ligamentous injuries and/or dislocations.

It is also important to perform a careful neurological examination as the subclavicular area contains not only the brachial plexus, but also the subclavian vessels. Neurovascular symptoms may range from mild dysesthesias or paresthesias to a full-blown thoracic outlet syndrome. Deficits in sensory and motor function of the shoulder and arm as well as vascular deficits should be documented. Brachial plexus palsies secondary to clavicle nonunion most often affect the medial cord, producing mostly ulnar nerve symptoms. The nonunions that are associated with brachial plexus palsies are most often hypertrophic and located in the midshaft where the medial cord crosses the clavicle **(Fig. 2–1)**.

Radiologic Evaluation

Plain anteroposterior (AP) radiographs generally are sufficient for radiographic diagnosis. Both the medial and lateral ends of the involved clavicle should be visualized on this film to rule out any associated pathology of the AC and/or the sternoclavicular (SC) joint. In case of shortening, an AP radiograph of both clavicles will allow determination of the length that must be regained. To better visualize the AC joint and lateral clavicle, a Zanca-view (aiming 15 degrees cephalad) can be helpful.

Computed tomography (CT) and/or magnetic resonance imaging (MRI) are seldom indicated, although for lateral and medial clavicle and/or SC injuries, a CT can better clarify intraarticular extension. Also, these methods may be helpful when dealing with a medial clavicle nonunion, which is often obscured by the sternum and ribs. Finally, MRI can be indicated when there is evidence of brachial plexopathy to precisely document the relationship between bone and brachial plexus.

Laboratory Studies

In addition to preoperative laboratory tests, we also obtain an erythrocyte sedimentation rate (ESR), C-reactive protein (CRP), and a complete white cell count to help rule out infection. We do not generally aspirate the nonunion to rule out infection at the site prior to surgery.

Treatment

Nonsurgical Treatment

Nonoperative treatment is seldom warranted. Although there are some anecdotal reports on the success of ultrasound on stimulating healing in a clavicle nonunion, we do not have any experience with this or other related techniques.

Surgical Treatment

Midshaft Clavicle Nonunion

Position the patient supine in the beach-chair semisitting position. A useful option is to use a Mayfield headrest rather than the standard broad headpiece of an operating table. The clavicle region and arm should be draped free so that the arm is freely mobile. The procedure can be done under interscalene block, but most often we use general anesthesia. This also allows harvesting of iliac

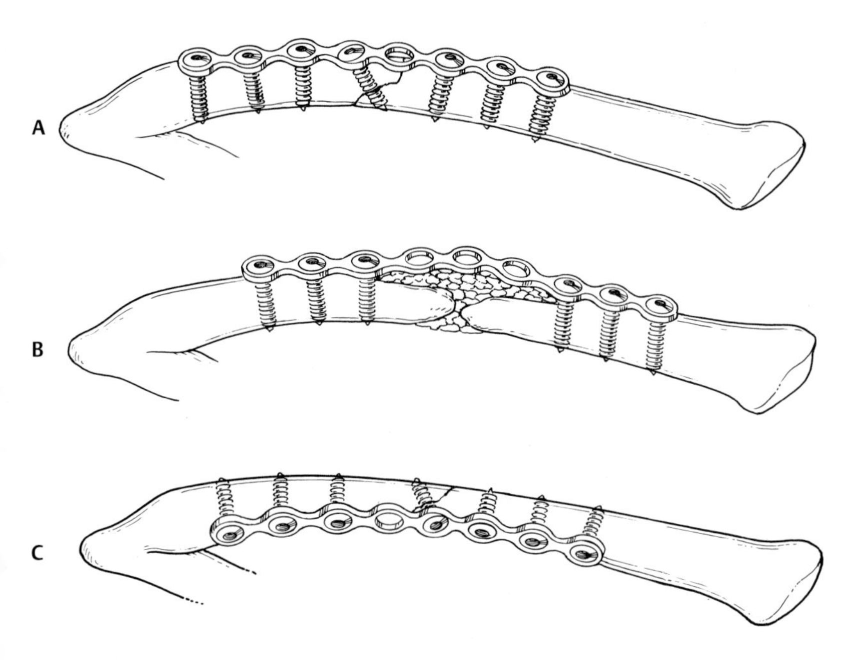

Figure 2–2 Optional plate positions: **(A)** superior, **(B)** wave-plate, and **(C)** anteroinferior.

crest bone graft. The head of the patient is turned away from the side of the clavicle that is to be operated upon, with the endotracheal tube positioned out the opposite corner of the mouth to maximize the operative field. Harvesting iliac crest bone from the same side is advantageous in terms of postoperative pain control, but using the contralateral iliac crest will allow two surgeons to work simultaneously.

Depending on the preferred plate position (anteroinferior,[3,11] superior,[9,10] or wave plate[9]) **(Fig. 2–2)**, the incision runs parallel to Langer's lines along the superior or inferior border of the clavicle overlying the nonunion. In case of a previous incision, we try to incorporate this into our incision. The incision is carried down to bone. Although others describe loupe dissection and preservation of the (cutaneous) supraclavicular nerves, we do not specifically isolate or protect these nerve endings.[10] In our experience, we have not had any postoperative complaints of dysesthesias or neuromas in the region of these nerves.

Once the nonunion is identified there is often a significant amount of intervening soft tissue and scar with displacement of the bony ends. With the underlying neurovascular components occasionally encased in this fibrotic tissue, it is much safer to proceed with the dissection from known to unknown territory. Using careful dissection the soft tissues are gently pried of the anteroinferior or anterosuperior (depending on the plate position you anticipate) aspect of the bony ends working toward the nonunion. At the level of the nonunion extending to ~1.5 cm on either side we decorticate using a sharp osteotome. This should be done with caution, taking care to avoid any potential damage to the anterior divisions of the brachial plexus and the subclavian vessels. Most surgeons place the plate on the superior aspect of the clavicle, and are strengthened in doing so by most reports that argue that the tension side of the nonunion is the superior aspect of the clavicle. The forces of distraction acting on the bone are thus converted into compression acting as a tension band.[10]

Recently, the placement of the plate on the anteroinferior side has been described.[3,11,12] The arguments in favor of this position are that the lateral fragment is often osteopenic and is now buttressed (like a shelf) by the plate rather than being suspended from it. In addition, screw length can be longer with a larger diameter from anteroinferior to superoposterior, and there is less risk of penetration of the drill into the subclavian neurovascular structures as opposed to drilling from superior to inferior. If placing the plate on the superior aspect, no dissection should be done on the anteroinferior side and vice versa. Deep tissue cultures are obtained and intravenous antibiotics can now be given.

The next step is based on the type of nonunion. In case of a *hypertrophic nonunion* there is generally no need to enter the nonunion itself for débridement. Excess callus prevents easy contouring of the plate and also places the neurovascular structures at risk of impingement or compression. Therefore, one should remove excess callus with an osteotome to allow apposition of the plate and to prevent prominence of the hardware under the skin when placing the plate superiorly and prevent impingement when placing the plate anteroinferiorly.

Occasionally, a fragment is rotated inward so that the excess callus is not appreciated easily. Both fragments should thus be rotated outward using a bone holding forces prior to reduction and fixation to make sure impingement of subclavian structures by callus is prevented.

In case of an *atrophic* or *oligotrophic nonunion*, all intervening tissue is removed with a knife or rongeur. Both ends of the nonunion should be inspected for the presence of a sclerotic end cap that would prevent contact between medullary canals of the two fragments. In case of an end cap, multiple holes are made with a small drill (2.0 or 2.5 mm) to reopen the medullary canal. The bone should be penetrated just enough to restore visible bleeding from both ends. We generally do not resect the sclerotic ends because this will lead to unnecessary shortening and/or a need for an intercalary graft.

For a true *synovial pseudarthrosis*, the entire fluid-filled cavity including the synovial lining is resected sharply. Meticulous technique is warranted here because the neurovascular structures are in close proximity to the back wall or inferior wall of the cavity.

For a so-called *gap* or *defect nonunion* where a small or large segmental defect is present (secondary to infection or resection), one has to decide whether to shorten the clavicle or to place some type of interposition graft. Shortening of the clavicle can theoretically lead to narrowing of the neurovascular space, creating a thoracic outlet syndrome and ipsilateral glenohumeral and/or scapulothoracic dysfunction. There are no clear guidelines as to what amount of shortening can be accepted. Recently, McKee et al[13] reported that residual shortening of ≥ 2 cm was associated with decreased abductor strength with a trend to greater patient dissatisfaction. Obviously, the placement of an intercalary graft implicates two healing sites as opposed to an end-to-end situation.

Once the nonunion is exposed and, if needed, débrided, small blunt Hohmann retractors are placed **(Fig. 2–3)**. The nonunion is then reduced with standard reduction clamps. This is easy for an oblique nonunion with little translation and/or displacement. When there is posterior displacement of the lateral fragment, however, this can be quite challenging. In this case, it might be helpful to grasp the lateral fragment with a pointed reduction clamp and gently tease it forward, carefully freeing it up by decortication, leaving small fragments of bone attached to the surrounding muscles. If there is relatively little shortening, the lateral fragment can be pulled medially to meet the medial fragment. A straight 3.5-mm plate (standard pelvic reconstruction, limited contact-dynamic compression plate [LC-DCP], DCP or reconstruction locking compression plate [LCP]) is contoured to fit the superior or anteroinferior aspect of the clavicle. Plate benders and twisters and the scalloping design of the 3.5-mm pelvic reconstruction type plates greatly facilitate the plate contouring. First, the plate is transfixed to the lateral fragment with at least two 3.5-mm screws. Rotating the lateral fragment upward with a reduction clamp facilitates placement of the screws when opting for an anteroinferior plate position. There is no need to keep the nonunion reduced at this time. Once the plate is attached

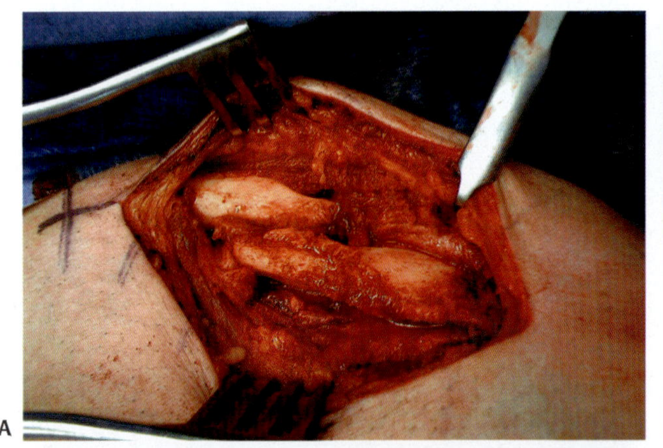

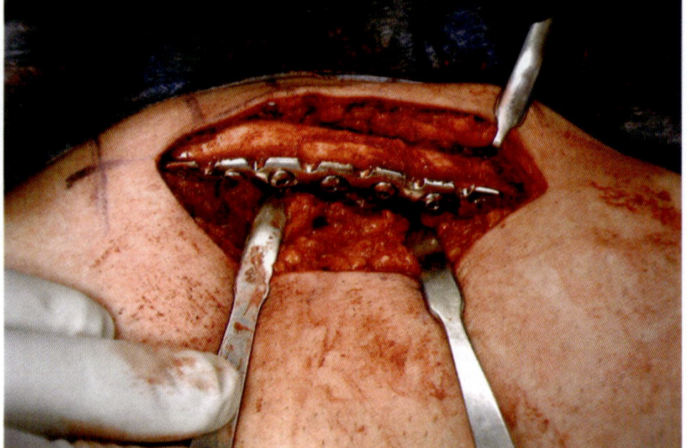

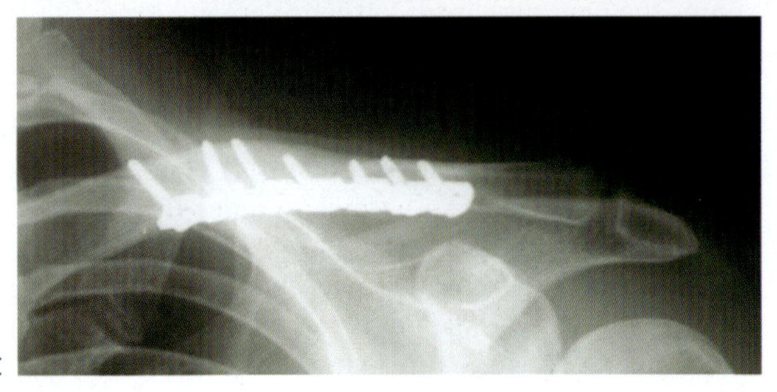

Figure 2–3 **(A)** Intraoperative view after exposure of a midshaft clavicle nonunion, and **(B)** after anteroinferior plate placement. **(C)** Final radiographic appearance. (Courtesy of David L. Helfet, MD, New York, NY.)

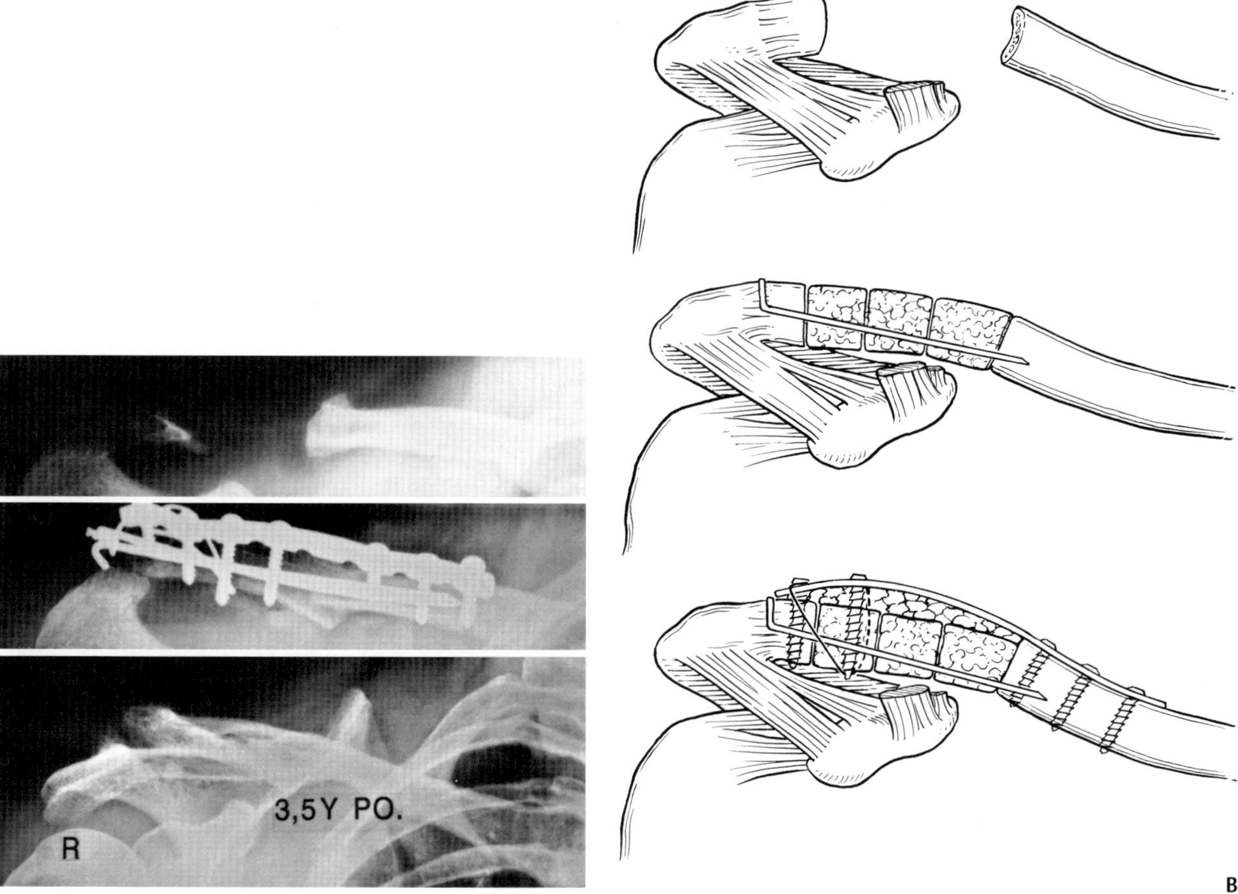

Figure 2–4 **(A)** Preoperative (*top*), postoperative (*middle*), and final follow-up (*bottom*) radiographs of a large gap nonunion of the clavicle treated with a combination of techniques: multiple intercalary grafts, intramedullary fixation with tension band, wave plate, and cancellous bone graft. **(B)** Schematic depiction of the reconstruction.

to the lateral fragment, the medial fragment is reduced to the plate by pushing the shoulder inward. If the obliquity of the nonunion allows it, a 3.5-mm cortical lag screw is placed across the nonunion through the plate. Subsequently, additional 3.5-mm cortical screws can be placed for a minimum of three screws on either side of the nonunion/fracture **(Fig. 2–3)**. This means that we usually use a 7- or 8-hole 3.5-mm plate. Although autogenous cancellous bone graft remains our gold standard, we have recently reported good results with a type of demineralized bone matrix with admixed allograft obviating the morbidity of iliac crest harvesting. In atrophic or oligotrophic nonunion, on both ends of the nonunion "petaling" or "shingling" of the cortex is done to stimulate graft incorporation and healing.

For a *nonunion with a defect and shortening* ($>$2 cm), a bicortical graft can be used to restore length. We prefer to harvest these grafts from the inner table so as not to change the outer (and most visible) contour of the iliac crest. We have used multiple intercalary grafts of up to 6.5 cm **(Fig. 2–4)**. Ideally, you should measure the needed length on a preoperative radiograph comparing the involved side with the opposite healthy side, but you can estimate reasonably well by palpating through the drapes. After harvesting the iliac crest graft, the medial and lateral aspects are sculptured into pegs and plugged into the medullary canals on either side. The cortical side of the graft is placed opposite the plate to increase biomechanical strength of the construct. At least one screw is placed through the plate and native bone on both ends of the graft. We generally do not place fixation through the midportion of the smaller size graft because this might disturb vascularization and weaken the graft. Additional cancellous graft around the nonunion is placed to promote healing. Assess the stability at the time of surgery to assure there is no residual micromotion. In addition, the upper extremity/shoulder needs to be tested for a gentle but full range of motion to assure no neurovascular compromise with position. Radiographs can also be obtained at the same time. Finally, after meticulous hemostasis drains are placed in the wounds. The deltoid and trapezial fascia are reconstructed using nonabsorbable suture, and the subcutaneous layer is closed using 2–0 absorbable suture. Skin closure is made using 3–0 monofilament suture after which Steri-Strips (3M Health Care, St Paul, MN) are applied. Local infiltration of a long-acting anesthetic can be very beneficial for the first 8 hours after surgery. The arm is placed in some type of sling.

Infected Midshaft Nonunion

Despite the subcutaneous position of the clavicle, open fractures are relatively unusual. Infected nonunion of the clavicle is most often the result of a failed attempt at surgical fixation. The combination of compromised soft tissues, osteopenia, failed hardware, and persistence of infection can present as an enormous challenge for the treating physician. The general principles for all infected nonunions hold true for the clavicle as well – aggressive débridement, antibiotics, and stabilization. Ideally, fixation of the infected nonunion is done with as little hardware inside as possible. We have treated infected nonunion with débridement, antibiotics, and an external fixation device customized from a DCP with standard screws that were stabilized with a nut and washer on the opposite site of the plate.[14] Later, we modified this by using a LCP, obviating the need for a bolt on the opposite site **(Fig. 2–5)**. Once the infection is under control and the soft tissues are healed, one can either maintain the external fixator in place until bony consolidation or convert to internal fixation and bone grafting if needed. Occasionally, if there is exposed hardware in situ with a nonunion and the fixation is deemed stable, one can try the "wait and see" approach.

Lateral Clavicle Nonunion

Make a vertical incision (saber cut) between the acromioclavicular joint and the nonunion. Skin flaps are easily raised, if necessary, to increase the surgical exposure. The

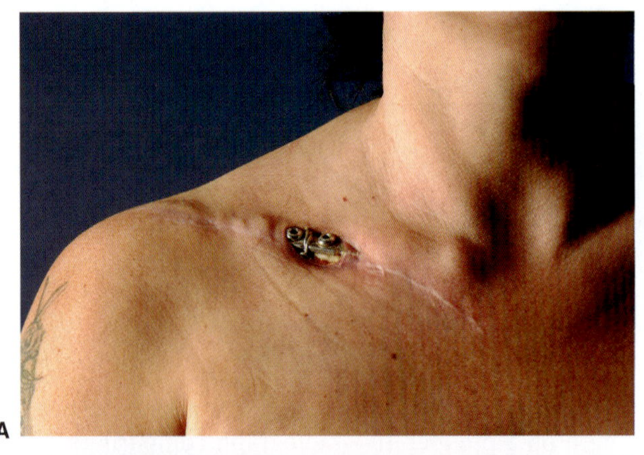

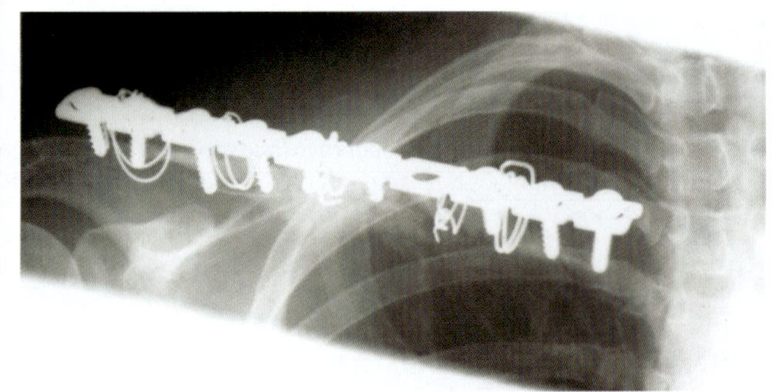

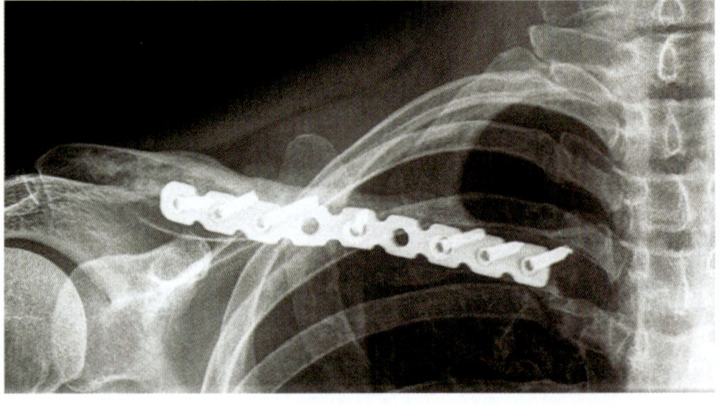

Figure 2–5 **(A)** Clinical appearance of infected nonunion of the midshaft clavicle after multiple failed surgical attempts. **(B)** Radiographic appearance. **(C)** After removal of all hardware, débridement, and temporary stabilization with 3.5-mm locking compression plate as external fixator. **(D)** After 8 weeks of antibiotics, the infection had been eradicated, and the wound had healed. Subsequent anteroinferior plating with cancellous autologous bone grafting led to rapid healing.

nonunion is now identified and utilizing sharp dissection the bone ends are exposed. A soft tissue elevator is needed to complete the dissection subperiosteally. The distal fragment is generally fairly small. Make sure not to compromise any soft tissue attachments, especially the ligaments. The nonunion is temporarily reduced with a small bone reduction clamp. Depending on the size of the fragment, various techniques for fixation are available. In case of a fairly large fragment, we have used a small fragment LCP T-plate. An alternative is a lag screw (in case of an oblique nonunion) with a neutralizing tension band with two Kirschner wires (K-wires) placed medially from the AC joint **(Fig. 2–6)**. Even with small lateral fragments, there is no need to compromise the AC joint with this type of fixation. We avoid bridging the AC joint with hardware as this will most likely lead to loosening and/or failure of hardware with the subsequent risk of hardware migration.[15,16] To support the reduction and fixation during bony healing, a cerclage wire can be placed around the clavicle and the coracoid prior to fixation, which is then tightened after fixation. In case of a combined lateral clavicle nonunion and acromioclavicular luxation, internal fixation and ligament reconstruction have to be combined. We have not used the Weaver–Dunn procedure (lateral clavicle resection and transposition of the acromial end of coracoacromial ligament onto the lateral clavicle) for this problem as we consider this a late salvage for failed nonunion treatment. The deltoid and trapezius fascia are repaired using a nonabsorbable suture. The subcutaneous layer is repaired using a 2–0 absorbable suture and the skin with a 3–0 monofilament-type suture reinforced by Steri-Strips.

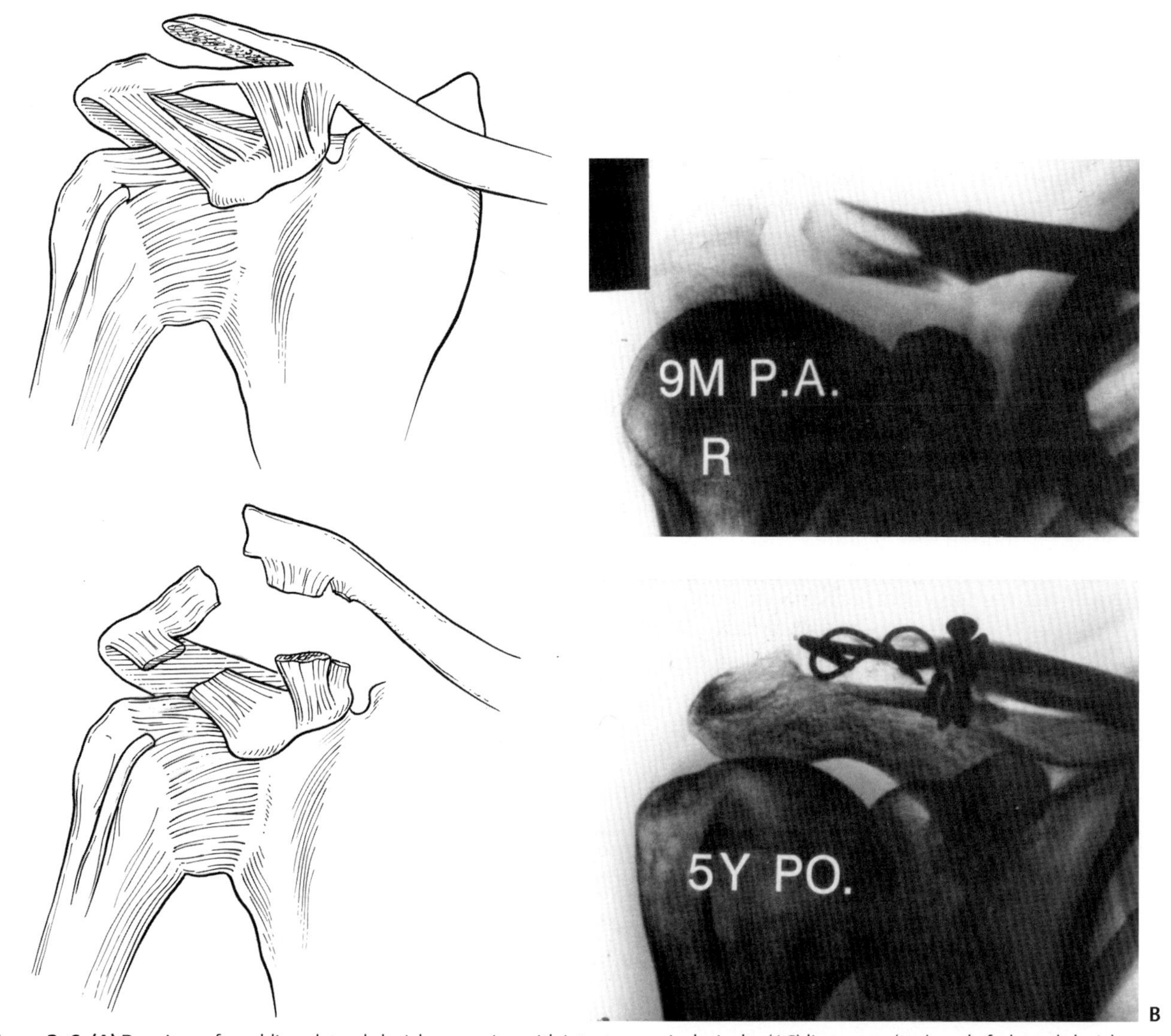

Figure 2–6 (A) Drawings of an oblique lateral clavicle nonunion with intact acromioclavicular (AC) ligaments (*top*), and of a lateral clavicle nonunion with torn AC ligaments (*bottom*). **(B)** Union in the former type was obtained after placement of a lag screw and neutralizing tension band.

Medial Clavicle Nonunion

These nonunions are extremely rare. The operative treatment we choose in these cases is similar as for acute fractures as described below. One should ensure a thoracic/vascular surgeon is available when operating on these medial displaced fractures in case intraoperative vascular and/or thoracic complications develop. To be prepared for an emergency sternotomy, the operative field should include the entire arm over the thoracic midline. The incision is horizontal traversing over the SC joint. There will most likely be scar formation "adhering" to the vascular structures behind the bone, making extreme care necessary during this procedure. There are no large series describing how to fix these medial nonunion and/or fractures. A method may be the utilization of cerclage wire to fix the fragment to the first or second rib or manubrium sterni. Case reports have increased the awareness of potentially life-threatening hardware migration.[15] Mersilene tape or nonabsorbable suture could be used as an alternative to metal wiring.

Postoperative Care and Rehabilitation

For nonunions, we maintain the patient on antibiotics until all intraoperative cultures are negative. A sling is worn until the wound is healed. Physical therapy is initiated on the first postoperative day with gentle active and active-assisted Codman's and pendulum exercises and the use of gentle overhead pulleys. In addition elbow flexion/extension range of motion (ROM) exercises without resistance can be initiated. The patient is advised to continue wearing a sling for 10 to 14 days, which is the time of the first postoperative visit. Radiographs are taken at 6 weeks, 3 months, and 6 months follow-up until crossing trabeculae confirm bony healing. At 3 weeks postoperatively, the patients are started on active and passive range of motion, as tolerated, but no lifting, throwing, or resistive activities until bony healing is confirmed. We do not routinely remove hardware unless indicated (e.g., in case of a previous infection) or requested by the patient. This should not be done earlier than 18 months after healing because of refracture risk. Our experience with the anteroinferior position of the plate is that patients seldom request removal.

Complications

Acute neurovascular injuries are unusual despite the proximity of the brachial plexus and the subclavian vessels. If these do occur they usually are seen in the more severe injuries of the shoulder girdle including scapular injuries. Compression of the neurovascular structures can be caused at the time of injury and as a result of a displaced fracture or malunion or even in some rare cases by the hypertrophic callus on the inferior aspect of the clavicle. Impingement, which usually is the result of a hypertrophic nonunion, most often affects the ulnar nerve distribution because of compression of the medial cord of the brachial plexus. In a recent series published on using a so-called wave plate (contoured from a regular 3.5 DCP) on the superior side of the clavicle, the results (no brachialgia and higher Constant scores) were better than for those patients treated with a regular (nonwave) plate.[9] It was felt that offsetting the wave on the superior surface would cause less hypertrophy (and risk of impingement of the brachial plexus) on the inferior side.

One of the clavicle nonunion patients treated with anteroinferior plating developed acute symptoms of a thoracic outlet syndrome secondary to hypertrophic callus that impinged upon the neurovascular structure after reduction and plating.[11] This necessitated removal of the callus and revisional internal fixation during the same hospital stay.

Although painful neuromas secondary to injury of the supraclavicular nerves that cause pain and/or dysesthesias on the anterior chest wall have been described, we have not encountered these.

Hardware problems are relatively common. Of these, the most worrisome complication has been the migration of pins, wires, and screws.[15] Not only can this lead to a life-threatening situation, but it also represents failed fixation. Hardware failure is not uncommon, especially in the elderly and longstanding nonunions with significant osteopenia. As far as plate choice we caution against use of one-third tubular plates as these are not strong enough for use in the adult clavicle. Although 3.5-mm pelvic reconstruction plates have the advantage of easy contouring, all other 3.5-mm plates (DCP, LC-DCP, and LCP) are adequate.

The prominence of the plate, wire, pin, and screw fixation on the superior (subcutaneous) aspect of the clavicle is often uncomfortable and sometimes disabling when wearing a bra or carrying a backpack. This is often a reason for hardware removal, requiring a second operation. Only two patients in our initial series of placing the plate on the anteroinferior aspect needed hardware removal because of discomfort. This pertained to the lag screw that was placed outside the plate from superior to inferior (the plate itself did not need removal), illustrating the benefit of the anteroinferior aspect plate and lag screws.[11]

Intraarticular fractures can lead to posttraumatic arthritis. This is more common for the AC than the SC joint. If nonoperative measures fail, then the patient might be a candidate for a resection of the medial or lateral aspect. The resection of the medial end of the clavicle should be carefully weighed because the reconstruction of the sternoclavicular joint is notoriously difficult.

Results

One of us (RKM) recently reported the results in 28 midshaft clavicle nonunions.[9] He introduced the technique of wave-plate fixation (as modified from use in the humerus and femur) using a 3.5-mm DCP. The theory behind "offsetting" the plate by a wave is that in addition to improved biomechanics, there is less callus formation on the undersurface of the clavicle, decreasing the risk of brachialgia postoperatively. For this technique, a longitudinal incision is made slightly inferior to the clavicle. By creating a flap, the wave plate is placed on the superior aspect and is thus well covered. Twelve patients had evidence of brachialgia preoperatively. Of these, 6 patients had their nonunion treated with a wave plate and 6 with a regular plate. All 6 with a wave plate had complete resolution of the brachialgia, whereas these symptoms only resolved in 2 patients in the other group. In 4 patients (all treated with a regular plate), brachialgia developed postoperatively.

The use of anteroinferior plating for midshaft clavicle nonunions using 3.5-mm standard stainless-steel pelvic reconstruction plating in 17 patients was recently described.[11] Autologous iliac crest bone or demineralized bone matrix was used as bone graft. All nonunions healed at an average 3.6 months (range: 2 to 8 months). Using the same techniques of anteroinferior plate positioning, one of the authors (PK) has now treated 20 midshaft clavicle nonunions in the last 6 years with a titanium 3.5-mm LCP reconstruction plate and autologous bone graft with comparable results. One plate failure was seen after 2 weeks, possibly due to increased mechanical demand in a patient who ambulated on crutches and/or early titanium fatigue after contouring/recontouring the plate. Of this latter group, only 1 patient has undergone hardware removal after she had lost ~40 pounds postoperatively and complained of an unsightly scar with stretch marks. She had initially been referred to us with an infected nonunion treated by us by débridement, antibiotics, and temporary stabilization using a 3.5-mm LCP as external fixator to allow soft tissue healing followed by a formal anteroinferior plating 6 weeks later **(Fig. 2–5)**.

Interestingly, it was recently shown that an anteroinferior plate position gave fewer symptoms when compared with a superior plate position.[12] This was, however, a nonrandomized, comparative study. A randomized study comparing the use of 3.5-mm DCP and 3.5-mm LC-DCP plates positioned on the superior aspect for fixation of midshaft clavicle nonunion showed improved results for the LC-DCP (better union rates and functional scores).[16] The clear advantage of the 3.5-mm LC-DCP, the standard 3.5-mm pelvic, and the 3.5-mm LCP reconstruction plates is that the plates can be easily contoured to fit on the serpentine-shaped clavicle; the 3.5-mm DCP reconstruction plate is more bulky and difficult to contour. The better holding power of locking (LCP) screws in osteopenic bone has an (at least theoretical) advantage in the osteopenic bone often associated with nonunions. Also, secondary screw loosening will not occur (especially important for anteroinferior plating). One-third tubular plates are not strong enough for fixation of clavicle nonunion. Whether to use the superior or anteroinferior plate position is still open to debate. The advantage of a superior plate position is its ease of surgical approach, whereas the advantage of an anteroinferior plate position is that patients seldom are bothered by the hardware and do not need hardware removal.

Summary

Fortunately, clavicle nonunions are very responsive to skilled operative treatment. Patients and their surgeon can typically expect an excellent outcome with improved function and relief of pain.[17,18]

References

1. Lazarus MD. Fractures of the clavicle. In: Bucholz RW, Heckman JD, eds. Fractures in Adults, 5th ed. Philadelphia: Lippincott Williams & Wilkins; 2001:1041–1078
2. Zlowodzki M, Zelle BA, Cole PA, Jeray K, McKee MD. Treatment of acute midshaft clavicle fractures: systematic review of 2144 fractures. J Orthop Trauma 2005;19: 504–507
3. Kloen P, Helfet DL. Open reduction and internal fixation of fractures and nonunions of the clavicle. In: Craig EV, ed. Master Techniques in Orthopaedic Surgery. The Shoulder (2nd ed). Philadelphia: Lippincott Williams & Wilkins; 2004:385–411
4. Goldfarb CA, Bassett GS, Sullivan S, et al. Retrosternal displacement after physeal fracture of the medial clavicle in children. J Bone Joint Surg Br 2001;83:1168–1172
5. Nordqvist A, Petersson C, Redlund-Johnell I. The natural course of lateral clavicle fracture. Acta Orthop Scand 1993;64:87–91
6. Allman FL. Fractures and ligamentous injuries of the clavicle and its articulation. J Bone Joint Surg Am 1967;49:774–784
7. Weber BG, Çech O. Clavicula-Pseudarthrose. In: Weber BG, Cech O, eds. Pseudarthrosen. Huber/Bern/Stuttgart: Verlag Hans Huber; 1973:108–111

8. Neer CS II . Fractures of the distal end of the clavicle. Clin Orthop Relat Res 1968;58:43–50
9. Marti RK, Nolte PA, Kerkhoffs GMMJ, Besselaar PP, Schaap GR. Operative treatment of mid-shaft clavicular non-union. Int Orthop 2003;27:131–135
10. Simpson NS, Jupiter JB. Clavicular nonunion and malunion: evaluation and surgical management. J Am Acad Orthop Surg 1996;4:1–8
11. Kloen P, Sorkin AT, Rubel IF, Helfet DL. Anteroinferior plating of midshaft clavicular nonunions. J Orthop Trauma 2002;16:425–430
12. Lim M, Kang J, Kim K, et al. Anterior inferior reconstruction plates for the treatment of acute midshaft clavicle fractures. Poster presented at: 20th Annual Meeting of the Orthopaedic Trauma Association; October 9–11, 2003; Salt Lake City, UT
13. McKee MD, Pedersen EM, Jones C, et al. Deficits following nonoperative treatment of displaced clavicular fractures. J Bone Joint Surg Am 2006;88:35–40
14. Marti RK, van der Werken C. The AO-plate for external fixation in 12 cases. Acta Orthop Scand 1991;62:60–62
15. Lyons FA, Rockwood CA. Current concepts review. Migration of pins used in operations on the shoulder. J Bone Joint Surg Am 1990;72:1262–1267
16. Kabak S, Halic M, Tuncle M, Avsarogullari L, Karaoglu S. Treatment of midclavicular nonunion: comparison of dynamic compression plating and low-contact dynamic compression plating. J Shoulder Elbow Surg 2004;13: 396–403
17. O'Connor D, Kutty S, McCabe JP. Long-term functional outcome assessment of plate fixation and autogenous bone grafting for clavicular non-union. Injury 2004;35: 575–579
18. Der Tavitian J, Davison JNS, Dias JJ. Clavicular fracture non-union surgical outcome and complications. Injury 2002;33:135–143

3 Treatment of Glenoid Fractures and Injuries to the Superior Shoulder Suspensory Complex

Michael J. Gardner, Bryan T. Kelly, and Dean G. Lorich

Injuries to the shoulder girdle can range from clinically insignificant avulsion fractures or partial ligament disruptions, to markedly displaced or comminuted fractures that may predispose to long-term shoulder dysfunction. Scapular fractures are relatively uncommon, comprising ~1% of all fractures,[1] and only between 10 and 30% of these involve the glenoid.[2–5] Because of the thick protective surrounding muscle envelope, the forgiving multiplanar ligaments, and the recoil of the chest wall, direct high-energy trauma is usually necessary to cause a scapular fracture. The significant energy imparted leads to a high incidence of concomitant head, thoracic, shoulder, and other injuries.[4,6,7] These multiple associated injuries often distract the surgeon from the scapular fracture, and these fractures are not always readily apparent on initial survey radiographs. Appropriate clinical suspicion, complete radiographic exam, and a thorough knowledge of the osseous and ligamentous anatomy of the shoulder girdle will allow for appropriate treatment to maximize the chance of a good outcome.

Patient Assessment

The initial evaluation of a patient with a potential glenoid or other shoulder girdle injury is a thorough history. For the multitrauma patient, details of the accident scene by emergency personnel or witnesses may give important clues about the mechanism of injury and level of energy involved, as well as any associated life-threatening injuries. A multisystem screening physical exam should be followed by a detailed upper extremity and neurovascular exam. Injuries to the shoulder girdle may reveal pain with passive or active motion, limited motion, ecchymosis and swelling, or gross crepitus. Visible deformity may be notably absent.

When the advanced trauma life support (ATLS) protocol has been completed and the patient is hemodynamically stable, a complete radiographic exam is performed. Plain radiographs must include anteroposterior and lateral views in the scapular plane, as well as axillary and West Point views. Ideally, tangential views of the glenohumeral joint should be obtained to evaluate articular displacement and concentricity of the glenohumeral joint. If doubt exists regarding shoulder stability in a small peripheral fracture, fluoroscopic stress views may be helpful.[8] Magnetic resonance imaging (MRI) may also be useful in assessing the critical ligament status in minimally displaced fractures. Additionally, several authors have reported on the use of arthroscopic evaluation and assisted reduction of intraarticular glenoid fractures.[9,10]

Because of the complex bony anatomy, and the often-overlapping cortical bone on x-ray views, complete fracture anatomy visualization can be difficult. Computed tomography (CT) and three-dimensional reconstructions are particularly useful to understand the multiplanar and multifragmented fractures, as well as articular comminution, both of which may affect surgical indications, surgical approach, or choice of instrumentation.[4]

Glenoid Fractures

Classification

Fractures of the glenoid may occur extraarticularly, at the neck at the junction of the glenoid and the scapular spine, or may occur through the articular surface. Intraarticular fractures may lead to shoulder instability acutely, or degeneration of the articular surface chronically. Glenoid neck fractures may involve both translational and angular deformity, and can also lead to chronic pain and weakness due to the alteration of glenohumeral biomechanics.

Glenoid Cavity Fractures

The most frequently used classification for fractures of the glenoid cavity is that proposed by Ideberg[11] and further modified by Goss[12] (**Fig. 3–1**). Type I fractures are the most common fracture pattern, and involve the anteroinferior or posterior articular margin. These fracture types often occur with a glenohumeral fracture-dislocation, and frequently lead to residual instability of the joint following reduction. Type I fractures are distinct from Bankart-type

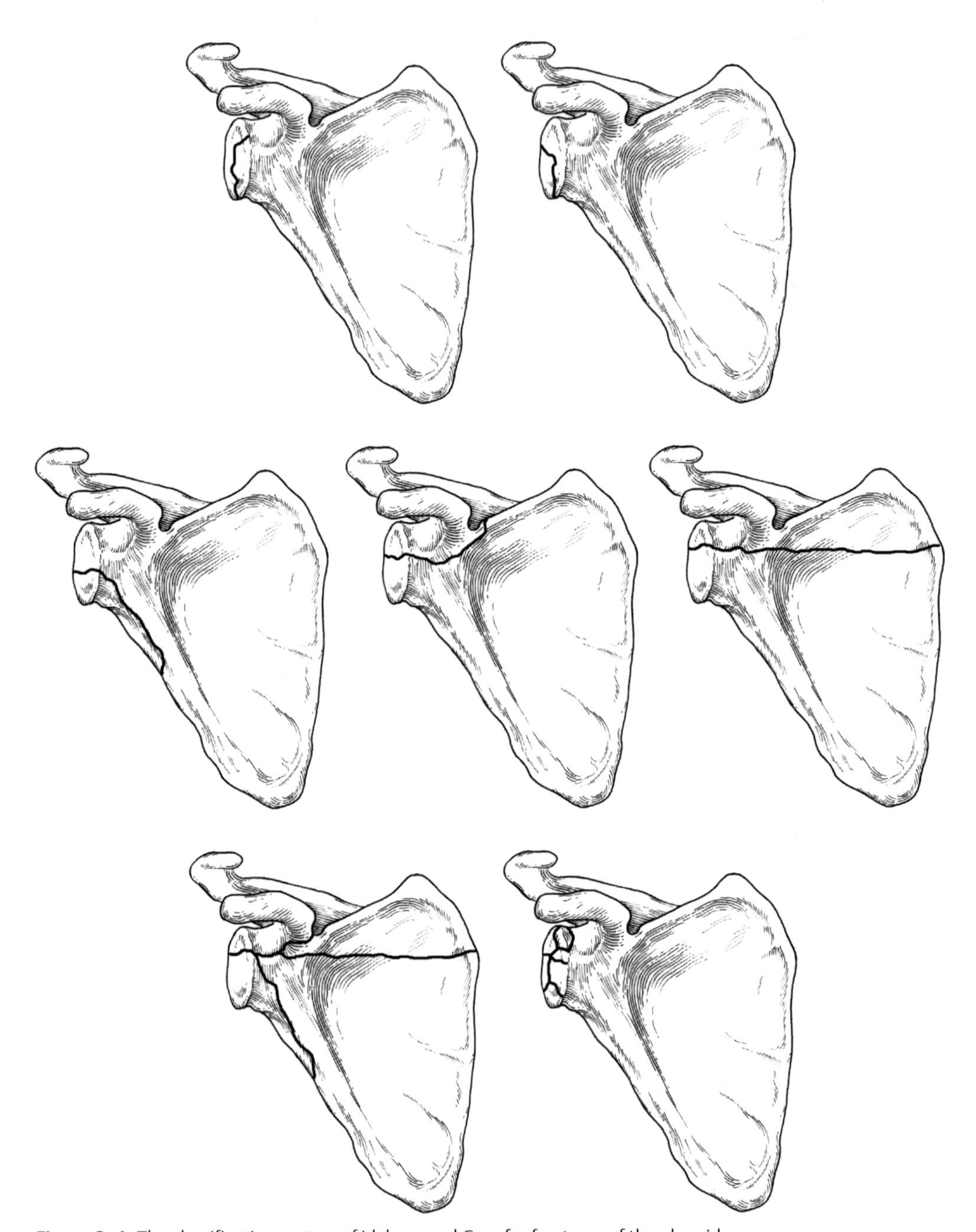

Figure 3–1 The classification system of Ideberg and Goss for fractures of the glenoid.

capsular avulsions seen in pure shoulder dislocations and typically involve a larger fragment due to humeral head impaction rather than a capsular avulsion. In type II fractures, the fracture line is transverse or slightly oblique at the articular surface, and exits the lateral border of the scapula inferiorly. When a significant portion of the articular surface is involved, inferior subluxation of the humeral head may be present. The inferior fragment may be pulled and angled distally by the long head of the triceps tendon. Type III fractures occur following a medially directed force with a cephalad component, and the superior one third of the glenoid fossa is affected. The fracture line courses superiorly and usually exits medial to the coracoid at the superior scapular border, and may follow the epiphyseal scar. The direction of the force vector in these injuries often disrupts the superior elements of the shoulder girdle, and may lead to fracture of the clavicle or acromion, or acromioclavicular (AC) separation. Type IV fractures result from a direct medial force. The glenoid is fractured centrally, and the fracture line extends medially to the medial border of the scapula. Type V fractures involve a type IV transverse fracture component with associated superior or inferior fragments as seen in types II and III fractures. Type VI patterns, added by Goss, are comminuted fractures of the glenoid fossa.

We have found this fracture classification useful for descriptive purposes only. The surgical approach follows common sense and logical biomechanical principles, and each fracture must be evaluated individually as no single approach applies for all fractures in a given class. Prognosis based on fracture type has also not been fully correlated, and most available data are anecdotal or small single-surgeon series.

Glenoid Neck Fractures

Fractures of the glenoid neck frequently occur following direct lateral impact on the humeral head, and may occur in concert with other bony or soft tissue disruptions around the shoulder girdle. When double disruptions of the superior shoulder suspensory complex (SSSC) occur, unique biomechanical issues must be considered. The first consideration when evaluating glenoid neck fractures is the inherent stability or lack thereof, for which associated lesions must be considered. These combination injuries are complex and will be discussed further in a later section. Additional specific factors relative to the glenoid neck have significant implications on treatment approaches, however, regardless of associated injuries. In particular, whether or not the fracture is deemed to be stable, malalignment of the glenoid neck may lead to permanent malunion and can have a detrimental effect on shoulder function. The force vector created by the deltoid during initial abduction is a shear force across the glenoid, which is stabilized by the compressive forces of the rotator cuff across an anatomically positioned glenoid. Alteration of this axis results in conversion of the rotator cuff force to shear in the case of inferior angulation, or in a shortened lever arm in the case of a medially displaced glenoid neck fracture.[13] For this reason, operative reduction and stabilization of glenoid fractures with evidence of inferior angulation or medial displacement is recommended.[13–17]

Measurements of angulation must be derived in relation to the scapular body. Some surgeons have advocated the threshold of 40 degrees of angulation or 10 mm of translational displacement as a surgical indication.[3,13,18,19] Despite these empiric recommendations, the clinical evidence supporting these indications is sparse. We have found the glenopolar angle (GPA) a useful tool for this purpose. In addition, several authors have correlated the GPA to outcomes after either conservative or operative treatment.[15,17,20,21] To obtain the GPA, an anteroposterior (AP) x-ray of the scapula is obtained. Two lines are drawn: the first between the superior and inferior margins of the glenoid, and the second

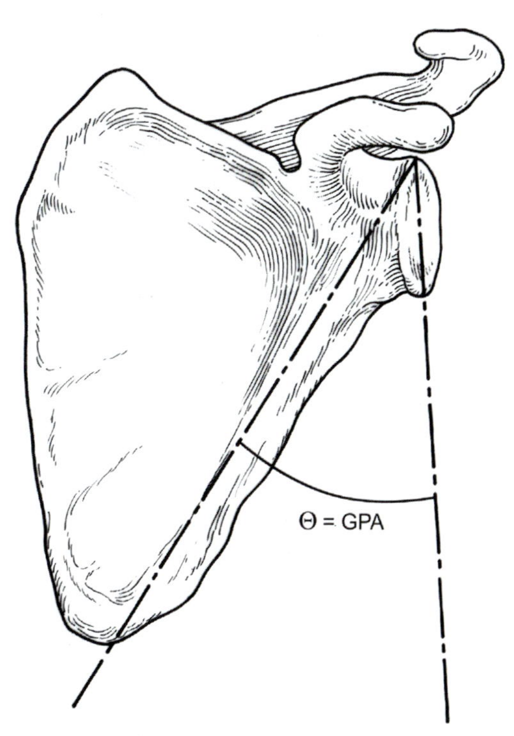

Figure 3–2 The glenopolar angle for assessing glenoid neck fractures accounts for the relative inferior tilt of the articular surface. Normal ranges from 30 to 45 degrees. Less than 20 degrees may be a good indicator for operative intervention.

between the superior glenoid and the most inferior point of the scapular body **(Fig. 3–2)**. The GPA is normally between 30 and 45 degrees, and as the glenoid becomes more misaligned inferiorly by the pull of muscular attachments and the weight of the extremity, the angle decreases. When the angle is 20 degrees or less, clinically significant angulation exists and we recommend operative intervention based on this angulation alone.

Treatment

Truly nondisplaced glenoid fractures, which have been adequately evaluated radiographically, may be successfully treated nonoperatively. In these cases, we recommend the use of a sling for comfort, and early dependent passive shoulder mobilization, such as pendulum exercises, to minimize posttraumatic shoulder stiffness. Frequent radiographic follow-up is required to ensure the fracture does not displace.

The goal of operative reduction and fixation is to correct bony deformity, to prevent chronic glenohumeral instability, and to restore articular congruity to minimize the risk of degenerative joint disease. Due to the relative paucity of long-term clinical outcome data, strict guidelines for operative indications do not exist.

Previous authors have advocated surgical treatment when at least 5 mm of articular displacement was present, or with persistent subluxation of the humeral head,[1,4,12,22,23] although these parameters are based on very little scientific data. Instability can be anticipated if at least one quarter of the anterior fossa or one third of the posterior fossa is displaced.

Authors' Recommended Treatment

The surgeon should not rely solely on the fracture classification to dictate surgical approach and fixation techniques. Each fracture should be evaluated for the optimal fixation construct based on ideal biomechanics, and the surgical approach tailored accordingly. However, the fracture type and location of the major fragments does allow for a general approach to the injury. Type Ia fractures are best visualized anteriorly through a deltopectoral approach, which gives adequate access to the anterior glenoid rim. In type Ib fractures, a limited posterior approach to the glenohumeral joint allows for reduction and fixation of the posterior glenoid fossa with small fragment screws.

The remainder of the fracture types (types II–VI) involve medial extension of the fracture into the scapular body, and require wider exposure for anatomic reduction and fixation individualized to the fracture. As a general rule, fractures that exit superiorly may be treated with an anterior approach, and inferior fractures are best treated with a posterior approach. For fractures with superomedial extension, a deltopectoral approach may be adequate to control and stabilize the fragment depending on its size. Due to the posterior position of the posterior border of the acromion, visualization of the superior fragment is usually better through an anterior approach. The deforming forces of the long head of the biceps and the conjoint must be counteracted during reduction. Interfragmentary 2.7- or 3.5-mm screws are used for final fracture stabilization. If plates are necessary for fixation, an anterior approach is suboptimal due to limited options of good bone stock for screw purchase posteriorly.

When the fracture line extends far medially, we prefer a posterior approach, often supplemented with an accessory superior approach. This technique involves placing a 4.0-mm Schanz pin in the coracoid as a joystick to facilitate reduction. Screws may then be placed from superior to inferior from the coracoid into the scapular spine (posteriorly) or distally into the stout glenoid neck and lateral body depending of the fracture pattern. The posterior approach for superior or medial fracture extension should involve reflecting the posterior head of the deltoid inferiorly and exposing the supraspinous fossa to directly address the fracture. Care must be taken to expose and protect the suprascapular nerve when performing this exposure, and mobilization of the nerve may be the limiting factor in the extent of exposure.

Most fractures with medial or inferior extension require a posterior approach to the scapula to visualize, reduce, and stabilize the inferior fragments through the scapular body. Position the patient in a lateral decubitus position with the affected extremity upward. Make a slightly oblique vertical incision, starting from the lateral one third of the scapular spine, angling slightly medially, and extending distally for 15 cm. The posterior head of the deltoid is then reflected from the scapula, and the interval between the infraspinatus and teres minor is identified laterally. The infraspinatus may be mobilized subperiosteally from the inferior scapular fossa as necessary, taking care to protect the suprascapular nerve on its undersurface. The infraspinatus insertion may be partially released from its tendinous insertion, and later repaired, to increase exposure. A T-shaped capsular incision is then made to expose the articular surface **(Fig. 3–3)**. If visualization and adequate control of all the fracture fragments are not possible through this interval, dissection superior to the spine may allow for complete exposure.

Reconstruction of the articular surface is performed under direct visualization, using Kirschner wires (K-wires) for provisional fixation followed by interfragmentary screws **(Fig. 3–4)**. A Schanz pin or threaded K-wire may be inserted into the dense lateral neck or subchondral bone to assist in reduction of the fracture if a large enough fragment is present. A 2.7-mm reconstruction plate placed along the solid bone stock of the lateral scapular is useful to maintain the reduction, and an additional 3.5-mm reconstruction plate may be contoured and placed on the posterior border of the lateral scapula to allow a 90–90 construct **(Fig. 3–5)**. It is important to recognize the optimal anatomic locations that allow for good screw purchase **(Fig. 3–6)**. Following internal fixation, the deltoid fascia should be repaired securely to its anatomic position using drill holes through the scapular spine.

When the fracture extends more directly inferiorly, we prefer a more limited posterior approach to the glenoid as described by Brodsky.[24,25] Abduction of the arm elevates the posterior head of the deltoid and may eliminate the need for extensive deltoid release. The interval between the infraspinatus and teres minor is developed, and release of the infraspinatus is limited to minimize the risk of denervation. The posterior glenoid is exposed and reduction and fixation proceeds as previously described. It is critical when using this limited approach to avoid injury to the axillary nerve, which migrates superiorly with humerus abduction.[26]

Glenoid neck fractures often occur in combination with injuries to other superior structures of the shoulder girdle, and the fracture infrequently extends more medially. Thus, a limited posterior approach usually affords

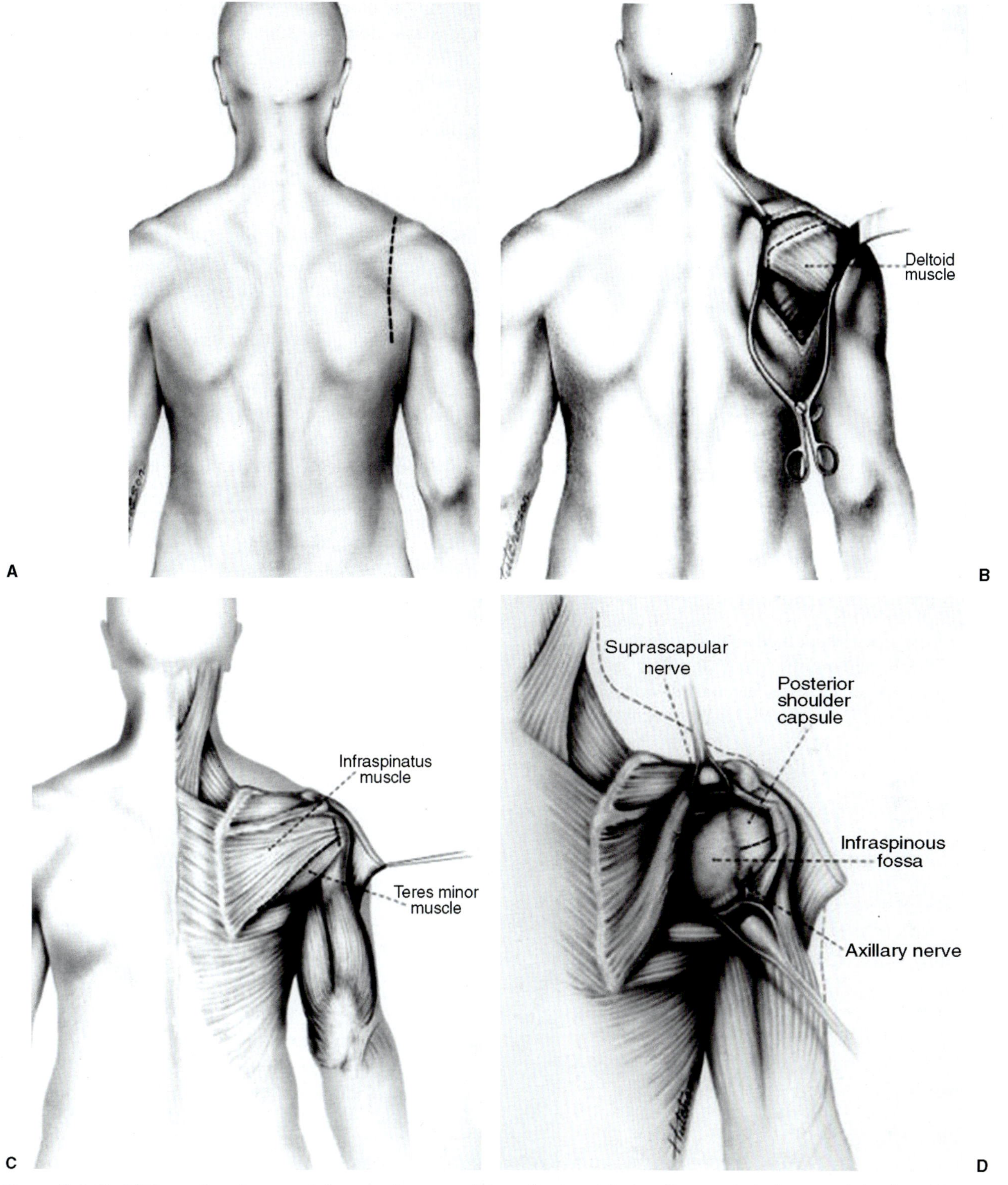

Figure 3–3 (A–D) The preferred approach for most fractures of the glenoid is posteriorly through the infraspinatus-teres minor interval. (From Kavanagh BF, Bradway JK, Cofield RH. Open reduction and internal fixation of displaced intra-articular fractures of the glenoid fossa. J Bone Joint Surg Am 1993;75:479–484. Reprinted by permission.)

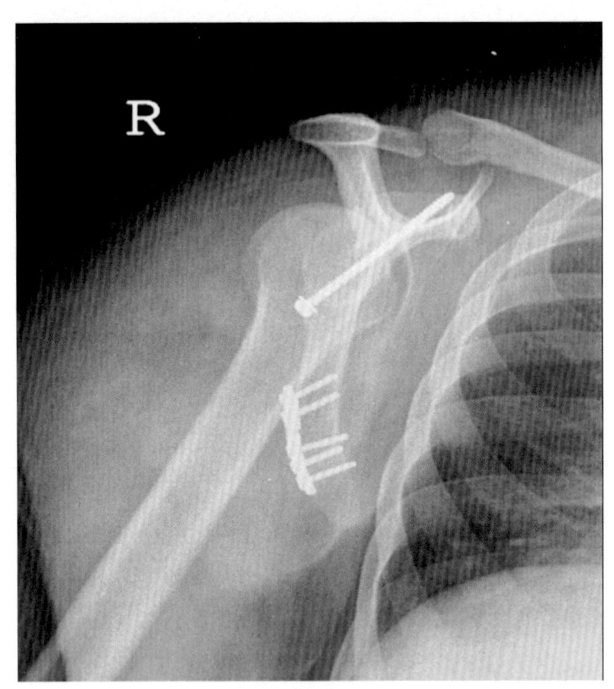

Figure 3–4 Case example showing articular reconstruction using a small fragment lag screw posteroinferiorly into the dense bone of the coracoid.

adequate exposure without medial dissection or extensive release of the deltoid or infraspinatus. With the fracture exposed, the neck can be disimpacted using a small elevator or bone tamp. A contoured 3.5-mm reconstruction plate may be placed on the posterior surface of the neck and distally along the lateral border of the scapula. If a significant defect remains after disimpaction, bone graft may be placed medially to the neck, and locking screws should be considered to buttress the reduced glenoid fragment.

Results

Scapular fractures are relatively rare injuries, and the variety of concomitant injury patterns about the shoulder girdle has led to a multitude of small heterogeneous case series in the literature.[1,3,4,7,12,27–29] Very few comparative trials exist, and it is still not completely clear which injuries are best treated by which method. It does appear that the majority of glenoid fractures, and particularly glenoid neck fractures, may be treated nonoperatively with the expectation of return of good shoulder function.[12,30–33]

When significant displacement of the articular surface is present, nonoperative treatment generally leads to poor results,[13,22,33,34] and surgical reconstruction is recommended. Leung et al[7] reported on 14 patients treated operatively using a deltopectoral or a limited posterior approach. All patients had good or excellent outcomes, both subjectively and objectively using the Rowe shoulder scoring system. In one of the largest series, Mayo et al[4] evaluated the functional outcomes after surgical treatment of 27 displaced glenoid fractures, and found 22 of 27 patients (81%) had good or excellent results. Eighteen

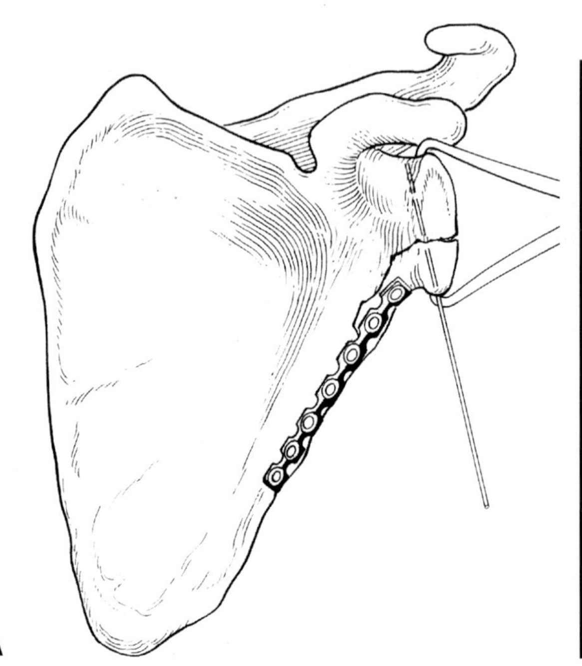

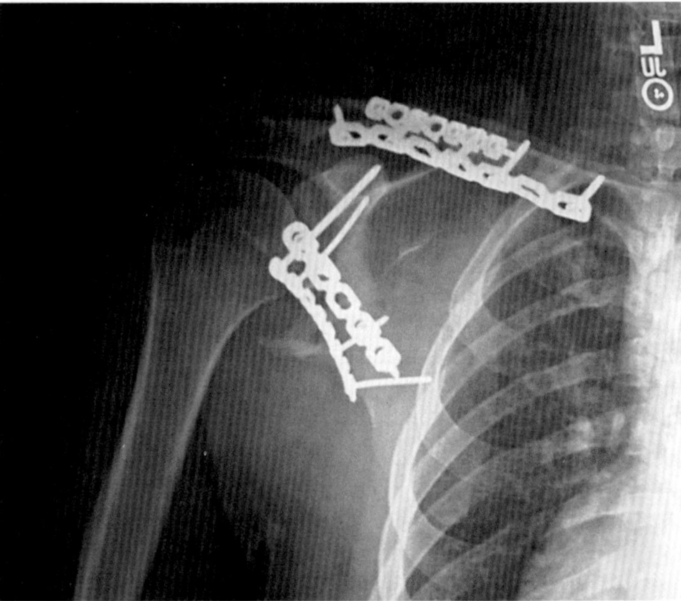

Figure 3–5 (A) Following a posterior approach, reduction and fixation may be performed with the use of a K-wire, a reduction clamp, and a reconstruction plate. **(B)** In this case, the fracture extended inferiorly and was stabilized with plate fixation along the lateral border and posteriorly with fixation into the spine and coracoid.

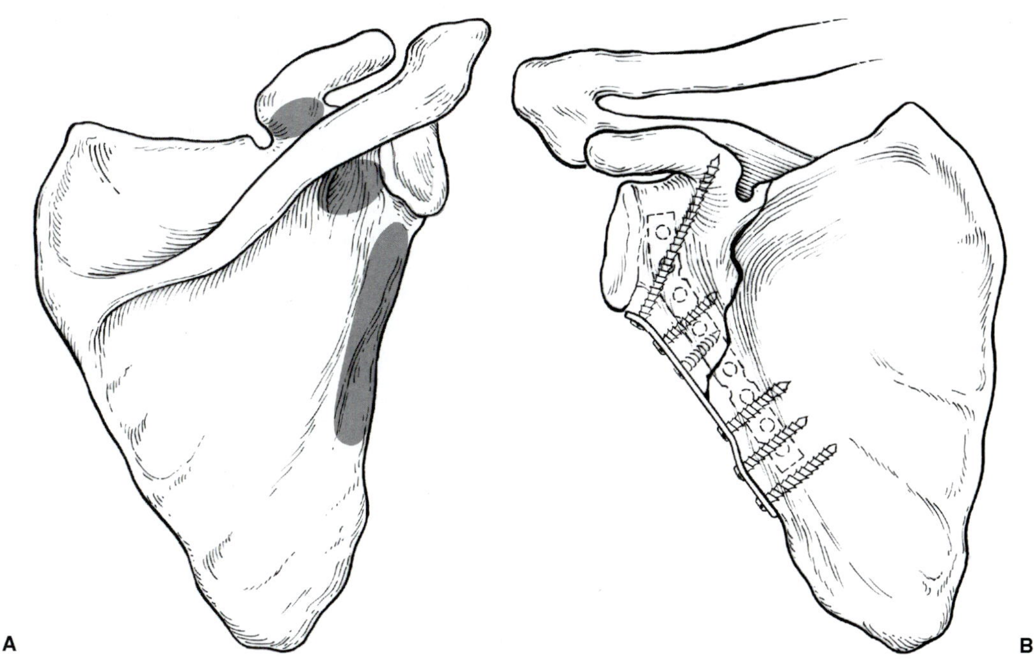

Figure 3–6 (A) Bone condensation regions are located in the glenoid neck, the acromion, the coracoid, and the lateral scapular border, **(B)** which are ideal for placement of fixation to optimize screw purchase.

patients (67%) had no pain, but only 6 (22%) regained full shoulder motion, and the most common deficit was in external rotation. Schandelmaier et al[23] evaluated 22 fractures treated operatively which were displaced at least 5 mm at an average follow-up of 10 years, and reported good overall results. Other series have generally found similarly good results following surgical treatment of displaced glenoid fractures.[1,3,28] Unfortunately, many studies of both conservative and surgical treatment do not, however, accurately quantify fracture displacement or stratify patients accordingly, and it is difficult to draw strong conclusions on treatment recommendations from the available literature.

Glenoid neck fractures often settle in an impacted and stable position. However, inferior angulation may lead to malunion and impair proper shoulder function. Romero et al[17] found significant differences in outcomes using an angulation threshold of a GPA of 20 degrees. Most patients who complained of moderate or severe pain had a GPA of less than 20 degrees, several of whom had severely limited range of motion. On the contrary, the majority of patients who had mild or no pain had a GPA of >20 degrees. Interestingly, half of the patients with malalignment (GPA <20 degrees) had no associated clavicle or AC joint injury, implying that fracture alignment or instability can occur and lead to a poor result without an associated clavicle injury.[17] Other authors have confirmed high correlations between the GPA and functional shoulder outcomes.[14,15]

Injuries to the Superior Shoulder Suspensory Complex

The superior shoulder suspensory complex is a biomechanical ring-link structure composed of both bone and soft tissue elements, suspended at the end of superior and inferior struts, as first described by Goss.[35] The classic components of the ring included the acromion, the glenoid, the coracoid process, the coracoclavicular (CC) ligaments, the distal clavicle, and the AC ligaments. Recently, the critical stabilizing role the coracoacromial (CA) ligament complex plays in disruptions of the ring has been recognized,[36] and this structure must be considered as part of the ring as well. The two suspension struts are the clavicle superiorly and the scapular spine and body inferiorly **(Fig. 3–7)**.

Unlike in the pelvis, the SSSC is composed of a greater number of more pliable ligaments, which allow for dissipation of force without gross failure. This allows the SSSC ring to be disrupted in a single location without loss of the mechanical support for the shoulder girdle.[18,37] When significant trauma to the shoulder occurs, two structures of the ring of the SSSC may be injured—the so-called double disruption.[35] Common injury patterns include type IIC and type V clavicle fractures and type III AC joint disruptions, as well as glenoid neck and clavicle fractures.[35]

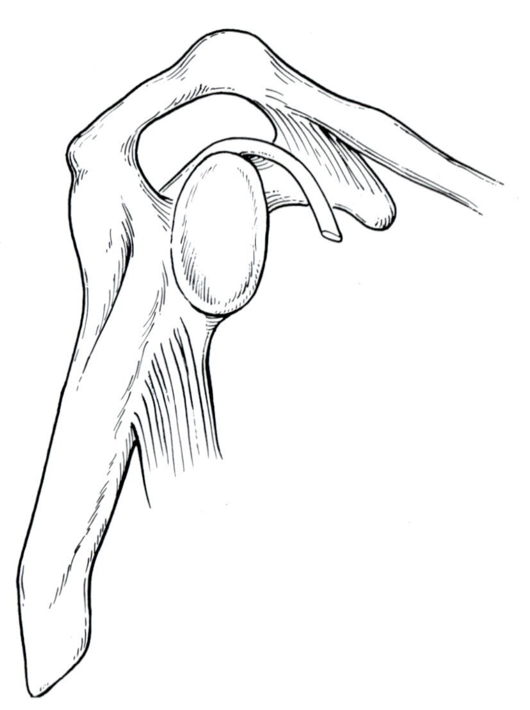

Figure 3–7 Structures of the superior shoulder suspensory complex.

Treatment

One specific double-disruption injury pattern, the combination of a clavicular and glenoid neck fracture, was originally termed the *floating shoulder* by Ganz and Noesberger.[38] Such fractures may result in an inferior displacement and internal rotation deformity of the distal fragment due to gravity and muscle forces, particularly the pectoralis major.[3,18] Hardegger et al[3] concluded that the stability of the scapular neck depended on an intact clavicle, and advocated operative fixation of all floating shoulder injuries. Subsequent authors have echoed these recommendations, adding that reduction and stabilization of the glenoid neck are often achieved indirectly following clavicle fixation alone.[16, 35,39–41]

These recommendations have been based on theoretical principles, not biomechanical evidence. Recently, Williams et al[36] created unstable glenoid neck fractures in cadaveric specimens, and found that only an additional 30% of medial displacement stability was lost following the addition of an associated midshaft clavicle fracture. In their model, complete transaction of both the AC and CA ligaments was needed to create true instability, or a floating shoulder. These authors emphasized that the vast majority of glenoid neck fractures occur through the surgical neck, exiting superiorly in the scapular notch medial to the coracoid.[13,37] This effectively keeps the glenoid fragment in continuity with the scapula, both directly through the CA ligament, and indirectly through the CC and AC ligaments.[36] Romero et al[17] found that displacement of the glenoid neck and instability was not dependent on the presence of a clavicle fracture, supporting the critical role the ligaments play in determining fracture stability.

Authors' Recommended Treatment

Patients with ipsilateral clavicle and glenoid neck fractures first require a complete history and physical examination, with assessment and treatment of any associated life-threatening injuries. The main challenge in treating these injuries is to first determine the necessity for open reduction and internal fixation. The main criterion in this decision is the perceived stability of the fracture. Although this can be a vague and subjective determination, evaluation of the glenoid fracture position and soft tissue integrity helps the surgeon clarify the personality of the fracture. If the glenoid has a GPA of <20 degrees or is medially displaced 1 cm or more, operative stabilization of both fractures is indicated, as this in itself indicates significant ligamentous incompetence. If the glenoid neck is minimally displaced, it is prudent to obtain weight-bearing films or an MRI, depending on the medical status and tolerance of the patient. If both the CA and AC or the CA and CC ligaments are ruptured, this again represents an unstable situation, and stabilization of both fractures is the preferred treatment.

The posterior approach allows excellent exposure of the glenoid neck. The interval between the infraspinatus and teres minor is developed, with variable release of the posterior deltoid and infraspinatus tendon, as detailed previously. K-wires placed in the glenoid fragment provide an excellent reduction aid, and definitive fixation is achieved with a 2.7-mm or 3.5-mm reconstruction plate along the lateral border of the scapula. A bone graft is seldom needed, but a tricortical autograft may be useful to reconstruct the inferior glenoid neck if significant medial impaction or osteoporotic bone is present. Clavicular fixation is performed using standard AO technique, using a reconstruction or limited contact dynamic compression (LC-DC) plate placed superiorly or anteroinferiorly.[42]

Results

Many authors have considered injury to any two structures of the SSSC to be biomechanically equivalent and equally unstable injuries, and thus have used this as an empiric indication for operative stabilization.[3,16,39,40] Much of the focus of double disruptions of the SSSC has been on the relatively common combination clavicular and glenoid neck fracture. This "floating shoulder" injury pattern has been treated by various methods. Herscovici et al[39] reported excellent functional results in patients with a floating shoulder treated with fixation of the clavicle alone, as have other authors.[16,35,41] Leung and Lam[40] reported similar results in 14 patients treated with open reduction and stabilization of both the clavicle and glenoid neck fractures. When initial glenoid neck displacement has been specifically quantified, however, it appears that operative clavicle reduction does not necessarily lead to indirect reduction of a displaced glenoid neck, which depends on the integrity of the supporting ligaments, and several authors have advocated internal fixation of both fractures when significant displacement is present.[15,16,43–45]

Several clinical studies have supported the feasibility of successfully treating glenoid neck and clavicle fractures nonoperatively. Ramos et al[46] reviewed 16 patients with these injuries who were treated conservatively, 14 (92%) of whom had a good or excellent result at a mean of 7.5 years postinjury. Edwards et al[47] treated 20 floating shoulders conservatively and had generally excellent results. Labler et al[15] treated a cohort of patients with floating shoulder injuries both surgically and conservatively, and found that minimally displaced fractures were stable and were successful treated nonoperatively. Oh et al[16] reviewed 13 floating shoulders treated both surgically and conservatively, but the treatment was dictated by the patient's medical condition, not fracture displacement. These and other authors have confirmed that all clavicle and glenoid neck injuries are not inherently unstable, and that surgical indications and outcomes are most dependent on the displacement of the glenoid neck fragment,[45,48] which further corroborates biomechanical evidence.[36]

Overall, it appears that the good clinical results reported after surgical treatment of ipsilateral clavicle and glenoid neck fractures may have been due to inherent stability in the injury pattern. These studies may have used unsubstantiated operative indications, and presumed that this combination of fractures unequivocally led to an unstable shoulder girdle, which has since been refuted biomechanically.[36] In addition, the lack of data regarding the displacement of the glenoid neck in some of these earlier studies makes it difficult to judge whether true instability was present in these patients. The successful nonoperative treatment of these injuries in later series indicates that additional criteria are necessary to assess instability, such as displacement of the glenoid neck, rather than simply the presence of these two fractures.

Postoperative Rehabilitation

Postoperative mobilization protocols ultimately depend on the quality of fracture fixation achieved. The patient is initially immobilized in a sling for comfort, but early mobilization is critical for a successful long-term outcome. Beginning in the first week postoperatively, gentle glenohumeral range of motion and scapular mobilization exercises are initiated. Active motion may begin as early as 2 weeks after surgery, with specific restrictions based on muscle detachments during the surgical approach (i.e., deltoid, infraspinatus, or subscapularis). Strengthening should be delayed until 6 to 8 weeks postoperatively.

Complications

Complications associated with surgical reduction and fixation of scapular fractures include superficial or deep infection. Patients with traumatic degloving soft tissue injuries are more prone to infection and skin slough. Denervation of the infraspinatus has been reported,[4] although it is not clear whether it was more likely a traumatic or iatrogenic injury. When the fracture line extends into the suprascapular or spinoglenoid notch, traumatic suprascapular nerve injury may occur.[49,50] Fixation failure has been rare in our experience, most likely due to the multiple regions of condensed bone at the scapular neck and lateral border available for screw placement. With high-energy fractures, chondral injuries are not uncommonly noted during surgery and may lead to degenerative joint changes. Following nonoperative treatment, initial or progressive displacement of the glenoid neck may alter glenohumeral mechanics, and may cause subcoracoid impingement[51] or abduction weakness,[52] and should thus be monitored closely with serial radiographs.

Summary

When glenoid neck fractures occur in association with a clavicle fracture or other disruption of the SSSC, the *potential* for instability exists. The assessment of stability is critical for treatment decisions, and may be more complicated than was once thought. Specifically, the presence of both a clavicle and glenoid neck fracture does not always result in an unstable shoulder girdle. Weight-bearing views and possibly an MRI may be necessary to fully assess the ligamentous injuries. When structural continuity exists between the distal fragment and the proximal fragment or thorax, which is implied by minimal glenoid displacement, conservative treatment with early rehabilitation has been successful. With fracture displacement under load, or with rupture of both the CA and AC ligaments seen on MRI, surgical reduction and stabilization of both the clavicle and glenoid neck should be performed. A thorough knowledge of the bony and ligamentous supporting structures of the shoulder girdle, coupled with adequate radiographic evaluation, is necessary to assess the stability of the various possible injury combinations.

Fracture instability in double disruptions of the SSSC is just one of the indications for surgical treatment. Angulation and translation of the glenoid neck must be corrected to ensure proper biomechanics of the glenohumeral joint and a good outcome. A GPA of less than 20 degrees or a medial displacement of 1 cm are useful guidelines for determining fracture displacement that necessitates open reduction.

Intraarticular glenoid fossa fractures should be treated like other articular fractures, and any incongruity should be anatomically reduced and stabilized to minimize the risk of posttraumatic degenerative arthrosis. In addition, the concentricity of the glenohumeral articular must be scrutinized for subtle subluxation, which is another indication for fixation of glenoid rim fractures.

When surgical treatment is indicated, the majority of glenoid fractures are adequately exposed using a posterior approach. Isolated anterior rim fractures (type IA) may be the exception. The interval between the infraspinatus and teres minor allows excellent visualization, and may be as extensile as necessary. Common constructs include interfragmentary screws for glenoid fossa fractures, and reconstruction plates along the lateral border for neck fractures. Regardless of the treatment approach, an early and aggressive supervised rehabilitation program is crucial to optimize outcome.

References

1. Adam FF. Surgical treatment of displaced fractures of the glenoid cavity. Int Orthop 2002;26:150–153
2. Ideberg R, Grevsten S, Larsson S. Epidemiology of scapular fractures. Incidence and classification of 338 fractures. Acta Orthop Scand 1995;66:395–397
3. Hardegger FH, Simpson LA, Weber BG. The operative treatment of scapular fractures. J Bone Joint Surg Br 1984;66:725–731
4. Mayo KA, Benirschke SK, Mast JW. Displaced fractures of the glenoid fossa. Results of open reduction and internal fixation. Clin Orthop Relat Res 1998;347:122–130
5. Thompson DA, Flynn TC, Miller PW, Fischer RP. The significance of scapular fractures. J Trauma 1985;25: 974–977
6. Papagelopoulos PJ, Koundis GL, Kateros KT, Babis GC, Nikolopoulos KE, Fragiadakis EG. Fractures of the glenoid cavity: assessment and management. Orthopedics 1999; 22:956–961; quiz 962–963
7. Leung KS, Lam TP, Poon KM. Operative treatment of displaced intra-articular glenoid fractures. Injury 1993;24: 324–328
8. Papilion JA, Shall LM. Fluoroscopic evaluation for subtle shoulder instability. Am J Sports Med 1992;20:548–552
9. Carro LP, Nunez MP, Llata JI. Arthroscopic-assisted reduction and percutaneous external fixation of a displaced intra-articular glenoid fracture. Arthroscopy 1999;15: 211–214
10. Cameron SE. Arthroscopic reduction and internal fixation of an anterior glenoid fracture. Arthroscopy 1998;14:743–746
11. Ideberg R. Fractures of the scapula involving the glenoid fossa. In: Bateman JE, Welsh RP, eds. Surgery of the Shoulder. Philadelphia: BC Decker; 1984:63–66
12. Goss TP. Fractures of the glenoid cavity. J Bone Joint Surg Am 1992;74:299–305
13. Ada JR, Miller ME. Scapular fractures. Analysis of 113 cases. Clin Orthop Relat Res 1991;269:174–180
14. Bozkurt M, Can F, Kirdemir V, Erden Z, Demirkale I, Basbozkurt M. Conservative treatment of scapular neck fracture: the effect of stability and glenopolar angle on clinical outcome. Injury 2005; 36(10):1176–1181
15. Labler L, Platz A, Weishaupt D, Trentz O. Clinical and functional results after floating shoulder injuries. J Trauma 2004;57:595–602
16. Oh W, Jeon H, Kyung S, Park C, Kim T, Ihn C. The treatment of double disruption of the superior shoulder suspensory complex. Int Orthop 2002;26:145–149
17. Romero J, Schai P, Imhoff AB. Scapular neck fracture–the influence of permanent malalignment of the glenoid neck on clinical outcome. Arch Orthop Trauma Surg 2001;121:313–316
18. Toro J, Helfet DL. Surgical management of the floating shoulder. Tech Shoulder Elbow Surg 2004;5:116–121
19. Nordqvist A, Petersson C. Fracture of the body, neck, or spine of the scapula. A long-term follow-up study. Clin Orthop Relat Res 1992;283:139–144
20. Bozkurt M, Can F, Kirdemir V, Erden Z, Demirkale I, Basbozkurt M. Conservative treatment of scapular neck fracture: the effect of stability and glenopolar angle on clinical outcome. Injury 2005;36:1176–1181
21. Ding X, Fan S, Zhang J. A comparative study on operation and non-operation in treating fractures of scapular neck. Zhongguo Xiu Fu Chong Jian Wai Ke Za Zhi 2005;19: 446–449
22. Kligman M, Roffman M. Glenoid fracture: conservative treatment versus surgical treatment. J South Orthop Assoc 1998;7:1–5
23. Schandelmaier P, Blauth M, Schneider C, Krettek C. Fractures of the glenoid treated by operation. A 5- to 23-year follow-up of 22 cases. J Bone Joint Surg Br 2002;84: 173–177
24. Brodsky JW, Tullos HS, Gartsman GM. Simplified posterior approach to the shoulder joint. A technical note. J Bone Joint Surg Am 1987;69:773–774
25. van Noort A, van Loon CJ, Rijnberg WJ. Limited posterior approach for internal fixation of a glenoid fracture. Arch Orthop Trauma Surg 2004;124:140–144
26. Burkhead WZ, Scheinberg RR, Box G. Surgical anatomy of the axillary nerve. J Shoulder Elbow Surg 1992;1:31–36
27. Aulicino PL, Reinert C, Kornberg M, Williamson S. Displaced intra-articular glenoid fractures treated by open reduction and internal fixation. J Trauma 1986; 26:1137–1141
28. Kavanagh BF, Bradway JK, Cofield RH. Open reduction and internal fixation of displaced intra-articular fractures of the glenoid fossa. J Bone Joint Surg Am 1993; 75:479–484

29. Kligman M, Roffman M. Posterior approach for glenoid fracture. J Trauma 1997;42:733–735
30. Imatani RJ. Fractures of the scapula: a review of 53 fractures. J Trauma 1975;15:473–478
31. Lindholm A, Leven H. Prognosis in fractures of the body and neck of the scapula. A follow-up study. Acta Chir Scand 1974;140:33–36
32. McGahan JP, Rab GT, Dublin A. Fractures of the scapula. J Trauma 1980;20:880–883
33. Wilber MC, Evans EB. Fractures of the scapula. An analysis of forty cases and a review of the literature. J Bone Joint Surg Am 1977;59:358–362
34. Ideberg R. Unusual glenoid fractures: a report on 92 cases. Acta Orthop Scand 1987;58:191–192
35. Goss TP. Double disruptions of the superior shoulder suspensory complex. J Orthop Trauma 1993;7:99–106
36. Williams GR Jr, Naranja J, Klimkiewicz J, Karduna A, Iannotti JP, Ramsey M. The floating shoulder: a biomechanical basis for classification and management. J Bone Joint Surg Am 2001;83-A:1182–1187
37. Goss TP. Scapular fractures and dislocations: diagnosis and treatment. J Am Acad Orthop Surg 1995;3:22–33
38. Ganz R, Noesberger B. [Treatment of scapular fractures] Hefte Unfallheilkd 1975;126:59–62
39. Herscovici D Jr, Fiennes AG, Allgower M, Ruedi TP. The floating shoulder: ipsilateral clavicle and scapular neck fractures. J Bone Joint Surg Br 1992;74:362–364
40. Leung KS, Lam TP. Open reduction and internal fixation of ipsilateral fractures of the scapular neck and clavicle. J Bone Joint Surg Am 1993;75:1015–1018
41. Rikli D, Regazzoni P, Renner N. The unstable shoulder girdle: early functional treatment utilizing open reduction and internal fixation. J Orthop Trauma 1995; 9:93–97
42. Reudi TP, Murphy WM. AO Principles of Fracture Management. Stuttgart: Thieme Medical Publishing; 2000
43. Oh CW, Kyung HS, Kim PT, Ihn JC. Failure of internal fixation of the clavicle in the treatment of ipsilateral clavicle and glenoid neck fractures. J Orthop Sci 2001;6: 601–603
44. Hashiguchi H, Ito H. Clinical outcome of the treatment of floating shoulder by osteosynthesis for clavicular fracture alone. J Shoulder Elbow Surg 2003;12:589–591
45. van Noort A, te Slaa RL, Marti RK, van der Werken C. The floating shoulder. A multicentre study. J Bone Joint Surg Br 2001;83:795–798
46. Ramos L, Mencia R, Alonso A, Ferrandez L. Conservative treatment of ipsilateral fractures of the scapula and clavicle. J Trauma 1997;42:239–242
47. Edwards SG, Whittle AP, Wood GW II. Nonoperative treatment of ipsilateral fractures of the scapula and clavicle. J Bone Joint Surg Am 2000;82:774–780
48. Egol KA, Connor PM, Karunakar MA, Sims SH, Bosse MJ, Kellam JF. The floating shoulder: clinical and functional results. J Bone Joint Surg Am 2001;83-A:1188–1194
49. Boerger TO, Limb D. Suprascapular nerve injury at the spinoglenoid notch after glenoid neck fracture. J Shoulder Elbow Surg 2000;9:236–237
50. Edeland HG, Zachrisson BE. Fracture of the scapular notch associated with lesion of the suprascapular nerve. Acta Orthop Scand 1975;46:758–763
51. Gerber C, Terrier F, Ganz R. The role of the coracoid process in the chronic impingement syndrome. J Bone Joint Surg Br 1985;67:703–708
52. Haraguchi N, Toga H, Sekiguchi Y, Kato F. Corrective osteotomy for malunited fracture of the glenoid cavity: a case report. Clin Orthop Relat Res 2002;404:269–274

4 Isolated Tuberosity Fractures

Frank A. Cordasco and Jonas R. Rudzki

Greater tuberosity involvement has been reported in 15 to 40% of proximal humerus fractures. Isolated tuberosity fractures, however, have a significantly lower reported incidence.[1–6] In a review of 930 operatively treated proximal humerus fractures at the AO Documentation Center (Davos Platz, Switzerland), fewer than 2% were isolated displaced tuberosity fractures.[7] Several authors have suggested that isolated greater tuberosity fractures may be underreported due to misdiagnosis caused by commonly encountered subtle radiographic findings.[1,8–12] The general consensus in the literature is that nondisplaced tuberosity fractures may be treated without operative intervention. However, treatment of displaced greater tuberosity fractures is a subject of controversy with regard to indications for operative management, surgical approach, and selection of optimal fixation to maintain an anatomic reduction. These injuries can be deceptively difficult to treat surgically as they frequently consist of suboptimal fragments for traditional internal fixation techniques and the muscle forces acting on the greater tuberosity may make obtaining and maintaining reduction more challenging than the preoperative images would suggest. Although acute anterior glenohumeral dislocations[13,14] and concomitant rotator cuff tears[15] are frequently associated with greater tuberosity fractures, in this chapter we will focus on the diagnosis and optimal treatment of isolated tuberosity fractures with an emphasis on the determination of surgical indications, operative techniques, and postoperative management.

Etiology and Mechanism of Injury

Isolated tuberosity fractures are most commonly caused by impaction or avulsion fractures. In the former, a direct blow from a fall or a hyperabduction injury results in impaction of the greater tuberosity against the acromion[16] or superior aspect of the glenoid with the transmission of a concomitant shear force to the tuberosity. Avulsion injuries of the greater tuberosity have been described as a result of forceful contraction of the rotator cuff in patients with osteopenic bone. More frequently, fractures of the greater tuberosity resulting from a combination of impaction, avulsion, and shearing mechanisms have been reported in association with anterior glenohumeral dislocations as a component of the commonly encountered two-part fracture dislocation.[8] McLaughlin[6] described these patients as having sustained a " posterior mechanism anterior dislocation" and included greater tuberosity fractures, as well as large full thickness rotator cuff tears in association with this group of anterior dislocations. Greater tuberosity fractures have been reported to occur in up to 15 to 30% of anterior glenohumeral dislocations.[13,14]

Anatomy

The greater tuberosity is the insertion site of the supraspinatus, infraspinatus, and teres minor. The tendinous insertions of the articular capsule, rotator cuff muscles, the coracohumeral ligament, and glenohumeral ligament complex blend into a confluent sheet prior to insertion into the humeral tuberosities. The tendons of the supraspinatus and infraspinatus muscles join 15 mm proximal to their insertion and are not readily separable by blunt dissection. Similarly, the infraspinatus and teres minor fuse near their musculotendinous junctions. The supraspinatus and subscapularis tendons join as a sheath that surrounds the biceps tendon at the entrance of the bicipital groove.[17,18] Displaced greater tuberosity fractures are pulled into a position of superior, posterior, and medial displacement by the posterior cuff muscles along the vector of their muscle forces **(Fig. 4–1)**. Knowledge of the regional anatomy of the rotator cuff and rotator interval between the supraspinatus and subscapularis is critical for mobilizing displaced, retracted greater tuberosity fractures to obtain an anatomic reduction.

The ramifications of displacement can more specifically be identified through a comprehensive knowledge of the relevant anatomical considerations. An anatomical study by Minagawa et al[19] described the supraspinatus insertion to be primarily (~75%) on the anterior half of the greater tuberosity. A subsequent study by Dugas et al[20] elegantly mapped the footprint (cuff insertion area) in 20 cadaveric specimens utilizing a 3-space digitizer. The mean medial-to-lateral insertion widths of the supraspinatus, infraspinatus, teres minor, and subscapularis tendons were 12.7, 13.4, 11.4, and 17.9 mm, respectively. The mean minimum medial-to-lateral insertion width of the entire rotator cuff insertion occurred at the midportion of the supraspinatus and was found to be

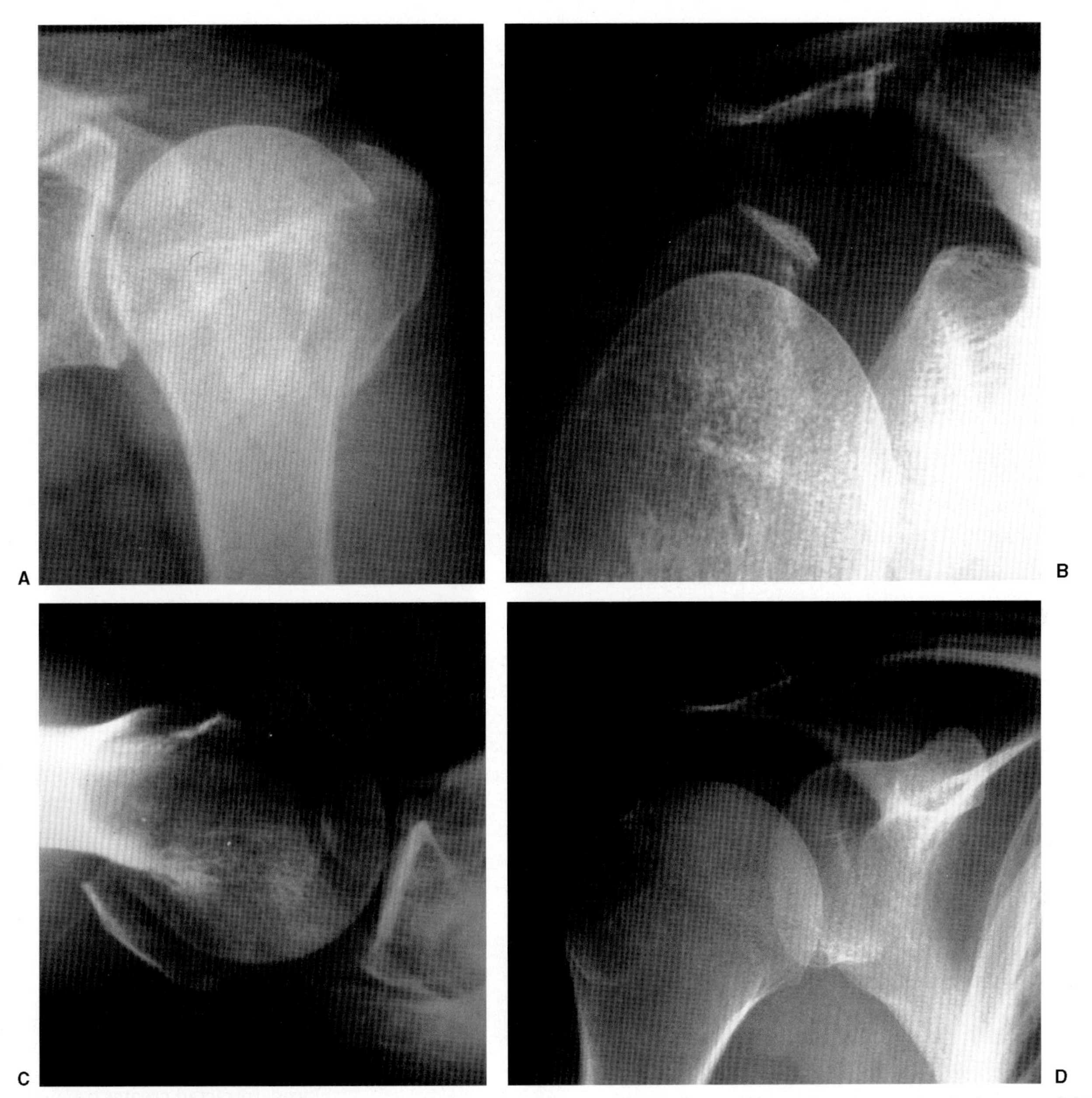

Figure 4–1 **(A)** Plain film true anteroposterior (AP) radiograph demonstrating a large fragment with posteromedial displacement. **(B)** Plain film AP radiograph demonstrating superior displacement. **(C)** Plain film axillary radiograph demonstrating posterior displacement. **(D)** Plain film radiograph demonstrating an impacted greater tuberosity fracture.

14.7 mm. The articular surface-to-tendon insertion distance was less than 1 mm along the anterior 2.1 cm of the supraspinatus/infraspinatus insertion. This distance progressively increased to an average distance of 13.9 mm at the inferior-most aspect of the teres minor insertion. The average anteroposterior distances of the supraspinatus, infraspinatus, teres minor, and subscapularis insertions were noted to be 1.63, 1.64, 2.07, and 2.43 cm, respectively.[20] Another cadaveric study by Ruotolo et al[21] examined 17 normal rotator cuffs and reported the supraspinatus tendon insertion was an average 1.7 mm from the articular margin. With regard to the osseous anatomy of the greater tuberosity, a three-dimensional analysis of the proximal humerus by Robertson et al[22] reported the mean vertical distance from the superior aspect of the greater tuberosity to the superior aspect of the humeral head was 6 ± 2 mm. Knowledge of the rotator cuff footprint dimensions and osseous anatomy is important for restoring the normal anatomical relationships when treating greater tuberosity fractures and may be of assistance when intraoperatively determining options for treatment of comminuted fracture patterns, fractures with concomitant rotator cuff tears, and fracture fragments with insufficient cortical density for stable fixation.

The primary blood supply to the proximal humerus is the anterior lateral branch of the anterior humeral circumflex artery.[23,24] The anterior humeral circumflex artery is derived from the third division of the axillary artery approximately 1 cm distal to the inferior border of the pectoralis minor. It then travels laterally posterior to the coracobrachialis and approaches the surgical neck of the humerus at the lower border of the subscapularis. The anterolateral branch of the anterior humeral circumflex artery travels superiorly in the lateral aspect of the intertubercular groove to penetrate bone as it approaches the greater tuberosity and this branch then becomes the arcuate artery. Multiple extraosseous anastomoses exist between the anterior humeral circumflex artery, the posterior humeral circumflex artery, the thoracoacromial artery, suprascapular artery, subscapular artery, and profunda brachii artery.[23] By selecting the most appropriate operative approach (see below), minimizing excessive dissection, and with a thorough knowledge of the regional vascular anatomy, the risks of nonunion, delayed union, and avascular necrosis may be minimized.

Patient Assessment

The rationale for more aggressive operative intervention in the treatment of displaced tuberosity fractures is predicated on concern for malunion resulting in symptomatic subacromial impingement, functional loss from decreased shoulder abduction, and an alteration in rotator cuff function due to a shortening of the lever arms for forward elevation and external rotation.[8,25–27] Hence, a rigorous approach to assessing the patient with an isolated tuberosity fracture is critical. After a thorough history and physical examination documenting the neurovascular status of the involved extremity, the initial plain radiographic evaluation consists of anteroposterior (AP), true AP, axillary, and scapular-Y or acromial outlet views. Plain radiographs may underestimate both the degree of displacement and extent of comminution. In addition, accurate assessment may be impaired by a small size fragment, comminution, or superimposition of the fragment on the humeral head.[1,11,28] A study by Parsons et al[1] was the first to examine the accuracy and reliability of image interpretation for known displacements of the greater tuberosity. In this cadaveric study, the authors reported that no one fluoroscopic view was significantly more accurate than any other and they noted a trend toward increased accuracy for imaging minimally displaced fragments (5 mm or less displacement) with the AP view in external rotation.

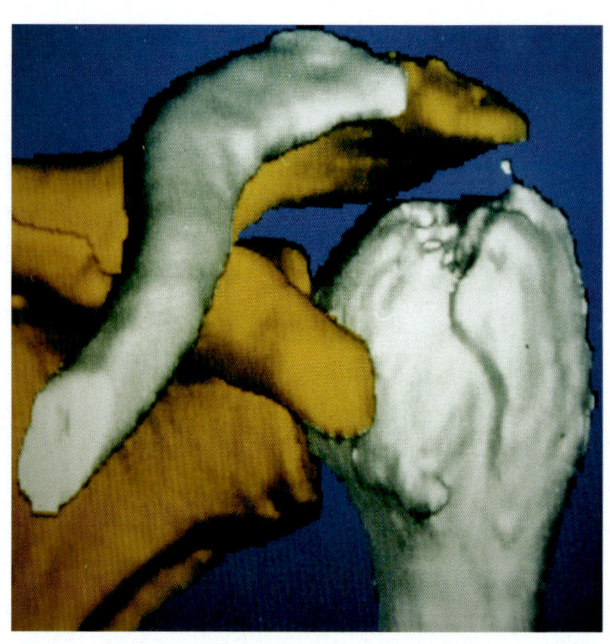

Figure 4–2 Three-dimensional computed tomography reconstruction image of a greater tuberosity fracture with superior displacement.

When a sufficient index of suspicion exists despite normal-appearing radiographs, consideration of further diagnostic imaging is appropriate. Computed tomography (CT) may be of assistance for its ability to accurately detail the osseous anatomy about the proximal humerus; however, its ability to adequately image the pertinent rotator cuff anatomy is limited **(Fig. 4–2)**.[28] As a result, magnetic resonance imaging (MRI) is more commonly employed and is a more practical modality **(Fig. 4–3)**.[9,26,29] Although

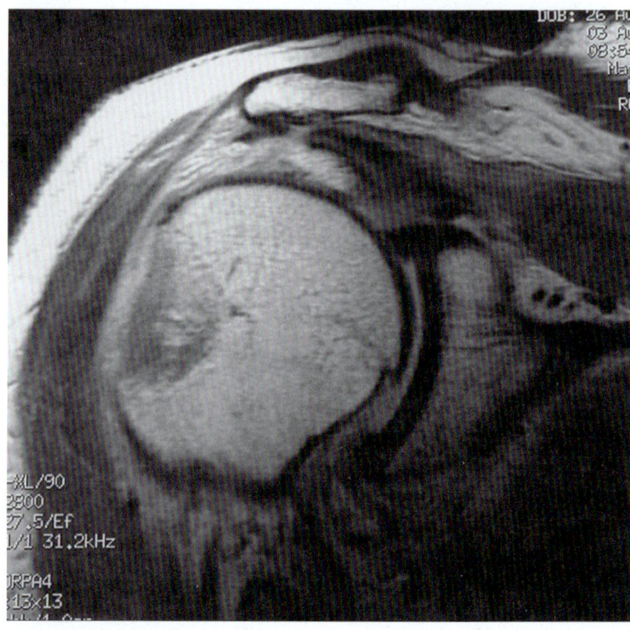

Figure 4–3 Magnetic resonance image of an impacted nondisplaced greater tuberosity fracture.

rarely used to evaluate for a possible greater tuberosity fracture, ultrasound has been reported as a method to diagnose occult nondisplaced greater tuberosity fractures.[30]

Treatment

Indications for Surgery

Classically, Neer[31] defined one centimeter as a threshold for displacement requiring operative treatment of proximal humerus fractures. Subsequently, Young and Wallace[32] reported good or acceptable results in 97% of cases with conservative treatment for minimally displaced greater tuberosity fractures. However, the authors of this study defined acceptable as abduction >60 degrees, a definition with which many contemporary orthopedic surgeons would not concur. In a case series of 79 pooled displaced and nondisplaced greater tuberosity fractures, Olivier et al[33] reported unsatisfactory results in 31%. Extrapolation of the historical literature on conservative treatment of greater tuberosity fractures is difficult due to small sample sizes, pooling of displaced and nondisplaced fractures, and nonstandardized, nonvalidated outcome measures. As described above, several investigators have advocated operative intervention for the treatment of displaced greater tuberosity fractures as malunion often results in symptomatic subacromial impingement, functional loss from decreased shoulder abduction, an alteration in rotator cuff function due to a shortening of the lever arms for forward elevation and external rotation, and the potential for capsular contracture restricting internal rotation and horizontal adduction.[8,25,26] As with any fracture or injury about the shoulder, tailoring operative indications to the patient's functional status, activity level, history of shoulder pain and function, and concomitant injuries is imperative. Nevertheless, the recent literature regarding operative indications for greater tuberosity fractures endorses the consideration of operative management of fractures displaced more than 5 mm superiorly or more than 0.5 to 1 cm posteriorly based on the concerns mentioned above.[11,26,34,35] Recent basic science studies have provided biomechanical data to further support these recommendations.

A study by Bono et al[26] employed a dynamic, cadaver-based biomechanical shoulder simulator to model greater tuberosity malunion and determine the change in deltoid force required for abduction with varying amounts of displacement. The authors demonstrated a statistically significant increase in abduction force for superior displacements of 0.5 cm (16%, $p = 0.006$) and 1 cm (27%, $p = 0.0001$). Combined together, posterior and superior displacements of 1 cm resulted in a 29% force increase ($p = 0.001$). Although there are limitations in any study employing a cadaveric biomechanical simulator, the biologic plausibility and statistical significance of the data reported support the clinical concerns of tuberosity displacement impeding normal glenohumeral kinematics through alteration of normal rotator cuff function.

Nonsurgical Treatment

As described above, nonoperative management is typically selected for patients with less than 5 mm of superior displacement or 0.5 to 1 cm of posterior displacement. The approach is similar to that of any periarticular fracture with a balance struck between immobilization to allow fracture healing and motion to prevent contracture, muscular atrophy, and disability. Most greater tuberosity fractures associated with glenohumeral dislocation are minimally displaced or nondisplaced after reduction of the glenohumeral joint and may be treated nonoperatively. In a study of glenohumeral fracture-dislocations, McLaughlin[6] reported that after closed reduction, the greater tuberosity was reduced in 24 of 34 cases (71%). As stated above, close follow-up is indicated for this patient population to prevent the treating physician from overlooking a concomitant acute, traumatic rotator cuff tear that would benefit from early operative intervention.[36] Patients should be advised and reassured that glenohumeral dislocations associated with greater tuberosity fracture have been reported to have a low risk of recurrent dislocation.[13,14]

Duration of immobilization is surgeon- and patient-dependent; however, general recommendations in the literature include shoulder immobilization for 2 weeks after confirmed anatomic reduction of the glenohumeral joint followed by initiation of passive motion to limit capsular contracture and subacromial adhesions. After approximately 6 weeks, and with radiographic confirmation of no additional displacement, active range-of-motion exercises are initiated followed by rotator cuff and periscapular muscle strengthening exercises once full passive shoulder motion is achieved.[8] The importance of low-weight (<2 lbs or 1 kg), high-repetition exercises along the vectors of the rotator cuff muscle bellies is emphasized with each patient and progressively increased. Great care is taken to prevent shoulder manipulation or aggressive shoulder mobilization techniques on the part of the physical therapist.

Greater tuberosity impaction fractures are typically nondisplaced and may be treated without surgical intervention as well. Some authors advocate earlier mobilization of these injuries based on an assumption of greater intrinsic stability of the injury pattern.[8] Although a reasonable recommendation, it is equally important to recognize the potential for displacement should patients inadvertently fire their posterior cuff muscles while participating in an early passive mobilization program. It would be optimal to determine treatment recommendations on a patient-specific basis as predicated by their cognitive and activity levels in conjunction with the radiographic appearance of the injury.

In summary, the goals of nonoperative management are to maximize motion while preventing further displacement. Complications of nonoperative management are typically due to shoulder stiffness and limited motion from subacromial adhesion formation, capsular contracture, or tuberosity displacement. Early appropriate passive motion exercises through a formal directed physical therapy program with a daily home program are critical to avoid these complications.

Surgical Treatment

Surgical Planning

Once operative management is indicated for a greater tuberosity fracture, the treating surgeon must carefully form a preoperative plan to obtain and maintain reduction through an approach that provides the most reliable means of achieving stable fixation. As these injuries may frequently consist of fragments with more comminution than appreciable on preoperative imaging, we recommend a preoperative plan with a primary and secondary strategy should the initial plan for fixation prove inadequate. The plan begins with selection of patient positioning and the selection of surgical approach and exposure. Several approaches have been described for operative management of greater tuberosity fractures including fragment excision and rotator cuff repair, percutaneous fixation, arthroscopic-assisted fixation, fixation through a mini-open lateral incision or anterolateral approach, and finally, via the deltopectoral approach. The rationales and limitations of each method will be discussed.

Percutaneous fixation techniques have gained greater popularity with the recent increasing enthusiasm for minimally invasive surgical procedures. These offer the benefits of smaller incisions with a theoretical decrease in disruption of fracture biology and violation of adjacent soft tissues that are critical to fracture healing.[37] It has been suggested that these techniques decrease postoperative pain; others believe that they allow for a more rapid recovery and return to normal function.[38] Although commonly used for two- and three-part proximal humeral fractures, percutaneous fixation techniques may be used for large tuberosity fracture fragments with less than 1 centimeter of displacement in physiologically young patients with dense cortical bone who undergo operative management within 7 to 10 days of injury (see Chapter 5). Limitations of the technique include its inability to directly visualize the fragment and remove interposed periosteal, tendinous, or fascial soft tissue. Excellent fluoroscopic imaging is mandatory and familiarity with patient positioning and fluoroscope positioning to obtain orthogonal views is beneficial.

Arthroscopically assisted reduction offers similar benefits to percutaneous techniques, but additionally provides significantly enhanced visualization of the fracture, articular surface, and rotator cuff. The techniques employed in mini-open or arthroscopically assisted rotator cuff repair are extremely useful and directly applicable to a combined treatment approach for the treatment of greater tuberosity fractures. Therefore, we favor an arthroscopically assisted approach in the treatment of greater tuberosity fractures, but our experience has led us to note that this method requires a greater degree of facility with shoulder arthroscopy on the part of the treating orthopedic surgeon. Limitations include the complex set-up in the operating room to facilitate the arthroscopic exam and allow for intraoperative fluoroscopic imaging, which may preclude some surgeons and facilities from employing this technique with ease. The large hematoma associated with a fracture may impair visualization and will be influenced by timing of surgery. Despite these potential limitations, the benefits of this approach are numerous, including the opportunity to visualize the rotator cuff directly to rule out a concomitant tear. Certain fracture patterns will allow for visualization of an anatomic reduction through placing the arthroscope in the subdeltoid space.[39,40] The arthroscope may be used to facilitate débridement of the fracture-site hematoma and adjacent fibrous scar, mobilization of the fracture fragment under direct arthroscopic visualization, and suture passage for a subsequent mini-open approach for internal fixation. Arthroscopy additionally allows for the concomitant treatment of associated pathology (the younger patient with an associated Bankart tear following dislocation) as well as an arthroscopic subacromial decompression as indicated. Finally, for greater tuberosity fractures with small fragments and significant comminution, fragment excision and rotator cuff repair in a single- or double-row construct may be more easily accomplished through an arthroscopic approach.

The mini-open lateral incision is frequently employed for the treatment of isolated greater tuberosity fractures for several reasons. Most orthopedic surgeons have great comfort in using this approach for rotator cuff repair and patient positioning and operating room set-up are familiar. In addition, direct visualization of the fracture fragment is possible with the ability to mobilize and manipulate the fragment for placement of stable fixation. Limitations include the inability to dissect greater than 5 centimeters below the lateral aspect of the acromion in concern for potential axillary nerve injury, the potential for difficulty in reducing fragments with significant posterior displacement, and the need for assistance with retraction of the deltoid. Some surgeons prefer to place this incision more posteriorly along the lateral border of the acromion to facilitate access to fragments with posterior displacement and then externally rotate the arm to "deliver" the humerus to the fragment and reduce it anatomically. A variation of this approach was recently reported in an anatomic study together with the initial results of an accompanying case series of 16 patients treated at our institution.[41] The extended anterolateral acromial approach as described by Gardner et al[41] facilitates exposure of the proximal humerus with less soft tissue dissection and muscle retraction to gain access to the lateral aspect of the humerus. In this study, 20 cadavers were dissected developing a plane through the anterior deltoid raphe. The authors reported that the anterior branch of the axillary nerve was reliably and predictably found approximately 35 mm distal to the prominence of the greater tuberosity deep to this raphe. They suggested that this approach allows for a minimally invasive approach with excellent exposure of the lateral aspect of the humerus, while minimizing adjacent soft tissue disruption.[41] An additional theoretical benefit of employing this approach for greater tuberosity fractures is the anterolateral location still allows for placement of a backup, secondary posterior incision in cases with more posterior displacement identified at surgery than recognized preoperatively.

Advantages of the deltopectoral approach are similar to the direct lateral mini-open approach in that most orthopedic surgeons feel comfortable with the dissection and exposure. Excellent visualization of the proximal humerus may be obtained and operating room set-up is familiar and straightforward. This approach is particularly useful in those patients with a nondisplaced surgical neck component. In that setting the anterolateral or direct lateral (mini-open) approaches will not offer adequate visualization in the event the surgical neck component needs to be addressed. Our preference in this type of fracture pattern is to wait 3 weeks for the surgical neck component of the fracture to heal enough to allow for an arthroscopic-assisted approach to the greater tuberosity fracture as described above. However, with fragments that are posteriorly displaced, it can often be exceedingly difficult to access and mobilize the greater tuberosity fracture fragment without extensive dissection and potential compromise of the blood supply. Additional concerns include the extent of anterior deltoid retraction and potential for compromise of deltoid integrity, a factor that is critical to any acceptable outcome with surgical intervention about the shoulder. Implant selection and secondary strategies will be discussed as they relate to the chosen approach.

Surgical Techniques

Arthroscopic-Assisted Techniques

Arthroscopy can be quite helpful in the evaluation of concomitant glenohumeral and subacromial pathology as noted above. Arthroscopic visualization of the subacromial and subdeltoid spaces can facilitate hematoma and scar débridement, fragment mobilization, and fracture reduction as described above while suture passage under arthroscopic visualization can be more accurate and secure **(Fig. 4–4)**. The direct lateral portal for rotator cuff repair is used to obtain reduction and achieve stable fixation with a cannulated screw in those cases with large fragments and good quality bone. Accessory portals allow for placement of tissue graspers or soft tissue elevators to débride soft tissue, facilitate reduction, and assist with subsequent guide-wire passage. Fluoroscopic confirmation of reduction and implant position is performed intraoperatively.

Comminuted fragments and/or poor bone quality preclude the use of screw fixation. In these cases, arthroscopic techniques employing suture passers to place sutures at the tendon/bone interface assist with mobilization of the fragments and will often allow a more limited open

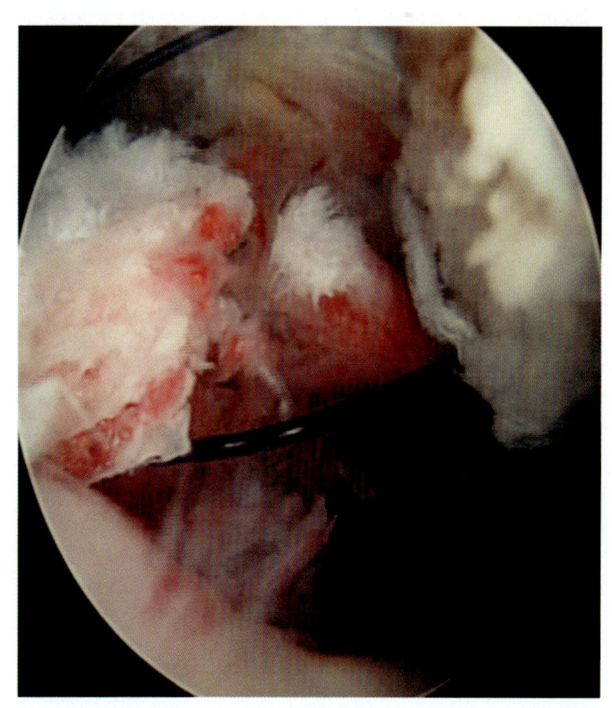

Figure 4–4 Intraoperative arthroscopic image of polydioxanone (PDS) suture placed through the greater tuberosity fracture fragment.

approach. The fragments can then be fixed to bone using the techniques noted above.

Open Techniques

With the patient under regional or general anesthesia and after the administration of intravenous antibiotics, the patient is placed in the beach-chair position with careful attention to the padding of all bony prominences and maintenance of stable, neutral cervical spine positioning. A beanbag mattress is utilized and the patient is lateralized as a unit to the edge of the operating room table. A direct lateral or anterolateral vertical incision is made for 5 to 8 cm extending from approximately 1 cm superomedial to the lateral aspect of the acromion extending distally. Full-thickness soft tissue flaps are developed above the deltoid fascia, and #2 braided polyester sutures are placed anteriorly and posteriorly as tagging stitches for later fascial repair. The deltoid is sharply incised in-line with its fibers and dissection carried to the level of the subdeltoid bursa, which is excised as necessary for visualization. A #0 Vicryl suture is then placed in a figure-eight fashion approximately 5 cm below the level of the acromion for the lateral approach as a stay suture to limit inferior dissection and the chance of iatrogenic axillary nerve injury. The rotator cuff is palpated, the fracture fragment identified and mobilized, and copious irrigation used to débride and visualize the fracture bed. Although adequate visualization for an anatomic reduction is important, it is equally important to minimize periosteal stripping and limit any unnecessary soft tissue dissection. To assist in obtaining anatomic reduction of the greater tuberosity fracture fragment, we will frequently place a #2 braided nonabsorbable polyester suture at the bone–tendon junction. Placing the suture in this location allows for tendon excursion without manipulating the potentially tenuous cortical bone and compromising fixation options.

Assessment of the fragment at this point determines the implant selection. For larger fragments with dense cortical bone or a subjective assessment of good bone stock, 4.5-mm AO/ASIF cannulated screws are well suited. Noncannulated screws may be used as well; however, we believe that placement of the cannulated screw guide-wire allows for multiplanar fluoroscopic imaging with minimal manipulation of the fracture fragment. Washers may be used in cases with amenable fragment size to distribute the compressive forces of interfragmentary compression over a greater surface area. When fragment comminution is present to an extent that screw fixation will not provide reliable compression, suture fixation may be considered. A more distally placed 3.5-mm AO/ASIF cortical screw may be used as[41] a post for heavy-suture fixation in a tension-band fashion. We prefer to use #2 FiberWire suture (Arthrex, Inc./Arthrotek, Inc., Warsaw, IN) for this purpose in figure-eight construct, which provides additional stability and assists in preventing tuberosity overreduction. Multiple sutures are placed in the bone–tendon junction and then distally through the humeral cortex distal to the fracture site. Alternatively, the parachute technique described by Cornell in 1994 can be used to secure the sutures to the humeral cortex using a post consisting of a screw and washer.[42] The reduction is confirmed with multiplanar fluoroscopy and the wound is copiously irrigated and closed in standard fashion.

Percutaneous Fixation Techniques

The patient is placed in a 30-degree beach-chair position on a beanbag to lateralize the entire body and facilitate intraoperative fluoroscopic imaging. The table is rotated such that the fluoroscope may be brought in and out from a cephalad position on the ipsilateral side of the operative procedure. Manipulating the rotational arc of the C-arm allows the surgeon to visualize anteroposterior and axillary views, and manipulating the tilt allows for converting between a true AP and a standard AP view. After the arm is prepped and draped in the usual sterile fashion, the fluoroscope is brought in for an AP view and a 1-cm incision is made along the lateral aspect of the acromion. A hemostat or straight Addison clamp is used to divide the deltoid in line with its fibers, and to triangulate the approach to the fragment. Placement of the guide-wire and screw are facilitated by gentle, small degrees of glenohumeral abduction or adduction to assist in achieving an optimal angle. Occasionally, an accessory anterolateral portal may be made for placement of a small freer elevator to assist in obtaining reduction. Knowledge of the anatomical details of the proximal humerus assists the surgeon in determining that a fluoroscopic reduction is indeed anatomic. The path along the guide-wire is then spread and cleared with a hemostat, and a 4.5- or 6.5-mm cannulated screw inserted with or without a washer as described above. Alternatively, one may use 2.5-mm terminally threaded AO pins placed percutaneously and cut off below the skin, which can be subsequently removed at 3 to 4 weeks pending radiographic evidence of healing. The wound is copiously irrigated and closed in standard fashion.

Complications

Complications of operative management are related to the nature of the injury, the surgical approach, and the technical methods employed to achieve reduction and fixation. For the purposes of clarification, these may be subdivided into perioperative and postoperative complications. Perioperative complications include infection, deltoid dehiscence, and axillary nerve injury. Postoperative complications include postoperative contracture, loss of reduction, malunion or nonunion, and rarely, avascular necrosis.[43]

Perioperative complications may be minimized through a proper selection of the surgical approach, which allows the surgeon to most reliably obtain and maintain reduction through minimal disruption to adjacent tissues. Perioperative antibiotics, meticulous skin handling technique, and thoughtful attention to the location of retractor placement and degree of force used to provide exposure will minimize the risks of infection, deltoid dehiscence, and axillary nerve injury. Anticipating the potential limitations and challenges with selection of the surgical approach will allow for maximal exposure through minimal dissection and retraction. In addition, a careful preoperative plan with a secondary strategy minimizes the duration of surgery and therefore the risk of perioperative complications.

Postoperative complications are minimized through the appropriate application of rehabilitation principals as discussed in detail below. Stable fixation is critical to allow early motion and prevent capsular contracture; however, active motion must be vigilantly prohibited in the early stages to minimize loss of reduction, malunion, and nonunion. Should capsular contracture develop and the patient fail to appropriately progress to obtain an acceptable range of motion, stiffness may initially be treated with aggressive active-assisted and passive range of motion exercises after union is confirmed. In the unusual case where these modalities are unsuccessful and the patient has a clinical picture consistent with the postoperative frozen shoulder, we advocate arthroscopic capsular release, which has proven quite successful to relieve pain and restore motion in the literature,[44] as well as subacromial débridement and acromioplasty when indicated. Malunion and nonunion of greater tuberosity fractures may be difficult to treat due to capsular contracture, subacromial scarring and impingement, and alterations in normal rotator cuff function. These issues are thoroughly addressed in Chapters 7 and 8.

Postoperative Care and Rehabilitation

Postoperatively the patient is placed in an abduction sling with the arm in neutral (not internal) rotation to minimize strain at the fracture site. Elbow, wrist, and digital range-of-motion (ROM) exercises with passive pendulums and Codman's exercises are begun immediately until 10 days when passive, supine external rotation and passive, supine forward elevation are initiated. Early internal rotation and horizontal adduction are avoided to limit tension on the operative fixation. At 6 weeks postoperatively, the sling is gradually discontinued and active-assisted ROM exercises are initiated to achieve full motion with an early emphasis on forward elevation and external rotation progressing to the addition of internal rotation and cross-body adduction. At 10 to 12 weeks, a program of rotator cuff and periscapular muscle strengthening is initiated and patients are again instructed to focus on a gradual low-weight high repetition progression. We counsel patients that recovery frequently takes 9 to 12 months for the full resumption of activities of daily living without mild occasional discomfort.

Results

There are few studies in the literature that clearly present the results of operative management of *isolated* greater tuberosity fractures. In 1924, Santee[45] suggested that even slight displacement of greater tuberosity fractures can result in significant disability. McLaughlin[6] presented a series of greater tuberosity fractures associated with glenohumeral dislocation in 1963 and reported that patients with 0.5 to 1.0 cm of displacement had a prolonged recovery and 20% required a reconstructive procedure. However, the concomitant dislocation may influence the results of this study; therefore, its pertinence to isolated tuberosity fractures is somewhat limited. Similarly, Young and Wallace[32] presented good and acceptable results of nonoperative management for 7 patients with a glenohumeral dislocation and associated tuberosity fracture; however, the results are difficult to interpret particularly because the criteria for shoulder motion were unclear. In a series of 930 proximal humerus fractures treated surgically, Jakob et al[7] reported only 17 isolated tuberosity fractures and did not report the results of treatment. Paavolainen et al[46] reported good results for the operative management of six displaced greater tuberosity fractures with screws. In a series of 141 two-part proximal humerus fractures, Chun et al[2] presented 24 cases of greater tuberosity fracture. Ten of these patients underwent open reduction and internal fixation; 8 patients were treated with screw fixation. At a mean follow-up of 5.1 years, 11 of the 24 patients were evaluated with Neer's criteria as follows: 1 – excellent, 7 – good, and 3 – fair (inclusion criteria for follow-up with regard to operative versus nonoperative management was unclear). The average forward elevation in this group at follow-up was 118 degrees and the average external rotation was 35 degrees. Perhaps the best data available in the literature were presented by Flatow et al.[11] In a series of 16 displaced greater tuberosity fractures treated with heavy nonabsorbable suture through a deltoid-splitting approach, the authors reported the results of 12 patients at an average of 4.5 years follow-up as follows: 6 – excellent and 6 – good. All patients in this series had at least 1 cm of posterior displacement.[11]

Summary

Isolated greater tuberosity fractures represent a challenging entity for the orthopedic surgeon with regard to optimal diagnosis,[47] operative indications,[11,26,34,35] and methods employed in surgical intervention. Although the historical literature suggests these injuries are relatively rare, recent studies have suggested that they may go undetected when a high index of suspicion is absent.[47] Improvements in our understanding of appropriate diagnostic plain film imaging[1] and the role of MRI will enhance our ability to identify these injuries. Knowledge of the biomechanical and clinical outcomes data will help to direct optimal treatment. Indications for operative management are influenced by the patient's physiologic age and level of vocational and recreational activity, as well as the physical exam and diagnostic imaging. The current general consensus in the literature suggests consideration of surgical intervention for fractures with more than 5 mm of superior displacement or more than 0.5 to 1 cm of posterior displacement. A careful preoperative plan with primary and secondary strategies for obtaining reduction and achieving stable fixation is critical as intraoperative findings may often present clinical scenarios that differ from the results of diagnostic imaging. Postoperative rehabilitation emphasizes early passive motion for optimal restoration of shoulder function with a subsequent focus on strengthening exercises when radiographic evidence of fracture site stability is confirmed. Opportunities for future research include determination of fragment size amenable to excision and rotator cuff repair versus suture fixation and the optimal implants to obtain interfragmentary compression without a risk of increasing comminution or fragment escape around a screw.

References

1. Parsons BO, Klepps SJ, Miller S, Bird J, Gladstone J, Flatow E. Reliability and reproducibility of radiographs of greater tuberosity displacement. A cadaveric study. J Bone Joint Surg Am 2005;87(1):58–65
2. Chun JM, Groh GI, Rockwood CA Jr. Two-part fractures of the proximal humerus. J Shoulder Elbow Surg 1994;3: 273–287
3. Lind T, Kroner K, Jensen J. The epidemiology of fractures of the proximal humerus. Arch Orthop Trauma Surg 1989;108:285–287
4. Rose SH, Melton LJ III, Morrey BF, Ilstrup DM, Riggs BL. Epidemiologic features of humeral fractures. Clin Orthop Relat Res 1982;168:24–30
5. Horak J, Nilsson BE. Epidemiology of fracture of the upper end of the humerus. Clin Orthop Relat Res 1975;112: 250–253
6. McLaughlin HL. Dislocation of the shoulder with tuberosity fracture. Surg Clin North Am 1963;43:469–473
7. Jakob RP, Kristiansen T, Mayo K, Ganz R, Muller ME. Classification and aspects of treatment of fractures of the proximal humerus. In: Bateman E, Welsh RP, eds. Surgery of the Shoulder. St. Louis: C.V. Mosby; 1984: 330–343
8. Green A, Izzi J Jr. Isolated fractures of the greater tuberosity of the proximal humerus. J Shoulder Elbow Surg 2003;12(6):641–649
9. Mason BJ, Kier R, Bindleglass DF. Occult fractures of the greater tuberosity of the humerus: radiographic and MR imaging findings. AJR Am J Roentgenol 1999;172(2): 469–473
10. Reinus WR, Hatem SF. Fractures of the greater tuberosity presenting as rotator cuff abnormality: magnetic resonance demonstration. J Trauma Inj Infect Crit Care 1998;44(4):670–675
11. Flatow EL, Cuomo F, Maday MG, Miller SR, McIlveen SJ, Bigliani LU. Open reduction and internal fixation of two-part displaced fractures of the greater tuberosity of the proximal part of the humerus. J Bone Joint Surg Am 1991;73:1213–1218
12. Ahovero J, Paavolainen P, Bjorkenheim JM. Fractures of the proximal humerus involving the intertubercular groove. Acta Radiol 1989;30:373–374
13. Rowe CR. Prognosis in dislocations of the shoulder. J Bone Joint Surg Am 1956;38:957–977
14. Rowe CR, Sakellarides HT. Factors related to recurrences of anterior dislocations of the shoulder. Clin Orthop Relat Res 1961;20:40–47
15. Keene JS, Huizenga RE, Engber WD, et al. Proximal humerus fractures. A correlation of residual deformity with long-term function. Orthopedics 1983;6:173–178
16. Kaspar S, Mandel S. Acromial impression fracture of the greater tuberosity with rotator cuff avulsion due to hyperabduction injury of the shoulder. J Shoulder Elbow Surg 2004;13(1):112–114
17. Clark JM, Harryman DT. Tendons, ligaments, and capsule of the rotator cuff. Gross and microscopic anatomy. J Bone Joint Surg Am 1992;74:713–725
18. Iannotti JP, Gabriel JP, Schneck SL, Evans BG, Misra S. The normal glenohumeral relationships. An anatomical study of one hundred and forty shoulders. J Bone Joint Surg Am 1992;74:491–500
19. Minagawa H, Itoi E, Konno N, et al. Humeral attachment of the supraspinatus and infraspinatus tendons: an anatomic study. Arthroscopy 1998;14:302–306
20. Dugas JR, Campbell DA, Warren RF, et al. Anatomy and dimensions of rotator cuff insertions. J Shoulder Elbow Surg 2002;11:498–503
21. Ruotolo C, Fow JE, Nottage WM. The supraspinatus footprint: an anatomic study of the supraspinatus insertion. Arthroscopy 2004;20:246–249
22. Robertson DD, Yuan J, Bigliani LU, Flatow EL, Yamaguchi K. Three-dimensional analysis of the proximal part of the humerus: relevance to arthroplasty. J Bone Joint Surg Am 2000;82-A(11):1594–1602

23. Laing PG. The arterial supply of the adult humerus. J Bone Joint Surg Am 1956;38:1105–1116
24. Gerber C, Schneeberger A, Vinh TS. The arterial vascularization of the humeral head. An anatomical study. J Bone Joint Surg Am 1990;72:1486–1494
25. Rasmussen S, Hvass I, Dalsgaard J, Christensen B, Holstad E. Displaced proximal humeral fractures: results of conservative treatment. Injury 1992;23:41–43
26. Bono CM, Renard R, Levine RG, Levy AS. Effect of displacement of fractures of the greater tuberosity on the mechanics of the shoulder. J Bone Joint Surg Br 2001;83(7):1056–1062
27. Craig EV. Operative treatment of tuberosity fractures, malunions, and nonunions. In: Craig EV, ed. Master Techniques in Orthopaedic Surgery: The Shoulder. 2nd ed. New York, NY: Raven Press; 2004:495-511
28. Morris ME, Kilcoyne RF, Shuman W, Matsen FH III. Humeral tuberosity fractures: evaluation by CT scan and management of malunion. Orthop Trans 1987; 11:242
29. Zanetti M, Weishaupt D, Jost B, Gerber C, Hodler J. MR imaging for traumatic tears of the rotator cuff: high prevalence of greater tuberosity fractures and subscapularis tendon tears. AJR Am J Roentgenol 1999;172(2): 463–467
30. Patten RM, Mack LA, Wang KY, Lingel J. Nondisplaced fractures of the greater tuberosity of the humerus: sonographic detection. Radiology 1992;182(1):201–204
31. Neer CS II. Displaced proximal humeral fractures. I. Classification and evaluation. J Bone Joint Surg Am 1970;52: 1077–1089
32. Young TB, Wallace WA. Conservative treatment of fractures and fracture dislocations of the upper end of the humerus. J Bone Joint Surg Br 1985;67:373–377
33. Olivier H, Duparc J, Romain F. Fractures of the greater tuberosity of the humerus. Orthop Trans 1986;10:223
34. Iannotti JP, Ramsey ML, Williams GR, Warner JP. Nonprosthetic management of proximal humeral fractures. J Bone Joint Surg Am 2003;85:1578–1593
35. Park TS, Choi IY, Kim YH, et al. A new suggestion for the treatment of minimally displaced fractures of the greater tuberosity of the proximal humerus. Bull Hosp Joint Dis 1997;56:171–176
36. Galatz LM, Rothermich SY, Zaegel M, Silva MJ, Havlioglu N, Thomopoulos S. Delayed repair of tendon to bone injuries leads to decreased biomechanical properties and bone loss. J Orthop Res 2005;23(6): 1441–1447
37. Herscovici D Jr, Saunders DT, Johnson MP, Sanders R, DiPasquale T. Percutaneous fixation of proximal humeral fractures. Clin Orthop Relat Res 2000;375:97–104
38. White RR. Percutaneous fixation of proximal humeral fractures. In: Craig EV, ed. Master Techniques in Orthopaedic Surgery: The Shoulder. 2nd ed. New York, NY: Raven Press; 2004:481–494
39. Kim SH, Ha KI. Arthroscopic treatment of symptomatic shoulders with minimally displaced greater tuberosity fracture. Arthroscopy 2000;16:695–700
40. Taverna E, Sansone V, Battistella F. Arthroscopic treatment for greater tuberosity fractures: rationale and surgical technique. Arthroscopy 2004;20(6):e53–e57
41. Gardner MJ, Griffith MH, Dines JS, Briggs SM, Weiland AJ, Lorich DG. The extended anterolateral acromial approach allows minimally invasive access to the proximal humerus. Clin Orthop Relat Res 2005;434:123–129
42. Cornell CN. Tension-band wiring supplemented by lag-screw fixation of proximal humerus fractures: a modified technique. Orthop Rev 1994;14(Suppl):19–23
43. Cordasco FA, Bigliani LU. Complications of proximal humerus fractures. Tech Orthop 1997;12(1):42–50
44. Warner JJ, Allen AA, Marks PH, Wong P. Arthroscopic release of post-operative capsular contracture of the shoulder. J Bone Joint Surg Am 1997;79:1151–1158
45. Santee HE. Fractures about the upper end of the humerus. Ann Surg 1924;80:103–114
46. Paavolainen P, Bjorkenheim JM, Slatis P, Paukku P. Operative treatment of severe proximal humeral fractures. Acta Orthop Scand 1983;54:374–379
47. Ogawa K, Yoshida A, Ikegami H. Isolated fractures of the greater tuberosity of the humerus: solutions to recognizing a frequently overlooked fracture. J Trauma Inj Infect Crit Care 2003;54(4):713–717

5 Percutaneous Pinning of Proximal Humeral Fractures

Kenneth J. Accousti and Evan L. Flatow

Proximal humerus fractures are common and occur at a rate of 4 to 5% of all fractures. This rate has increased since the 1970s and is expected to continue to rise. The major risk factors are old age, female gender, and osteoporosis.[1] The vast majority (85%) of these fractures are not displaced or minimally displaced and can be treated with nonoperative means. The remaining 15% present a challenge to the clinician in terms of the best treatment option.

There are many surgical options including open reduction and internal fixation with locked or nonlocked plates, tension-band wiring, intramedullary nail fixation with solid or flexible nails, humeral head replacement, and percutaneous reduction and pinning. Hagg and Lundberg[2] reported a doubling of the rate of avascular necrosis with open reduction. The advantages of percutaneous pinning include decreased soft tissue stripping and a decreased risk of vascular compromise to the fracture fragments. In addition, there is less adhesion formation with closed reduction, which makes any subsequent revision surgery easier secondary to decreased scarring. The major disadvantages are technical difficulty and risk to neurovascular structures around the proximal humerus. These risks can be decreased with strict attention to anatomic principles, careful dissection, and soft tissue protection during placement of hardware.

Patient Assessment

It is important to perform a thorough history and physical examination when the patient first presents to the office or emergency room. Most patients are elderly and may have other comorbid conditions, which may help guide the physician to an operative or nonoperative course. The preinjury functional level of the patient is important to assess and may help guide expected outcomes.

The surgeon must document a complete neurologic and vascular assessment of the extremity preoperatively. Axillary artery and nerve dysfunction is common after proximal humerus fractures and may prolong the recovery time.[3] It is important to assess both the sensory as well as the motor function of the axillary nerve. Injuries to the axillary artery may not present with a dysvascular limb secondary to the vast collateral circulation around the shoulder. If a vascular injury is suspected, an angiogram should be performed. An electromyogram (EMG) should be obtained at 3 weeks postinjury if a patient has any residual neurological symptoms.

Standard radiographic evaluation includes an anteroposterior (AP) and lateral (Y-view) in the plane of the scapula as well as an axillary view. This shoulder trauma series is usually sufficient to determine the fracture configuration. If the fracture pattern cannot be determined from plain films, computed tomography (CT) with reconstructions may aide in the determination of the position and displacement of the fracture fragments.

Fractures are classified using the Neer system, which describes the fracture as the number of parts that are displaced 10 mm or angulated 45 degrees. Greater than 5 mm of superior displacement of the greater tuberosity has recently been felt to require reduction and fixation, especially in younger, active patients.

The majority of two-part fractures have surgical neck displacement. Isolated fractures of the greater or, less commonly, the lesser tuberosity also occur. Three-part fractures have a displaced surgical neck component as well as a displaced fracture of either the greater or lesser tuberosity. In a classic four-part fracture-dislocation both tuberosities are separated from the dislocated head and the shaft. Valgus-impacted four-part fractures are a specialized subset of four-part fractures because they usually have a medial periosteal sling, which connects the head fragment to the shaft and preserves the ascending branches of the anterior and posterior circumflex arteries to the head.[4] This periosteal hinge also aids in reduction of the fragments via ligamentotaxis. The head segment itself is fragmented in the "head splitting" fractures.

Fracture fragment displacement varies depending on the fracture configuration. The deforming forces around the shoulder include the subscapularis, which will displace a lesser tuberosity or head fragment medially. The supraspinatus, infraspinatus, and teres minor will displace the head or greater tuberosity fragment superiorly and posteriorly. The pectoralis major will medialize the proximal aspect of the humeral shaft with respect to the head. Understanding these deforming forces will facilitate proper reduction based on fracture configuration (**Fig. 5–1**).

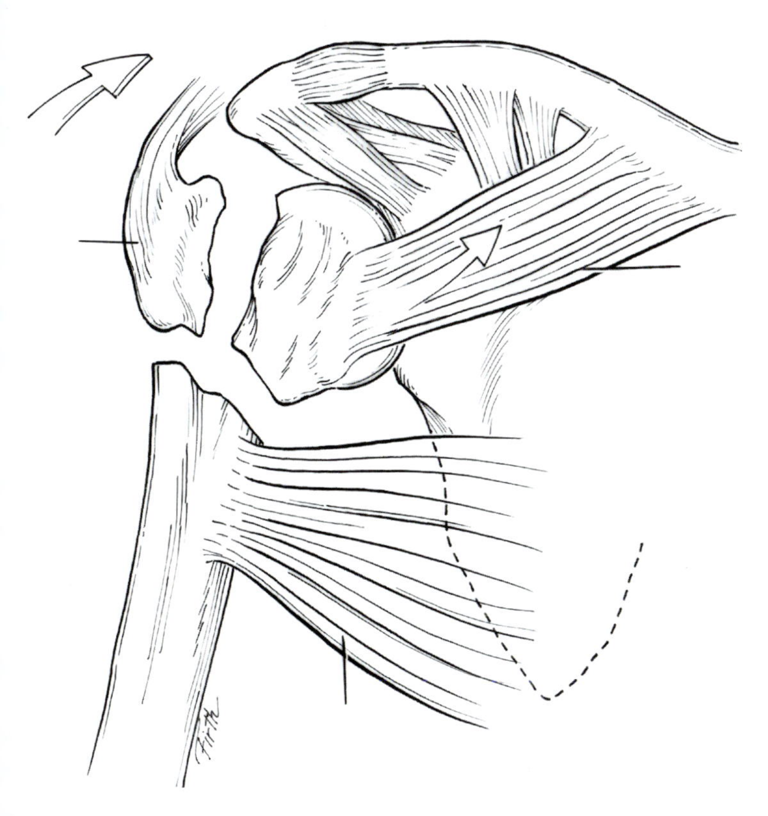

Figure 5–1 Deforming forces on proximal humeral fracture fragments include the pectoralis major pulling the humeral shaft medially, the subscapularis pulling the lesser tuberosity medially, and the supraspinatus, infraspinatus, and teres minor displacing the greater tuberosity fragment superiorly and posteriorly.

Treatment

Nonsurgical Treatment

The majority of fractures can be treated nonoperatively with short-term immobilization followed by range of motion (ROM) exercises once the fracture begins to heal.

Surgical Treatment

Most displaced fractures will require reduction and operative fixation. Although closed reduction and percutaneous fixation is a good treatment for two- and three-part displaced fractures, other methods can be effective, including intramedullary rods, fixed-angle plates, and tension-band wiring. Percutaneous repair is especially well suited, however, to the treatment of impacted-valgus four-part fractures, as the reduced soft tissue stripping leads to a lower rate of avascular necrosis compared with open treatment.[2] Minimally invasive repair also leads to less stiffness and reduced adhesions, making revision, if needed, easier. Classic four-part fracture-dislocations generally require humeral head replacement given the high rate of avascular necrosis due to the disruption of the blood supply to the humeral head. Fractures with severe comminution or patients with osteoporotic bone are not ideal candidates for percutaneous pinning. Head splitting fractures usually require arthroplasty given the high rate of avascular necrosis and posttraumatic arthritis. The results of revision hemiarthroplasty after failed open reduction are poorer than for primary arthroplasty for fracture.[5]

Technique for Percutaneous Pinning

At our institution, we routinely perform percutaneous fixation under interscalene regional anesthesia and place the patient in the beach-chair position. The patient is placed as far lateral on the table as possible so that the affected arm can move freely and the image intensifier, placed cranially at the head of the table, can move from an AP (over the top position) to an axillary view with ease. Prior to prepping the patient, we will attempt a closed reduction, assessing the position of the fracture fragments using the image intensifier **(Fig. 5–2)**. It is important to make sure that the image intensifier is positioned properly to obtain both AP and axillary views to assess both the quality of the reduction and the position of the pins and screws. The surgical site is then prepped and placed into a hydraulic arm holder that helps position and fix the arm in space.

For two-part fractures involving the surgical neck, we will reduce the fragments with gentle traction on the adducted arm with slight internal rotation to properly align the head to the shaft noting that there is usually

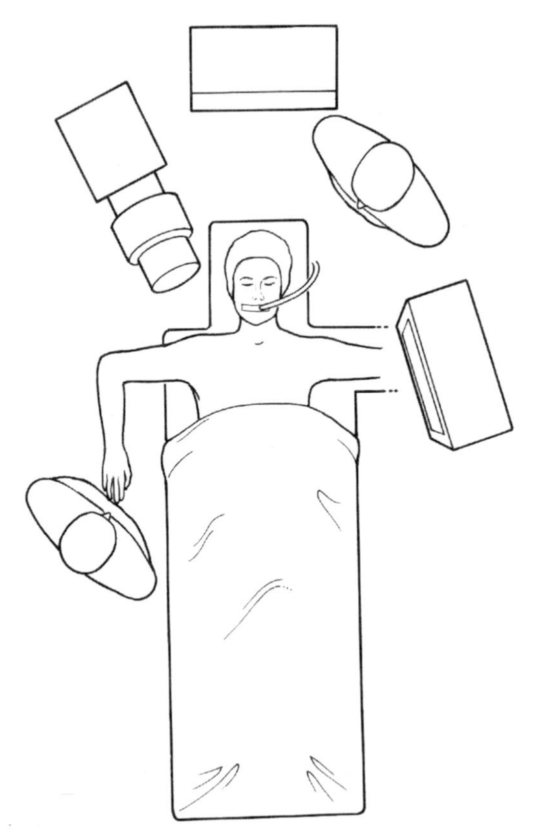

Figure 5–2 Operating room layout with the image intensifier placed cranially, with the monitor across the patient to act as an "arthroscopy" monitor.

30 degrees of retroversion of the humeral head with respect to the epicondylar axis of the distal humerus. A bolster of surgical towels can be placed in the axilla to help hold the proximal shaft laterally, counteracting the pull of the pectoralis major as well as serving as a counterforce to the push on the humeral shaft when advancing the 2.5-mm terminally threaded Schantz pins. A small stab incision is then made on the lateral aspect of the arm proximal to the deltoid tuberosity. The soft tissues are carefully dissected with a straight Adson clamp down to bone in a proximal direction. Soft tissue protectors are used to help hold the entry position on the humeral shaft as well as to protect the anterior branch of the axillary nerve on the undersurface of the deltoid. A Schantz pin is then inserted into the humeral head at a 30- to 40-degree angle from the axis of the humeral shaft. The entry point should be twice the distance from the superiormost aspect of the articular cartilage to the inferiormost margin of the humeral head **(Fig. 5–3)**.

It is important to enter the lateral cortex of the humeral shaft at least 2 cm below the fracture line to help hold the integrity of the pin in the distal shaft fragment. The Schantz pin is slowly advanced to the subchondral bone of the humeral head. It is important not to penetrate into the articular surface because these threaded pins cannot be backed out without losing their fixation. If penetration has occurred, the pin must be removed and a new pin is inserted at a slightly different angle to avoid the tract of the previous pin. At a minimum, two orthogonal views are needed and we routinely will image the pin through a range of motion in both the AP and axillary planes once stability of the fragments has been achieved to assess for joint penetration. A second Schantz pin is inserted in a proximal direction from the lateral cortex of the shaft into a different area of the humeral head. Again, the position is checked with multiple views of the image intensifier.

When the fracture involves displacement of the greater or lesser tuberosity, a small hook can be inserted percutaneously to reduce the tuberosity to the head fragment. The tuberosities must be brought back to their anatomic positions to prevent subacromial or subcoracoid impingement and to restore the mechanical lever arm of the muscle-tendon unit. It is important to direct the hook toward the bone to prevent injury to any neurovascular structures. Once the tuberosity is reduced, it is held with a Kirschner wire (K-wire) prior to fixation with either two 4.0 cannulated screws (Synthes, Inc., West Chester, PA) or 2.5-mm terminally threaded Schantz pins **(Fig. 5–4)**. One is placed lateral to medial into the head; the other is inserted in a proximal to distal direction from the greater tuberosity into the medial cortex of the humeral shaft. It is important to get bicortical fixation because the pins will not achieve purchase in the medullary canal of the humerus. It is also essential to prevent overpenetration on the medial side to avoid injury to the main branch of the axillary nerve and posterior humeral circumflex artery as it passes posteriorly underneath the subscapularis, inferior capsule, and glenoid **(Fig. 5–3)**. In an anatomic study by Rowles and McGrory,[6] the greater tuberosity pins were a mean distance of 6 to 7 mm from the axillary nerve and posterior circumflex artery. The distance from the pin tip to the nerve increased with external rotation of the arm **(Fig. 5–5)**.

Valgus-impacted four-part fractures present a challenge to achieve an anatomic reduction. Open reductions can be performed at first with gradual progression to an all-closed method once the surgeon becomes comfortable with the reduction and fixation technique. A 1-cm incision is made on the anterior lateral aspect of the shoulder at the level of the surgical neck fracture line and an elevator is used to lift the head fragment above the greater tuberosity. The elevator is placed on the anterolateral aspect of the head fragment and is tapped up gently with a mallet to disimpact the fragment **(Fig. 5–6)**. It is important to restore the height, inclination, and retroversion of the humeral head. If reduction cannot be achieved by

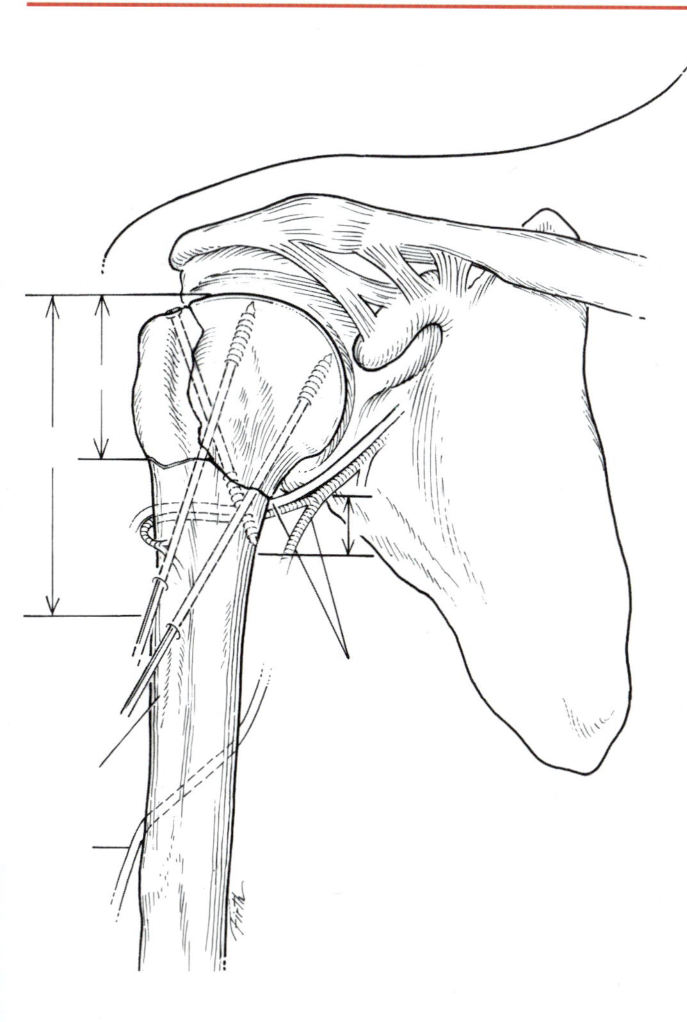

Figure 5–3 Anatomic risks include the posterior humeral circumflex artery and the axillary nerve (both the main branch medially and the anterior branch on the undersurface of the deltoid laterally). Laterally the nerve is ~6 cm distal to the lateral border of the acromion. The inferior pins should enter the lateral cortex of the humerus at twice the distance from the superior aspect of the humeral head to the inferiormost medial margin of the humeral head. The superior to inferior pins should penetrate the medial cortex at least 20 mm or more from the inferior articular margin to avoid the main branch of the axillary nerve and posterior humeral circumflex artery. External rotation with insertion of these pins will move the pins away from the nerve.

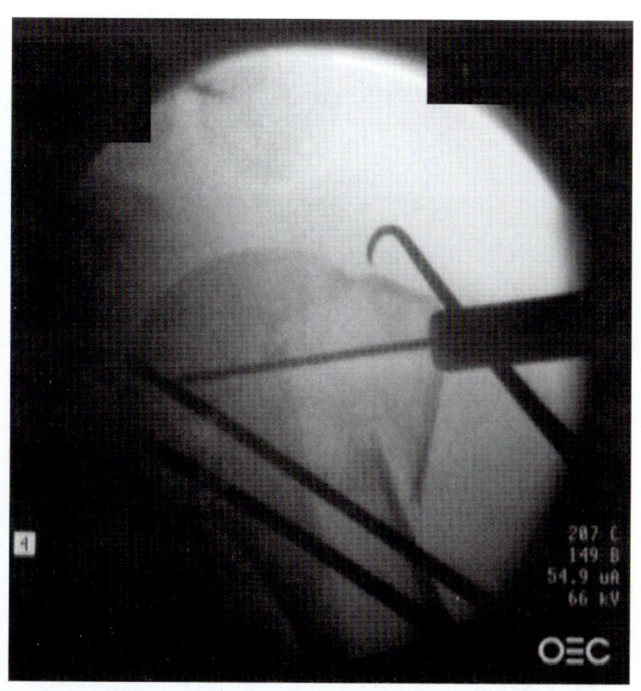

Figure 5–4 The greater tuberosity is reduced with a small bone hook while a K-wire is used to fix it to the head fragment.

elevating the head fragment, it is likely that the medial periosteal hinge is disrupted along with the blood supply to the head fragment. Head fragments with significant lateral displacement will have disruption of the medial periosteum. The superiormost aspect of the articular cartilage is, on average, 8 to 10 mm higher than the top of the greater tuberosity. Once the head is elevated, the shaft is then fixed to the head with two Schantz pins as described earlier. The greater tuberosity is then fixed to the head and shaft with either pins or cannulated screws **(Fig. 5–7)**. The lesser tuberosity piece is fixed to the head with a posteriorly directed screw through the tuberosity into the head fragment.

All pins are cut as low as possible to prevent pressure on the skin once the swelling subsides at around 2 weeks and the incisions are closed with sutures. This also decreases the risk of pin tract infections that are associated with pins left through the skin. Patients are held in a sling postoperatively and shoulder ROM is begun once the pins have been removed in the clinic or at 3 to 4 weeks postoperatively. Gentle passive ROM is then begun. No lifting or strengthening is allowed until 6 weeks postoperatively.

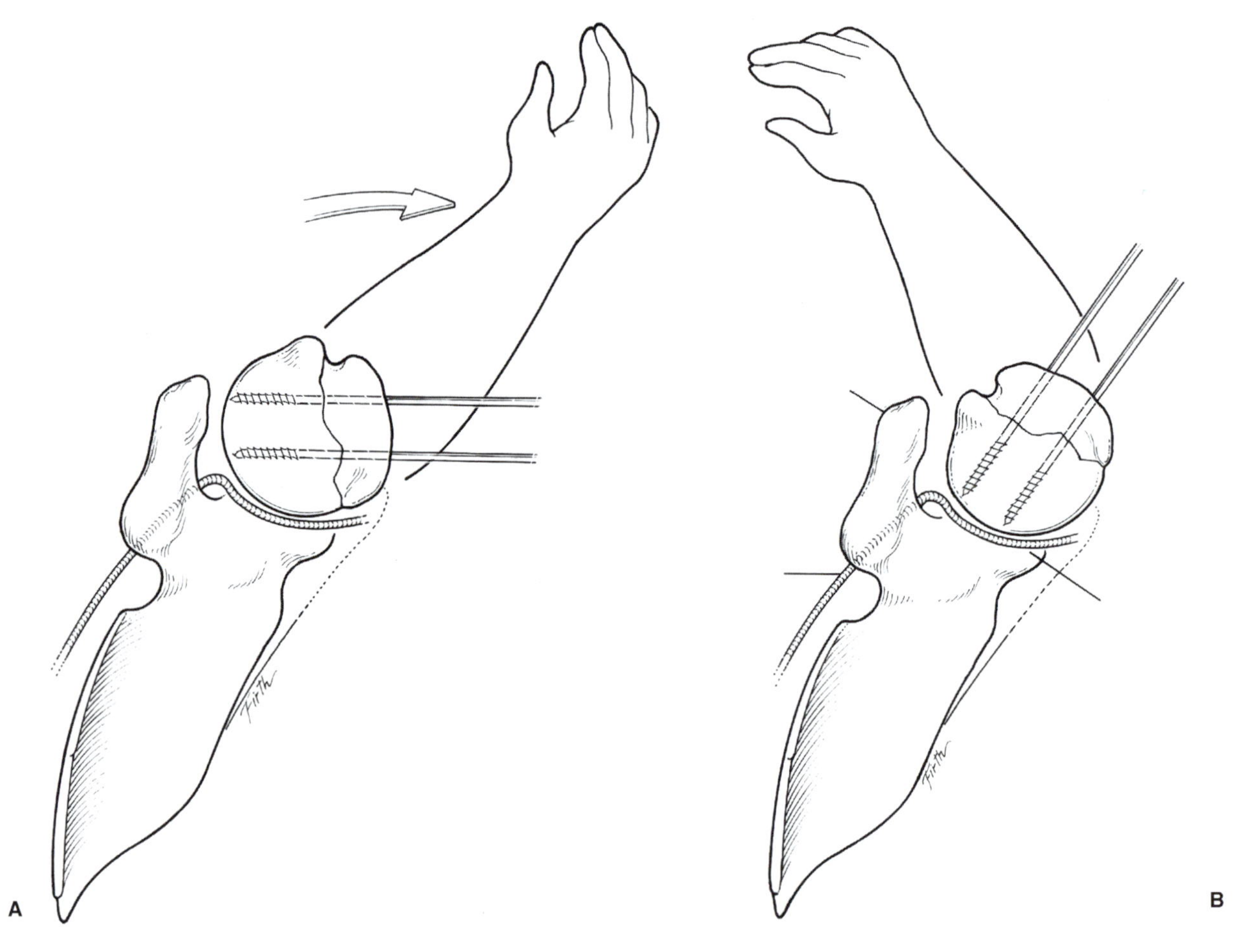

Figure 5–5 External rotation increases the distance from the pin tips to **(A)** the axillary nerve and **(B)** the posterior humeral circumflex artery as they pass under the inferior joint capsule and glenoid.

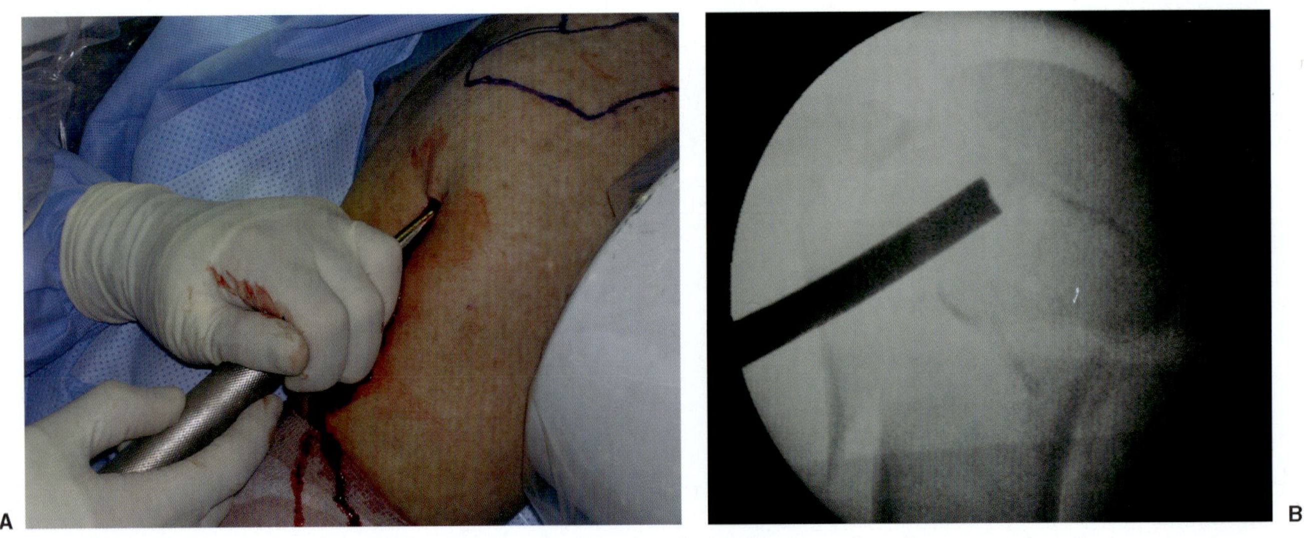

Figure 5–6 **(A,B)** Through a small stab incision, an elevator is used to reduce the head fragment above the greater tuberosity.

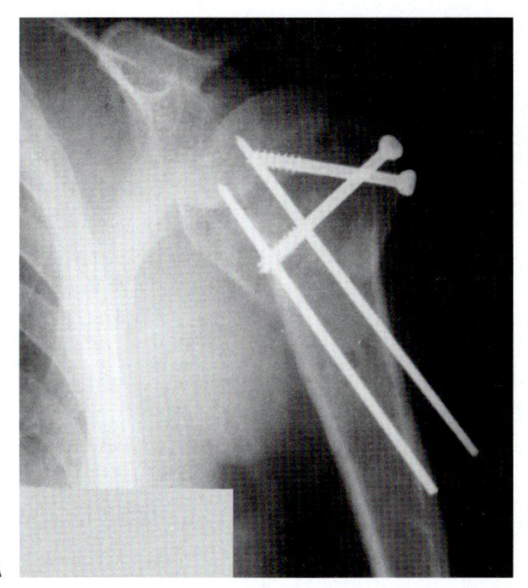
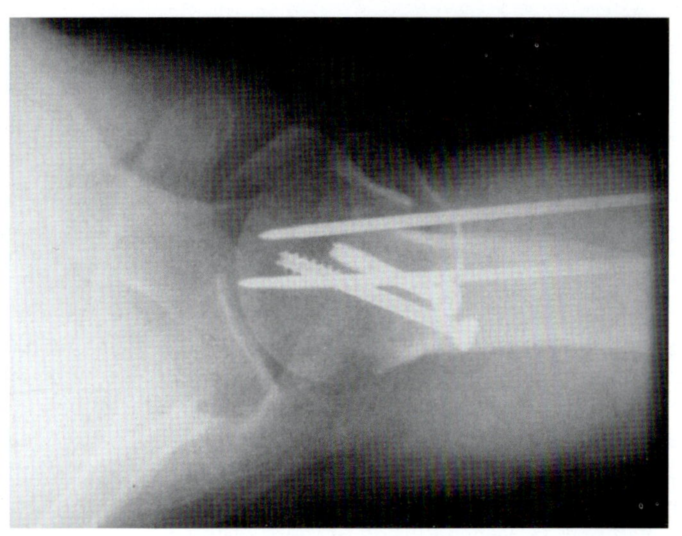

Figure 5–7 Postoperative **(A)** anteroposterior and **(B)** axillary x-rays demonstrating fixation of the shaft to the humeral head with two 2.5-mm terminally threaded Schantz pins and two 4.0-mm partially threaded cannulated screws through the greater tuberosity fragment.

Complications

Hagg and Lundberg[2] reported avascular necrosis rates of 3 to 14% for displaced three-part fractures treated by closed methods. This rate increased to 12 to 25% with open reduction of three-part fractures. The rate of avascular necrosis for four-part fractures was nearly double for fractures treated openly versus closed, ranging from 41 to 59% for fractures treated by open methods. Resch et al[7,8] reported no avascular necrosis for three-part fractures and 11% for all four-part fractures treated with closed reduction and percutaneous pinning. Their rate of avascular necrosis for valgus impacted four-part fractures was 8%, which was one case of asymptomatic partial necrosis. They had no nerve palsies or infections in their series.

Herscovici et al[9] noted failure of fixation in all fractures treated with smooth k-wires but had no failures of fixation with terminally threaded Schantz pins. They also reported two cases of pin tract infections which both resolved with antibiotic treatment. One patient required operative débridement.

Nonunion is rare and was seen in 2 patients out of 48 in a series by Jaberg, Warner, and Jakob.[10] Four patients had loss of fixation that required a repeat operation with only 1 patient having a poor result from malunion. They had two cases of complete avascular necrosis, and eight cases of partial necrosis, which subsequently resolved over a 1- to 2-year period.

Results

Chen et al[11] reported good or excellent results in 84% of patients with two- and three-part proximal humerus fractures. They had no incidents of avascular necrosis with 18 of 19 patients obtaining a solid union at a mean follow-up of 21 months. There was no difference in outcomes between two- or three-part fractures. Resch et al[8] had good or very good functional results for all AO type B1 and B2 fractures with an average Constant score of 91% with no cases of avascular necrosis. Type C1 and C2 fractures had an average Constant score of 87% (not including two failures).

We recently evaluated our experience with percutaneous pinning of proximal humerus fractures. Twenty-two patients were followed for an average of 30 months (range of 12 to 69 months). There were 8 valgus four-part fractures, 8 three-part fractures, 4 two-part surgical neck fractures, and 2 two-part greater tuberosity fractures. A good result was obtained in 86% of the patients and the average ASES and Constant scores were 81 and 73, respectively. There were two cases of avascular necrosis (both in four-part fractures) with 1 patient undergoing a hemiarthroplasty 2 years after the index procedure. The other patient refused treatment. There was no incidence of infection and one case of pin loosening, which was removed without incident. One patient had significant postoperative stiffness, which was treated by arthroscopic capsular release with a good result. The average active ROM for forward flexion and external rotation was 141 and 51 degrees, respectively.[12]

Summary

Percutaneous pinning offers a minimally invasive method of treating two-, three-, and valgus-impacted four-part fractures of the proximal humerus. The technique is demanding, but with proper patient selection, good results can be expected. Decreased soft tissue disruption compared with open procedures better preserves the tenuous blood supply to the humeral head and also decreases scarring within the subdeltoid and subacromial bursa. This helps make revision surgery easier if subsequent avascular necrosis develops and humeral head replacement becomes necessary. Strict attention to anatomic principals and surgical technique decrease the likelihood of neurovascular injury.

References

1. Kannus P, Palvanen M, Niemi S, Parkkari J, Jarvinen M, Vuori I. Increasing number and incidence of osteoporotic fractures of the proximal humerus in elderly people. BMJ 1996;313:1051–1052
2. Hagg O, Lundberg B. Aspects of prognostic factors in comminuted and dislocated proximal humeral fractures. In: Bateman JE, Welsh RP, eds. Surgery of the Shoulder. Philadelphia, PA: BC Decker;1984:51–59
3. Visser CP, Coene LN, Brand R, Tavy DL. Nerve lesions in proximal humeral fractures. J Shoulder Elbow Surg 2001;10:421–427
4. Brook CH, Revell WJ, Heatley FW. Vascularity of the humeral head after proximal humeral fractures – an anatomical study. J Bone Joint Surg Br 1993;75:132–136
5. Norris TR, Green A, McGuigan FX. Late prosthetic shoulder arthroplasty for displaced humerus fractures. J Shoulder Elbow Surg 1995;4:271–280
6. Rowles D, McGrory D. Percutaneous pinning of the proximal part of the humerus. J Bone Joint Surg Am 2001;83(11):1695–1699
7. Resch H, Povacz P, Frohlich R, Wambacher M. Percutaneous fixation of three- and four-part fractures of the proximal humerus. J Bone Joint Surg Br 1997;79:295–300
8. Resch H, Hubner C, Schwaiger R. Minimally invasive reduction and osteosynthesis of articular fractures of the humeral head. Injury 2001;32(Suppl 1):SA25–SA32
9. Herscovici D, Saunders D, Johnson M, Sanders R, DiPasquale T. Percutaneous fixation of proximal humeral fractures. Clin Orthop Relat Res 2000;375:97–104
10. Jaberg H, Warner JJ, Jakob RP. Percutaneous stabilization of unstable fractures of the humerus. J Bone Joint Surg Am 1992;74(4):508–515
11. Chen CY, Chao EK, Tu YK, Ueng S, Shih CH. Closed management and percutaneous fixation of unstable proximal humerus fractures. J Trauma 1998;45(6):1039–1045
12. Galatz L, Williams G, Keener J, Parsons B, Braman J, Flatow EL. Percutaneous pinning of proximal humerus fractures. Poster presented at: Annual Meeting of the American Academy of Orthopaedic Surgeons; February 23–26, 2005; Washington, DC

6 Open Reduction and Internal Fixation of Proximal Humeral Fractures Using Locking Plates

Norbert P. Südkamp and Peter C. Strohm

Fractures of the proximal humerus, representing 5% of all extremity fractures, are common fractures. Apart from the distal fracture of the radius and fractures adjacent to the hip joint, the proximal humerus fracture is the most common fracture in elderly people. The incidence in the total population is 70 per 100,000 per annum, but this rises in women over 70 years to 400 per 100,000 per annum.[1] In contrast to the more common indirect type of accident experienced by older people, injury in younger people is likely to be the consequence of high-energy trauma.

Operative stabilization of fractures of the humeral head is still a surgical challenge and remains the subject of many clinical and experimental investigations. The large number of implants currently available on the market and the different recommendations for operative stabilization procedures reflect the problems involved with this injury and its treatment. From the point of view of evidence-based medicine, it is still not possible to define the gold standard for stabilization of fractures of the humeral head.[2,3]

New findings about the biomechanics and pathophysiology of bones and soft tissue have influenced and directed the design and function of new forms of osteosynthesis. In particular, the development of locking implants has strongly influenced modern surgical techniques.

Anatomy of the Proximal Humerus

Due to blood flow dynamics in the area of the proximal humerus, the risk of a necrosis developing in the humeral head because of surgical manipulation is high, and can result from the fractures alone. The blood supply of the proximal humerus is provided mainly by the circumflex humeral arteries, which branch off the axillary artery. The ascending branch running through the area of the bicipital groove is significant as it also flows through a substantial part of the calvaria.[4,5] Recently, using more refined preparation and drainage techniques, additional periosteal irradiating vessels were identified in the area of the lesser tubercle in the humeral head. This periosteal blood flow is only disturbed when the humeral head suffers gross dislocation and usually continues to ensure residual blood flow to the calvaria. Studies also show that the periosteal blood flow plays an important role in the area of the calcarine spur and that the size of the fracture fragment and the extent of the dislocation permit conclusions to be drawn about the risk of necrosis developing in and around the humeral head.[6] Manipulation during surgery can also slightly upset or even destroy the blood flow. Blood flow is usually further reduced by the pressure of conventional plates/screws on the periosteum. This problem is eliminated by the use of locking implants.

Classifications of Proximal Humeral Fractures

Codman drew up a classification in 1934, which was based on the four segments: the greater tubercle, the lesser tubercle, calvaria, and shaft. Neer compiled the classification most widely used now; it is based on Codman's four-fragment classification and is divided into six groups. According to the Neer classification, surgery is indicated when all four fragments are involved, with a dislocation of the fragments of at least 0.5 to 1 cm or with more than a 45-degree tilt.[7,8] Various studies, however, have shown that there are difficulties with the practical application of this classification.[9–12] It has not been possible to generally implement the AO classification according to Müller et al.[12–14]

The low reliability of these classifications causes difficulties in the numerous clinical comparative studies. According to accident records, which often lack technical details but must used as a main basis for classification, the question arises whether it is possible at all to make a precise assessment of the degree of dislocation of the individual segments using these initial records. However, taking conventional x-rays in one to three planes is still the standard diagnostic procedure for the proximal humerus. If the extent of the fracture cannot be assessed a computed tomography (CT) scan is indicated.[10] This is especially helpful if there is a possibility of a comminuted fracture of the calvaria and of so-called head split fractures, which the classifications do not describe adequately. Codman's classification is still practical because it is not based on the dislocation of the individual fragments that is difficult to assess, but focuses on the instability of the fragments affected.

Treatment

In principle, both surgical and conservative treatment can be considered for fractures of the proximal humerus. Although Neer intended his classification to be an aid for determining the indications for conservative or surgical treatment of proximal humerus fractures,[7,8] it has not resulted in a gold standard for the treatment of proximal humerus fractures according to the criteria of evidence-based-medicine.[12,15] The advantages and disadvantages of conservative and surgical procedures are still controversial; very good as well as poor outcomes for both procedures are described.[16,17] However, there are still not many prospective or even randomized studies with locking implants. Our own prospective trial is in progress.

In our clinic, we tend to advocate a surgical procedure–we have had good results with locking implants even when the bone quality is poor. In our opinion, shoulder function profits from early functional rehabilitation.

Surgical Treatment

In past decades, various methods of surgical stabilization were used. Until the 1980s, the standard technique was to use various conventional plates such as T-plates or one-third tubular plates, which are still used in some cases today.[3,18–21] The use of angled blade plates is also described in the recent literature.[22] However, these nonlocking plate fixations cause damage to soft tissue and allow extensive bone exposure. Many cases also result in typical complications such as implant failure, loss of reduction, and necroses of the humeral head.[3,18,23] Problems have also arisen from the choice of implant–plates with higher stability are bulkier, which further compromises the soft tissue. Smaller implants, such as one-third tubular plates, show too little stability and are often unsuitable, particularly in cases of low bone quality.

Because of these problems, the future trend is toward minimal fixation procedures.[3,18,24] This term applies to stabilization procedures that offer fixation using a minimally invasive approach. The procedures include Kirschner wire (K-wire) fixations in (partially) open or closed technique, cerclage wire fixation or PDS (polydioxanone) sutures, and isolated percutaneous screws, which have been used as conventional small fragment screws or inserted as cannulated screws over guide wires.[23–27]

These changes in surgical technique are revealing the problems of stabilization procedures at the proximal humerus and the need for the development of new implants. The priority is the preservation of the soft tissue; to this end, blood flow must be maintained to the greatest possible extent.

Locking Plates

In the past, the aim of internal fixation was to achieve the best possible anatomical reduction and then to fix the bone in this position. If conventional plates were used as implants, a relatively large approach with complete exposure was necessary.[28] This resulted in additional damage to the soft tissue, which encouraged infections and impaired healing of the bone as well as the soft tissue.[29,30] The stabilizing principle of conventional plates results from the friction between plate and bone.[28] The pressure exerted by the plate through the strong application of the screws on the bone suppresses the blood flow of the periosteum, which further impairs healing of the fracture.

Accordingly, to avoid this additional alteration in blood flow, the principle of internal fixation was developed and initially implemented in the form of the point contact fixator (PC-Fix) and the LISS (less invasive stabilization system).[31] Using the principle of internal fixation, reduction can be maintained through implants–analogous to external fixation–without suppressing the blood flow by the pressure applied. Hence, the locking compression plate (LCP) was developed and modified for different anatomic regions (for example, the distal tibia plate, the pilon plate, the locking proximal humerus plate [LPHP], the distal humerus plate, etc.).[32] This new generation of locking plates combines the advantages of the conventional techniques of dynamic compression (DC plates) with the advantages of the internal fixator.[31] The plate is no longer being pulled toward the bone by the screws; therefore, the periosteal blood flow is no longer compromised. In addition, comminuted fractures can also be bridged with the locking plates and reduction maintained without risking a secondary loss of reduction through collapse of the fracture parts, as nothing in the locking system changes in terms of the plates and/or screw angles. Retention by the implant is therefore maintained. The biological insertion of the implants by the so-called minimally invasive percutaneous osteosynthesis technique (MIPO) is possible with these plate systems, which guarantees less damage to the soft tissue and better bone healing. Locking implants are also very well suited for use in osteoporotic bones.

Advantages of Locking Plates at the Proximal Humerus

The new locking plates, designed especially for fixation procedures on the proximal humerus, have been developed giving special consideration to the specific characteristics of this anatomic region. The plates have a low profile and are not very bulky. Thus, the soft tissue is only slightly compromised during the procedure, and the danger of a postoperative impingement syndrome by the plate is lower.

The plates are also biomechanically not as stiff as other implants designed for this region, which has a positive effect on load capacity and is also better suited to osteoporotic bones. Furthermore, the plates sit very firmly in the bone due to the (converging/diverging) screw orientation and the locked screw anchorage.[33] The locking head screws ensure that the periosteal blood flow is not too severely impaired, which stimulates the healing of the fracture and counteracts the danger of a necrosis of the humeral head. In addition, functional physiotherapy can be started directly after the operation because of the locked fixation of the fragments, without the risk of the screws becoming loose and/or secondary loss of reduction.

Locking Plate Systems

In our department, we use the LPHP **(Fig. 6–1)** and the PHILOS (proximal humerus internal locking system) **(Fig. 6–2)** as the standard implants for the stabilization of proximal humerus fractures. There are only slight differences between both plates. The long PHILOS plate is preferred for long fractures, which may still have comminuted areas. The LPHP, being slightly less thick, puts even less pressure on the soft tissue and it is more likely that a postoperative impingement syndrome will be avoided. The PHILOS plate may possibly provide greater stability as it has a greater number of screws in the head area, greater variability, and perhaps higher stability for certain fractures.

The form of both plate systems is anatomical and shaped to accommodate the junction of the humeral head and the shaft. In the area of the humeral head the plate has, in addition to the holes for the locking head screws, small holes to fix the rotator cuff with sutures or cerclage wires. The screw holes of the plates in the area of the humeral head have been designed exclusively for the insertion of locking head screws for safer fragment fixation. The holes are drilled either with an aiming device or through the LCP drill sleeves; after length measurement, the locking head screws are inserted. The special arrangement of the locking head screws ensures a high level of stability. This does not result from the angular stability alone, but also from the partly converging (and also diverging) angulation of the screws. Due to its flat profile the plate can also be fixed in a very proximal position, without causing impingement later when the range of motion is good. With the locking system, the plate may also be inserted via a minimally invasive approach in the manner of a biological osteosynthesis. In our experience, however, this technique is still reserved for more simple types of fractures, although good results have been reported for more severe fracture patterns.[34–36]

In the shaft area different plate fixation techniques are possible due to the combination holes provided by the LCP, permitting insertion of different types of screw. Conventional small fragment screws can also be introduced as compression screws, lag screws, or to hold individual fragments.

Longer versions of the plate can stabilize complex fractures long term, or fractures where shorter implants have pulled out. Good results are likewise envisaged with other locking plates such as, for example, the Königseeplatte,[37] the humerus fixator plate,[38] the humeral suture plate,[39] and the NCB-PH (noncontact bridging proximal humerus) plate,[40] but we have not used these implants as yet.

Indications and Contraindications for Use of Locking Plates at the Proximal Humerus

The locking plates mentioned are suitable for the stabilization of fractures requiring surgery in the area of the proximal humerus as well as for the stabilization of pseudarthroses. Their superiority in comparison with traditional fixation techniques and implants becomes increasingly apparent with the severity of the fracture. According to the classifications of Codman and Neer for fractures of the humeral head, the indications for application of these locking plates is primarily for dislocated three- and four-part fractures of the humeral head. We also use them for tilted or strongly dislocated, subcapital fractures of the humerus. The limit of reconstruction procedures is reached when the surgeon is confronted with so-called head split fractures, in which case the indication for primary, prosthetic treatment is clear.

In the end, the only contraindications for the use of locking plates are for pediatric fractures with open growth plates and cases of acute infection.

Techniques

The patient can be placed in the beach-chair position or supine. In our clinic, the supine position has gained acceptance because fluoroscopy during the operation is easier in this position. It is worthwhile to perform nonsterile screening in both planes before the start of the operation to eliminate problems caused by positioning.

If it is still not possible to make a definitive decision preoperatively for stabilization with a plate or for replacement

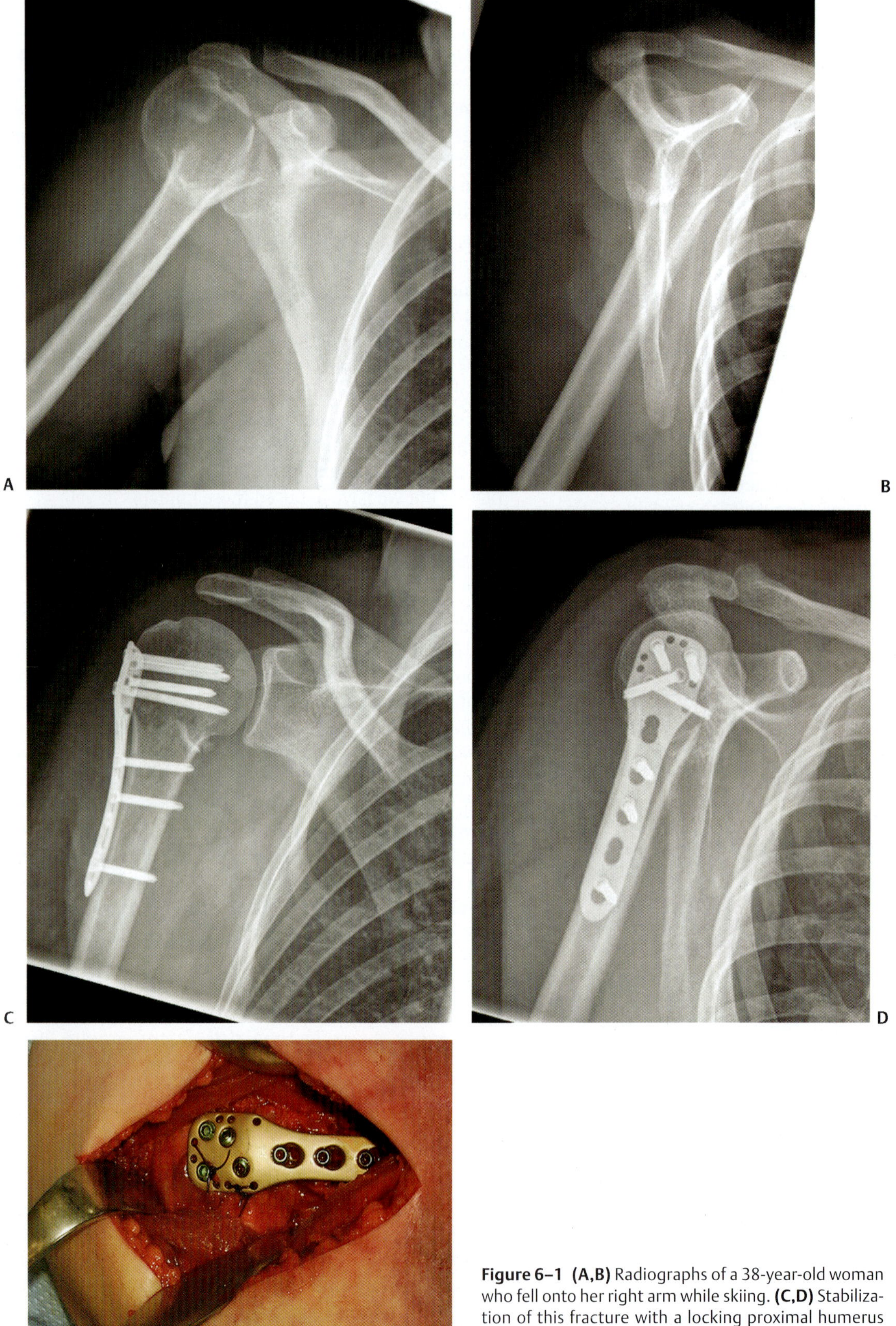

Figure 6–1 **(A,B)** Radiographs of a 38-year-old woman who fell onto her right arm while skiing. **(C,D)** Stabilization of this fracture with a locking proximal humerus plate (LPHP). **(E)** Intraoperative position of a LPHP; the tubercula are fixed with polydioxanone (PDS) sutures.

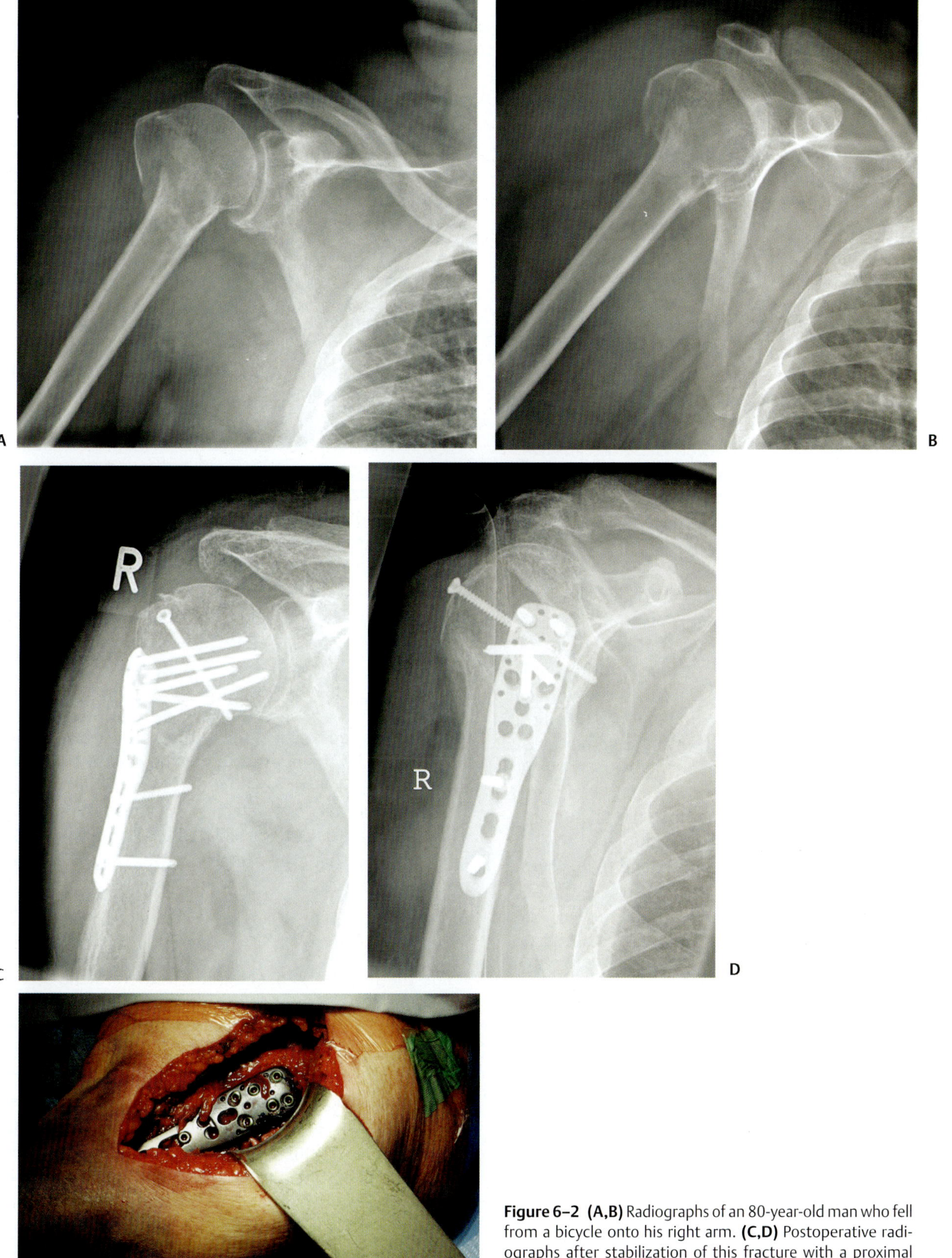

Figure 6–2 **(A,B)** Radiographs of an 80-year-old man who fell from a bicycle onto his right arm. **(C,D)** Postoperative radiographs after stabilization of this fracture with a proximal humerus internal locking system (PHILOS) plate. **(E)** Intraoperative position of a PHILOS plate.

of the humeral head with a prosthesis, the beach-chair position is recommended as it is not easy to perform prosthesis implantation properly in the supine position.

Approach, Reduction, and Retention

The standard approach to the proximal humerus is normally chosen as the approach, the incision is made in an imaginary line between the coracoid process and the capitulum humeri, entry is then made into the deltopectoral groove, and the cephalic vein is prepared and retracted intact laterally. Reduction is performed as carefully as possible, indirectly via the arm. In the case of multifragmentary fractures, a bone rasp can be introduced into the fracture, to reduce the fragments in the anatomical position. If there is avulsion of the tubercles, it is often helpful to hold these, together with the tendons of the rotator cuff, with absorbable sutures (for example, PDS, which can make reduction easier. These threads can also be knotted later into the available holes in the plate blade.

If necessary the reduction can now be temporarily held with cerclage wires, to avoid a loss of reduction when attaching the plate. The plate should be placed in the most lateral position to support a careful inward rotation of the arm. When placed in a cranial position, possible subacromial impingement by the plate must be considered.

The plate can now be initially fastened to the shaft with a screw, a conventional screw being the best for this, making it easier to correct the position of the plate later. The screws should then be gradually introduced in a locking position into the humeral head; alternatively, this can also be the first step. In the case of humeral head fractures or subcapital fractures, fixation to the shaft with two screws is sufficient as a locking procedure.

As has been reported in the literature and in our own cases of defects in the cancellous bone of the humeral head, the use of bone cement, for example, Norian SRS (Skeletal Repair System; Norian Corp., Cupertino, CA), has proven successful.[41]

As an alternative to the standard approach, a minimally invasive approach can also be chosen, in which case the longitudinal incision is in the direction of the fibers above the deltoid muscle, while taking care not to injure the axillary nerve.[34–36] Reduction can be supported by the use of percutaneous K-wires and a bone rasp.[42]

Postoperative Care and Rehabilitation

Immediately after the operation, we apply a Gilchrist bandage to the operated arm. Physiotherapy/physical therapy begins on the first or second postoperative day. Both passive movements and active physiotherapy are performed, provided that the patient can tolerate them. In practice, the use of continuous passive motion devices has proven worthwhile. Lifting of weights should be avoided until the sixth week.

Complications

Despite the use of locking plates, complications do still occur. These are caused partly by fractures, but are also often the consequence of surgical technique.

Necrosis of the Humeral Head

It can be assumed according to the normal classifications of Codman and Neer that the greater the number of fragments and the more severe the dislocation, the higher the risk of necrosis of the humeral head. A further factor is the line of the fracture in relation to the calcarine spur, as it is here that both the extent of the residual blood supply via the periosteum and the probability of damage to the anterior branch of the circumflex humeral artery can be assessed. A dislocation of the head in relation to the calcarine spur >8 mm gives an unfavorable prognosis.[6] Incidentally, it can be established that the rate of humeral head necroses is clearly lower after conservative treatment than after surgical treatment.[43,44] In addition, damage to the soft tissue during surgery can be significant.

Screw Loosening

In most cases, loosening of the screws is caused by locking head screws not being inserted at the correct predrilled angle. An angle deviation of up to 5 degrees can be tolerated, although significant loss of stability can already be expected where there are deviations of 5 degrees.[45] For this reason, strict attention should be paid to ensuring that the LCP drill sleeves are correctly screwed onto the hole.

Screw Perforation

While the fracture is healing, the humeral head screws may penetrate the joint. In many cases, this is the consequence of a (partial) necrosis of the humeral head. In our experience, it is helpful not to penetrate the cartilage-covered cortex of the humeral head when inserting the screws. It is also important to confirm the length and position of the screws during the operation, which means possibly even checking them by fluoroscopy. If screw penetration is suspected during the operation, this should be clarified promptly because as movement increases, screws that have penetrated the shoulder joint will quickly destroy the glenoid and the joint. We use fluoroscopy or CT to ensure diagnosis. However, shoulder arthroscopy has been presented as the method of choice for the safe diagnosis of screw penetration, thus directing a change of screws or their removal. This method seems very invasive to us; nevertheless, definite penetration should certainly be corrected quickly.

Secondary Dislocations

In secondary dislocations, mainly the tubercles are affected; they have not been sufficiently grasped by the screws. Dislocation of the tubercles may be avoided by fixation with PDS sutures.

Malalignments

Varus, valgus, and rotational deformities can be tolerated to a certain extent. An important indicator when considering a revision operation will always be the general condition of the patient and the complaints of each individual. Otherwise, varus and valgus malalignments of up to 45 degrees can be compensated by movement of the scapula without substantial functional loss. The compensation mechanisms for rotational deformities are less efficient; therefore, correction of malalignments of 30 degrees and above is recommended. Surgical intervention is indicated for severe malalignment, depending on the restriction of movement and the complaints of the patient. In these cases, the derotation osteotomy described by Weber can be considered; in rare cases, the implantation of a shoulder prosthesis is necessary.[43,46]

Formation of Pseudarthroses

The etiology of the formation of pseudarthroses can be approached in several different ways. It is frequently due to a local disruption of blood flow; incomplete fragment contact and insufficient stability of the fixation procedure can also stimulate the development of a pseudarthrosis. In addition, exogenic factors such as alcoholism or pharmacotherapy are named as causes. The treatment of pseudarthrosis is described in most publications as urgently requiring surgery. On occasion, it is recommended not to wait for the formation of a pseudarthrosis, but to aim for operative intervention if there is delayed fracture healing.

Different surgical procedures may be used for treatment. If the formation of the pseudarthrosis is due to residual motion at the fracture site or insufficient bone contact, the insertion of cancellous bone graft with a more stable, locking fixation procedure is sufficient.[47,48] The transplantation of a corticocancellous graft is sometimes indicated for larger defects.[49] Good outcomes have also been reported for stabilization with a nail alone; however, we have no experience with this method.[50] If the cause of the pseudarthrosis is damage to the local blood flow, stabilization in combination with a vascularized bone graft is necessary. For example, a free, microvascular bone graft from the iliac crest may be used.[43] Osteo-septocutaneous fibular graft has been described for large defects where pseudarthroses have formed.[51] Depending on the developmental stage of the pseudarthrosis, and the age and general condition of the patient, the implantation of a hemiarthroplasty or of a complete shoulder joint replacement is also to be considered.[52]

Bending of the Plates

Different mechanical stresses can also result in bending of the inserted implant. In our patient sample, this occurred due to the excessive exertion of force during treatment for alcohol withdrawal and during fixation, as well as due to falls following recent osteosynthesis.

Incorrect Plate Position

Similar to dislocation of the greater tubercle, improper positioning of the plate can result in restriction of movement or pain. If the plate is in a superior position, subacromial impingement may develop; if the plate position is too dorsal, it may prevent external rotation. In our own patient sample, there was postoperative impairment of function of the long biceps tendon in some cases, which resulted from fixation by the implant. During preparation, its relationship to the tubercles should be identified and retracted in a vessel loop to avoid this complication. It is of prime importance that the plate be positioned correctly.

Summary

The first published results for locking plates at the proximal humerus together with our own experiences are very promising.[34,53–56] Where there is a relevant indication, stabilization with a locking plate fixation procedure is our treatment of choice for dislocated multifragmentary fractures of the proximal humerus. In our clinic, we are currently running a prospective study with the LPHP for cases of fresh multifragmentary fracture of the humeral head.

Operative stabilization of this injury, especially in view of its frequency, will certainly remain a topic of discussion. At the moment, however, the LPHP and the PHILOS plates are the standard implants for injuries of the proximal humerus in our clinics and in many others. However, it is likely that locking implants will also gain acceptance for use in this anatomical region.

References

1. Hessmann M, Gehling H, Gotzen L. Proximal humerus fracture in advanced age. Langenbecks Arch Chir Suppl Kongressbd 1996;113:907–909
2. Gibson JN, Handoll HH, Madhok R. Interventions for treating proximal humeral fractures in adults. Cochrane Database Syst Rev 2001;1:CD000434
3. Tingart M, Bäthis H, Bouillon B, Tiling T. Die dislozierte proximale humerusfraktur: gibt es gesicherte therapiekonzepte? Chirurg 2001;72:1284–1291
4. Duparc F, Muller JM, Freger P. Arterial blood supply of the proximal humeral epiphysis. Surg Radiol Anat 2001;23: 185–190
5. Gerber C, Schneeberger AG, Vinh TS. The arterial vascularization of the humeral head. An anatomical study. J Bone Joint Surg Am 1990;72:1486–1494
6. Hertel R, Hempfing A, Stiehler M, Leunig M. Predictors of humeral head ischemia after intracapsular fracture of the proximal humerus. J Shoulder Elbow Surg 2004;13:427–433
7. Neer CS. Displaced proximal humeral fractures. I. Classification and evaluation. J Bone Joint Surg Am 1970;52: 1077–1089
8. Neer CS. Displaced proximal humeral fractures. II. Treatment of three-part and four-part displacement. J Bone Joint Surg Am 1970;52:1090–1103
9. Bernstein J, Adler LM, Blank JE, Dalsey RM, Williams GR, Iannotti JP. Evaluation of the Neer system of classification of proximal humeral fractures with computerized tomographic scans and plain radiographs. J Bone Joint Surg Am 1996;78:1371–1375
10. Brien H, Noftall F, MacMaster S, Cummings T, Landells C, Rockwood P. Neer's classification system: a critical appraisal. J Trauma 1995;38:257–260
11. Kristiansen B, Andersen UL, Olsen CA, Varmarken JE. The Neer classification of fractures of the proximal humerus. An assessment of interobserver variation. Skeletal Radiol 1988;17:420–422
12. Siebenrock KA, Gerber C. The reproducibility of classification of fractures of the proximal end of the humerus. J Bone Joint Surg Am 1993;75:1751–1755
13. Kostler W, Strohm PC, Sudkamp NP. New techniques for bone synthesis on the humerus. Chirurg 2002;73:969–977
14. Müller M, Nazarian S, Koch P, Schatzker J. The Comprehensive Classification of Fractures of the Long Bones. Berlin/Heidelberg/New York: Springer; 1990
15. Tingart M, Bathis H, Bouillon B, Tiling T. The displaced proximal humeral fracture: is there evidence for therapeutic concepts? Chirurg 2001;72:1284–1291
16. Fjalestad T, Stromsoe K, Blucher J, Tennoe B. Fractures in the proximal humerus: functional outcome and evaluation of 70 patients treated in hospital. Arch Orthop Trauma Surg 2005;125:310–316
17. Olsson C, Nordquist A, Petersson CJ. Long-term outcome of a proximal humerus fracture predicted after 1 year: a 13-year prospective population-based follow-up study of 47 patients. Acta Orthop 2005;76:397–402
18. Kuner EH, Siebler G. Dislocation fractures of the proximal humerus–results following surgical treatment. A follow-up study of 167 cases. Unfallchirurgie 1987;13:64–71
19. Speck M, Lang FJ, Regazzoni P. Proximal humeral multiple fragment fractures–failures after T-plate osteosynthesis. Swiss Surg 1996;2:51–56
20. Strohm PC, Kostler W, Sudkamp NP. Locking plate fixation of proximal humerus fractures. Tech Shoulder Elbow Surg 2005;6:8–13
21. Wanner GA, Wanner-Schmid E, Romero J, et al. Internal fixation of displaced proximal humeral fractures with two one-third tubular plates. J Trauma 2003;54: 536–544
22. Hintermann B, Trouillier HH, Schafer D. Rigid internal fixation of fractures of the proximal humerus in older patients. J Bone Joint Surg Br 2000;82:1107–1112
23. Weber E, Matter P. Operative behandlung proximaler humerusfrakturen - internationale multizenterstudie. Swiss Surg 1998;4:95–100
24. Wijgman AJ, Roolker W, Patt TW, Raaymakers EL, Marti RK. Open reduction and internal fixation of three and four-part fractures of the proximal part of the humerus. J Bone Joint Surg Am 2002;84-A:1919–1925
25. Rowles DJ, McGrory JE. Percutaneous pinning of the proximal part of the humerus. An anatomic study. J Bone Joint Surg Am 2001;83-A:1695–1699
26. Speck M, Regazzoni P. 4-fragment fractures of the proximal humerus. Alternative strategies for surgical treatment. Unfallchirurg 1997;100:349–353
27. Zyto K, Ahrengart L, Sperber A, Tornkvist H. Treatment of displaced proximal humeral fractures in elderly patients. J Bone Joint Surg Br 1997;79:412–417
28. Wagner M. General principles for the clinical use of the LCP. Injury 2003;34(Suppl 2):B31–B42
29. Broos PL, Sermon A. From unstable internal fixation to biological osteosynthesis. A historical overview of operative fracture treatment. Acta Chir Belg 2004;104: 396–400
30. Frigg R, Ulrich D. Innovative implants–a prerequisite for biological osteosynthesis. Ther Umsch 2003;60:723–728
31. Frigg R. Development of the locking compression plate. Injury 2003;34(Suppl 2):B6–B10
32. Frigg R. Locking compression plate (LCP). An osteosynthesis plate based on the dynamic compression plate and the point contact fixator (PC-Fix). Injury 2001;32 (Suppl 2):63–66
33. Lill H, Hepp P, Korner J, et al. Proximal humeral fractures: how stiff should an implant be? A comparative mechanical study with new implants in human specimens. Arch Orthop Trauma Surg 2003;123:74–81
34. Gallo RA, Zeiders GJ, Altman GT. Two-incision technique for treatment of complex proximal humerus fractures. J Orthop Trauma 2005;19:734–740
35. Gardner MJ, Griffith MH, Dines JS, Lorich DG. A minimally invasive approach for plate fixation of the proximal humerus. Bull Hosp Joint Dis 2004;62:18–23
36. Lill H, Hepp P, Rose T, Konig K, Josten C. The angle stable locking-proximal-humerus-plate (LPHP) for proximal humeral fractures using a small anterior-lateral-deltoid-splitting-approach - technique and first results. Zentralbl Chir 2004;129:43–48

37. Lungershausen W, Bach O, Lorenz CO. Locking plate osteosynthesis for fractures of the proximal humerus. Zentralbl Chir 2003;128:28–33
38. Mückter H, Herzog L, Becker M, Vogel W, Meeder P, Buchholz J. Die winkel- und rotationsstabile osteosythese proximaler humerusfrakturen mit der humerus-fixateurplatte. Chirurg 2001;72:1327–1335
39. Wiedemann E, Zeiler C. Winkelstabile Plattenosteosynthesen - Die Humeral Suture Plate. In: Lill H, ed. Die Proximale Humerusfraktur. Stuttgart: Thieme; 2006:112–117
40. Kinzl L, Gebhard F. Winkelstabile Plattenosteosynthesen - Die NCB-PH Winkelstabile Humerusplatte. In: Lill H, ed. Die Proximale Humerusfraktur. Stuttgart/New York: Thieme; 2006:108–112
41. Robinson CM, Page RS. Severely impacted valgus proximal humeral fractures. Results of operative treatment. J Bone Joint Surg Am 2003;85:1647–1655
42. Gerber C, Werner CM, Vienne P. Internal fixation of complex fractures of the proximal humerus. J Bone Joint Surg Br 2004;86:848–855
43. Habermeyer P, Schweiberer L. Corrective interventions subsequent to humeral head fractures. Orthopade 1992; 21:148–157
44. Kollig E, Kutscha-Lissberg F, Roetman B, Dielenschneider D, Muhr G. Complex fractures of the humeral head: which long-term results can be expected? Zentralbl Chir 2003;128:111–118
45. Kaab MJ, Frenk A, Schmeling A, Schaser K, Schutz M, Haas NP. Locked internal fixator: sensitivity of screw/plate stability to the correct insertion angle of the screw. J Orthop Trauma 2004;18:483–487
46. Maurer H, Resch H. Schultergelenk. In: Kremer K, Lierse W, Platzer W, Schreiber H, Weller S, eds. Chirurgische Operationslehre. Stuttgart/New York: Thieme; 1995:61–128
47. Duralde XA, Flatow EL, Pollock RG, Nicholson GP, Self EB, Bigliani LU. Operative treatment of nonunions of the surgical neck of the humerus. J Shoulder Elbow Surg 1996;5:169–180
48. Galatz LM, Williams GR Jr, Fenlin JM Jr, Ramsey ML, Iannotti JP. Outcome of open reduction and internal fixation of surgical neck nonunions of the humerus. J Orthop Trauma 2004;18:63–67
49. Walch G, Badet R, Nove-Josserand L, Levigne C. Nonunions of the surgical neck of the humerus: surgical treatment with an intramedullary bone peg, internal fixation, and cancellous bone grafting. J Shoulder Elbow Surg 1996; 5:161–168
50. Lin J, Hou SM. Locked-nail treatment of humeral surgical neck nonunions. J Trauma 2003;54:530–535
51. Heitmann C, Erdmann D, Levin LS. Treatment of segmental defects of the humerus with an osteoseptocutaneous fibular transplant. J Bone Joint Surg Am 2002;84-A:2216–2223
52. Antuna SA, Sperling JW, Sanchez-Sotelo J, Cofield RH. Shoulder arthroplasty for proximal humeral malunions: long-term results. J Shoulder Elbow Surg 2002;11:122–129
53. Bjorkenheim JM, Pajarinen J, Savolainen V. Internal fixation of proximal humeral fractures with a locking compression plate: a retrospective evaluation of 72 patients followed for a minimum of 1 year. Acta Orthop Scand 2004;75: 741–745
54. Fankhauser F, Boldin C, Schippinger G, Haunschmid C, Szyszkowitz R. A new locking plate for unstable fractures of the proximal humerus. Clin Orthop Relat Res 2005; 430:176–181
55. Hente R, Kampshoff J, Kinner B, Fuchtmeier B, Nerlich M. Treatment of displaced 3- and 4-part fractures of the proximal humerus with fixator plate comprising angular stability. Unfallchirurg 2004;107:769–782
56. Plecko M, Kraus A. Internal fixation of proximal humerus fractures using the locking proximal humerus plate. Oper Orthop Traumatol 2005;17:25–50

7 Proximal Humeral Malunions

Joshua S. Dines, Edward V. Craig, and David M. Dines

As the average age of the population increases, the prevalence of proximal humerus fractures and the late sequelae of such fractures increase. The majority of fractures of the proximal humerus can be treated nonoperatively with good expected results. Yet there is a subset of patients treated, either nonoperatively or surgically, who go on to develop malunions. These patients often develop debilitating pain and dysfunction from their deformity, prompting them to seek further treatment.

The surgical treatment of such problems is particularly challenging due to disruption of the normal tuberosity–humeral shaft architecture, excessive scar formation, adhesions, and stiffness. In addition, concomitant neurologic impairment, rotator cuff pathology and poor bone quality make surgical repair technically demanding. Successful treatment of proximal humerus malunions requires a thorough preoperative evaluation, a meticulous preoperative plan, a comprehensive understanding of the necessary surgical techniques, and a well-developed postoperative rehabilitation protocol.

Etiology and Mechanism of Injury

Malunion can occur after open or closed treatment of a proximal humerus fracture, though it more frequently develops in cases treated nonoperatively. In many cases, the treating physician willingly accepts a nonanatomic alignment due to the age or underlying medical problems of the patient. On occasion, surgeons adopt a " wait and see" approach, allowing the fracture to heal prior to assessing the patient's functional limitations. In rare instances, a proximal humerus fracture or the extent of the injury is not fully appreciated. An unfortunate example of this involves a missed posterior dislocation associated with a fracture because appropriate radiographs were not obtained. Axillary view radiographs should be included in any trauma series of the shoulder. It is important to remember that the results of late reconstruction are often inferior to those of acute anatomic restoration, so nonoperative treatment may not be indicated as often as it is.[1]

Other causes of malunions, or nonunions, include soft tissue interposition at the fracture site, inadequate immobilization, and overly aggressive rehabilitation. Rarely, the long head of the biceps tendon, capsule, or deltoid muscle interpose at the fracture site, blocking reduction and eventuating a non- or malunion.

Proximal humerus malunions can occur secondary to failure of internal fixation. It is often difficult to gain good screw purchase in the cancellous bone of the humeral head or tuberosity, and displacement may occur.

Types of Proximal Humeral Fractures

When evaluating a proximal humerus fracture, four parts are usually assessed: humeral head and articular fragment, greater tuberosity, lesser tuberosity, and humeral shaft. An understanding of the various types of proximal humerus fractures and the corresponding deforming forces on each fragment is helpful, as the position of malunions usually relates to these forces.

Two-Part Surgical Neck Malunions

Anterior displacement of the shaft secondary to the pull of the pectoralis major and possible abduction of the head by the rotator cuff result in anterior angulation and a varus or valgus deformity.[2] When severe, these deformities can cause limitation of forward flexion, and, in some cases, loss of abduction. The work of Keene et al showed that increased anterior angulation greater than 45 to 55 degrees causes limited forward elevation.[3] In addition, in malunions of this type, the greater tuberosity impinges on the superior aspect of the glenoid, preventing sufficient external rotation to allow the arm to elevate properly. With each degree of varus angulation, one degree of overhead elevation is lost.[4]

Two-Part Tuberosity Malunions

Reports by Mclaughlin and Craig indicate that displacement of the greater tuberosity >5 mm may result in a symptomatic nonunion.[5,6] Two-part fractures involving the greater tuberosity may heal with the tuberosity fragment displaced posterosuperiorly secondary to the deforming forces of the rotator cuff muscles. In this fracture pattern, the normal architecture of the articular segment, humeral shaft, and glenoid are maintained. Malunions of this nature present with limited abduction and external rotation and possible secondary subacromial impingement.[7] Relative losses of forward elevation or external rotation relate to the degree of superior and posterior malunion, respectively.

Isolated lesser tuberosity malunions result from pulling of the fragment medially due to the subscapularis pull. This displacement causes a spread in the anterior fibers of the rotator cuff at the rotator interval producing a bony prominence. Clinically, this is usually insignificant, though rarely a mechanical block to internal rotation or elevation develops and may result in coracoid impingement.[2,8]

Three- and Four-Part Malunions

Three- and four-part malunions result in severely impaired function. Three-part fracture malunions with displacement of the greater tuberosity and surgical neck can cause deformity, avascular necrosis, and posttraumatic arthritis.[4] When the lesser tuberosity remains intact, the humeral head is brought into internal rotation due to the pull of the subscapularis. The greater tuberosity is displaced posterosuperiorly, and the humeral shaft is pulled anteromedially. In these settings, the articular fragment often faces posteriorly. The end result is severely impaired abduction and loss of rotation.

Three-part fractures with displacement of the lesser tuberosity and surgical neck result in more severe limitation of internal rotation. In this situation, the articular segment externally rotates and abducts, causing it to face anteriorly and give the appearance of being dislocated (*false fracture dislocation*). Because the greater tuberosity remains attached to the humeral head, the supraspinatus, infraspinatus, and teres minor all act as deforming forces.

In four-part fractures, the blood supply to the humeral head is frequently compromised leading to high incidences of avascular necrosis. The head may be displaced laterally and may not even contact the glenoid.[2] Malunions of four-part fractures result in soft tissue contractures and adhesions and joint incongruity. Patients present with pain and severely restricted range of motion (ROM). In addition, these patients may suffer from chronic nerve injuries.[7]

Fracture-Dislocation Malunions

Malunions of fracture dislocations are extremely challenging cases to manage. The humeral head is no longer concentric within the glenoid, and the resultant displacement of the head may cause injury to the neurovascular bundle.[9] Extensive soft tissue contractures are often present, and there is an increased incidence of myositis ossificans.[4] In addition, the head location may be in close proximity to the brachial plexus and major vessels.

Patient Assessment

The patient with a proximal humerus malunion may present in a variety of ways. A thorough history and physical exam is crucial to determine the main disability. Is the primary complaint pain or lack of function? As the pain or disability associated with proximal humerus malunions varies, an assessment of the patient's lifestyle and activity level is necessary. This will allow the physician to advise the patient of the relative benefits of surgical reconstruction. Successful treatment of these malunions demands that patients have realistic expectations of surgical reconstruction. Details of the initial injury should be elicited including mechanism, treatments received, and associated injuries. Previous injuries to the shoulder, hand dominance, and potentially complicating medical issues are all pertinent.

An overall sense of the patient's health should be assessed during the physical exam. If the patient is dependent on the affected upper extremity to remain ambulatory and independent, one might have a lower threshold to indicate a reconstruction. The converse is also true. If it seems that a patient may not be able to participate in the extensive postoperative rehabilitation process, the threshold to operate might be raised.

On inspection, atrophy of the shoulder musculature can be expected, but signs of infection, including erythema, fluctuance, and wound drainage necessitate further infection work-up. Previous scars should be noted, as these might affect the choice of surgical approach.

Loss of motion is often the primary problem after proximal humerus malunions. ROM, especially passive ROM, allows assessment of soft tissue contractures and joint congruity. External rotation should be checked with the arm at the side and at 90 degrees of abduction. A classic finding on exam of patients with greater tuberosity malunions is the absence of external rotation with the arm maximally abducted.[6] Impingement may also limit motion.

Rotator cuff injury may have occurred during the initial injury and should be addressed at the time of reconstruction.[7] External rotation strength allows evaluation of the infraspinatus and teres minor. Supraspinatus function can be tested with opposed abduction at 90 degrees. Both the "lift off" test and the abdominal compression test can help assess the integrity and strength of the subscapularis. When the tuberosities are displaced there is less mechanical advantage to the rotator cuff muscles. In these instances, even with the rotator cuff intact, weakness may result. Instability is sometimes present, and should be evaluated. It is important to remember that in cases when the greater tuberosity is malunited posteriorly, it may lever the humeral head from the glenoid, simulating anterior instability.[6]

Neurologic injuries may have occurred secondary to the initial trauma, or even during the initial treatment. Careful evaluation of the motor strength of the axillary, musculocutaneous, and suprascapular nerves should be performed. Axillary nerve injury is often associated with inferior subluxation of the proximal humerus. It is important to remember that sensory deficit at the lateral border of the deltoid is not a reliable indicator of axillary nerve injury. Brachial plexus involvement may also be seen in patients with proximal humerus malunions. Fracture-dislocations have the highest incidence of accompanying neurologic injuries. In patients older than 50 with proximal humerus fractures, the incidence of electromyography- (EMG) diagnosed neurologic injuries is 50%.[6] Thus, in patients with suspected nerve injury, preoperative EMG studies should be obtained.

Radiologic Assessment

Appropriate imaging assessment of patients with malunions begins with a plain radiograph trauma series of the shoulder. This includes an anteroposterior and lateral view in the plane of the scapula and an axillary view. These views usually provide sufficient information regarding the position of the fragments as well as the bone quality; however, supplemental internal and external rotation views can provide more information if necessary. In patients previously treated with internal fixation, radiographic evidence of loosening may be an indication of infection. In these cases, one should consider aspiration and culture of the joint.

Computed tomography (CT) is often essential to evaluate the full extent of injury. The degree of tuberosity displacement and certain fracture patterns, such as head splitting fractures, articular impression fractures, and chronic fracture-dislocations are best visualized with CT scans that allow three-dimensional evaluation of the fragments.[10,11] Morris et al reported that CT identified axial malposition of the greater tuberosity that was not appreciated on plain x-ray in 10 of 18 patients. Furthermore, plain films were inadequate in assessing displacement of the lesser tuberosity in all 18 patients.[11] Three-dimensional CT reconstructions also aid in the understanding of the position of malunited fragments.[12]

Other imaging modalities that can be useful to the surgeon include magnetic resonance imaging (MRI) and scanograms. MRI helps delineate soft tissue pathology, especially with regard to the rotator cuff and labrum. MRI also allows earlier identification of avascular necrosis than is provided by plain films. In patients with hardware from previous surgery, artifact can diminish the information available from MRI. Scanograms aid in determining the proper length of the humerus and are especially useful in proximal humerus reconstruction with hemiarthroplasty. The scanogram can establish the proper height for the prosthesis; thereby allowing the surgeon to reestablish the appropriate tension of the soft tissues.

Classification

To date, no universally accepted classification system for proximal humerus malunions exists. Many authors have simply modified the commonly used classification of acute proximal humerus fractures developed by Neer and applied it to their series of malunions.[1,9,12] Other authors have attempted to develop original classification systems useful in determining the treatment approach to the malunion.

Beredjiklian et al[13] proposed a system of categorizing osseous and soft tissue defects. Osseous abnormalities were categorized as malposition of the greater or lesser tuberosities by more than 1 cm (type I malunion); intraarticular incongruity or a step-off of the articular surface of >5 mm (type II malunion); and malalignment of the articular segment by more than 45 degrees in any of the three planes (type III malunion). They categorized soft tissue abnormalities more broadly: soft tissue contracture, rotator cuff tear, and subacromial impingement. Although not all-inclusive, this classification system is useful in providing an overview of the involved pathology with the goal of treating each component.

Boileau et al[12] developed a general classification system relating to sequelae of proximal humerus fractures that included proximal humerus malunions. Category 1 included intracapsular/impacted fracture sequelae: type I – cephalic collapse and necrosis; type II – chronic dislocation or fracture-dislocation. Category 2 dealt with extracapsular/disimpacted fracture sequelae: type 3 – surgical neck nonunions; type 4 – severe tuberosity malunions **(Fig. 7–1)**. Category 1 fractures can be reconstructed with a proximal humerus arthroplasty without a greater tuberosity osteotomy with predictably good results. Category 2 fractures require a greater tuberosity osteotomy and yield less predictable, usually poorer results. Boileau's system does not account for malunions treated with osteotomy and internal fixation without the use of proximal humerus arthroplasty.

Treatment

The appropriate treatment of proximal humerus malunions depends on myriad factors. The patient's overall state of health, physiologic age, degree of pain, and loss of function relative to his or her needs all warrant consideration prior to embarking on a treatment course. Patients

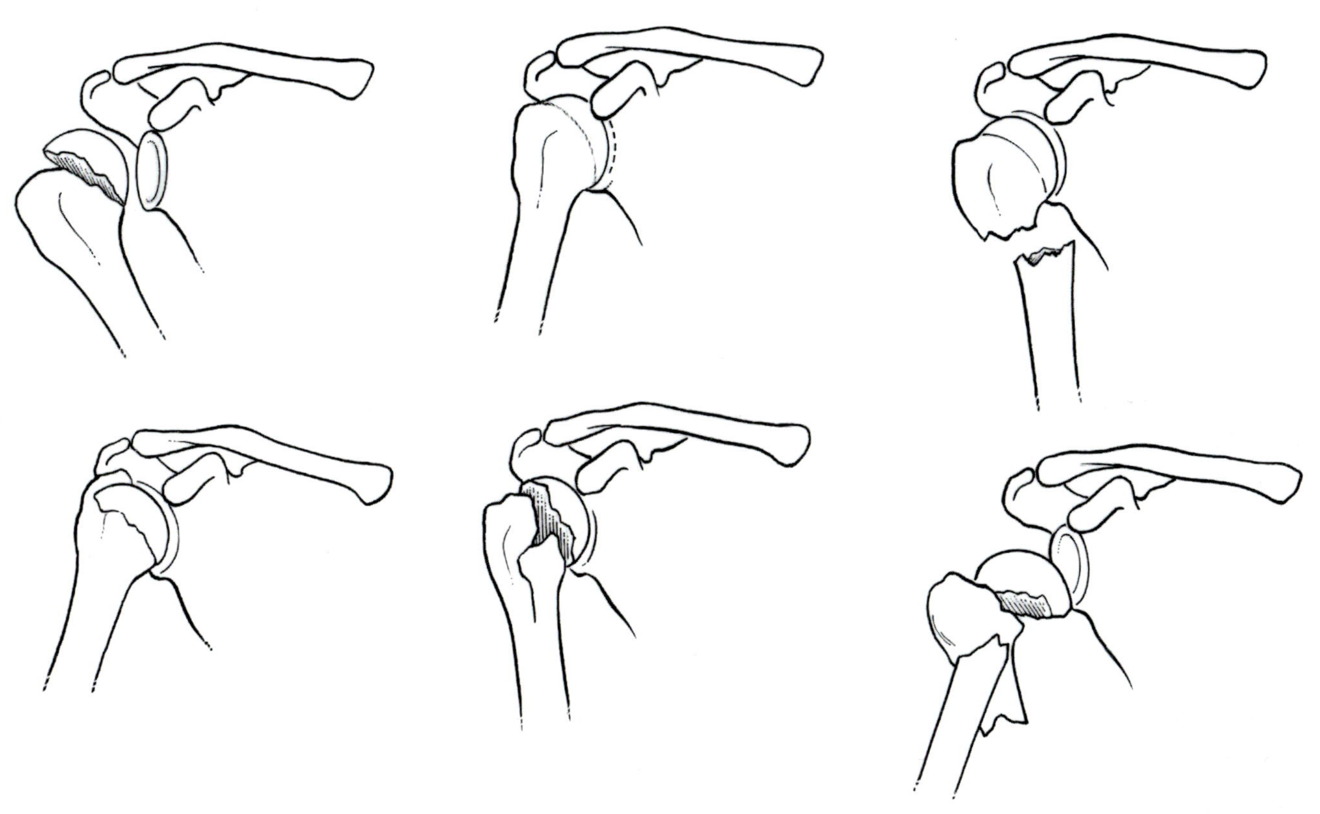

Figure 7–1 Surgical classification of sequelae of proximal humerus fractures as defined by Boileau et al.[12]

with a low activity level, whose pain is tolerable, and who are able to remain independent despite the injured shoulder can reasonably be treated conservatively. Others for whom conservative treatment would be reasonable include those with medical conditions that put them at severe risk for surgery and patients who are not able to participate in postoperative rehabilitation.

Nonsurgical Treatment

Physical therapy and pain control are the cornerstones of conservative treatment. The goal of therapy is to maximize and maintain the shoulder's ROM and to strengthen the shoulder musculature. Scapular strengthening can help regain functional strength and some ROM. It is important to remember that in some patients, glenohumeral motion may be limited by bony impingement.

The use of nonsteroidal antiinflammatory medications and intraarticular steroid injections can decrease the secondary inflammatory changes that cause pain. Modalities, including heat or cold compresses, electrical stimulation, ultrasound, and phonophoresis, may decrease some of the pain in these patients. At times, patients who are not surgical candidates benefit from consultation with a chronic pain doctor. These specialists often use antidepressants, biofeedback, and/or nerve root injections to help with difficult pain management problems.

Surgical Treatment

There are two categories of surgical treatments for proximal humerus malunions: humeral head preserving and humeral head sacrificing. When the blood supply to the humeral head is viable, the articular surface is preserved, and if the patient has good bone quality, humeral head preserving procedures are indicated. These are usually cases of two-part and some three-part malunions. Reconstruction in these cases primarily involves osteotomies and fixation of the tuberosities or the surgical neck along with soft tissue reconstruction. In the cases of surgical neck malunion or tuberosity fractures, removal of bone protuberances and soft tissue releases can significantly improve outcome, especially in the presence of a supple glenohumeral joint. Arthroscopic releases have been considered in these difficult cases, especially when associated with posttraumatic arthritis; however, Holloway and Iannotti[14] reported that the only successful results were in primary cases of posttraumatic arthritis without an element of significant malunion. Arthroscopy can be considered in cases where posttraumatic bursitis and

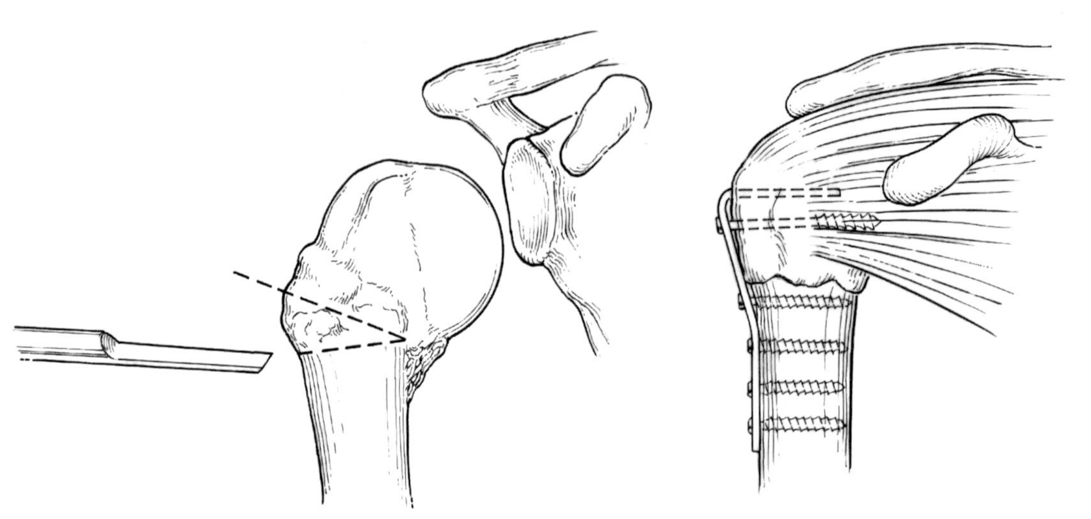

Figure 7–2 Varus surgical neck malunion treated with valgus derotational osteotomy and secured with proximal humerus locking plate.

secondary outlet impingement are significant causes of pain and disability. Tuberosity spur removal and capsular releases do not correct the underlying problem.

Humeral head sacrificing procedures are indicated when the head has developed or is likely to develop avascular necrosis. They are also indicated when extensive damage to the articular surface is present. These procedures, which include hemiarthroplasty or total shoulder replacement (TSR), are usually reserved for some three-part malunions, most four-part fractures, head splitting injuries, and humeral head impression defects involving more than 40% of the articular surface.[15] The indications for hemiarthroplasty versus TSR depend on the condition of the articular surface of the glenoid and the integrity of the rotator cuff.

Techniques

Humeral Head Sparing Techniques

Two-part surgical neck malunions, with resultant varus deformity and loss of forward elevation and internal and external rotation, are rare. As mentioned above, increased anterior angulation >45 to 55 degrees causes decreased forward elevation, which correlates with Beredjiklian's classification system in which 45 degrees of angulation in any plane warrants surgical reconstruction. Because the incidence of these malunions is low, there is not much in the literature discussing the methods and results of treatment. Solonen and Vastamaki[16] preformed a valgus wedge derotational osteotomy through as standard deltopectoral incision. The osteotomy was secured with a T-shaped AO plate. During this approach, the axillary nerve must be dissected free and protected. Soft tissue adhesions and contractures need to be addressed, and humeral height needs to be reestablished. With the advent of locked plating, rigid fixation can be achieved, allowing for early ROM **(Fig. 7–2)**. In certain cases in which the joint remains supple despite severe deformity on x-ray, soft tissue contracture releases and removal of prominent bone provide good results.

The procedure for treatment of two-part greater tuberosity malunions is similar to that used for acute tuberosity fractures. Often these malunions are addressed through an anterosuperior approach, with the arm draped free and the patient in a modified beach-chair position.[6] The authors recommend releasing a portion of the anterior deltoid in addition to the usual deltoid split, which helps mobilize the soft tissues. Because of the extensive disease in the subacromial space, an acromioplasty and release of the coracoacromial ligament are often performed. The greater tuberosity is then osteotomized **(Fig. 7–3A)**. As opposed to lesser tuberosity, osteotomies that are usually uniplanar, greater tuberosity osteotomies are often biplanar. Distinguishing fracture callus from the tuberosity fragment is often difficult; thus, it is safer to err on osteotomizing too large a piece of bone. Most of these fractures originate at the bicipital groove, so the biceps tendon is a useful landmark for osteotomy orientation. It is very important to protect the axillary nerve, especially as it courses through the quadrilateral space, during the osteotomy. To help control the free fragment, heavy nonabsorbable sutures are placed at the insertion of the rotator cuff into the greater tuberosity. A crucial part of the procedure involves lysis of contractures and mobilization of the soft tissues. A superior and posterior capsulotomy may help, as will lysis of extra- and intraarticular adhesions. The rotator cuff should be mobilized as well. We have found that, in these patients, subacromial decompression alone rarely works. One may consider arthroscopic subacromial decompression, tuberoplasties, and capsular release, as these can provide a successful outcome. Again, with significant displacement of the tuberosity, osteotomy is necessary.

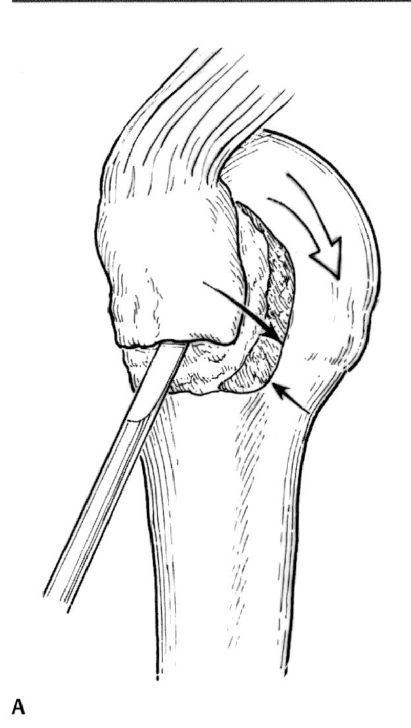

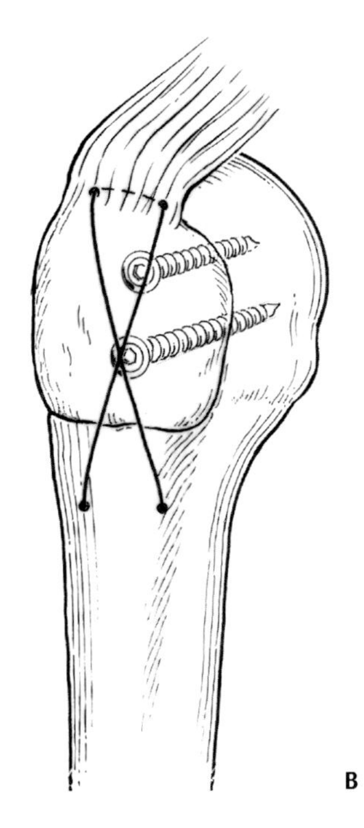

Figure 7–3 (A) Greater tuberosity malunion osteotomized with circumferential release of adhesions around the tuberosity-tendon unit. The fragment is then shifted anteroinferiorly into an area that has been decorticated. **(B)** Fixation of the tuberosity with two cancellous screws and a figure-eight tension band.

At this point, the greater tuberosity should be able to be mobilized to the donor site (external rotation of the humerus may be necessary). In some lesser tuberosity malunions, the piece is very small and may benefit from excision followed by repair of the subscapularis tendon. Prior to reapproximating the tuberosity fragment to the donor site, the site needs to be decorticated to a bed of bleeding cancellous bone. In addition, the anterior glenoid rim should be examined through the invariable rent in the rotator interval between the supraspinatus and subscapularis. There might be an associated Bankart lesion, especially if the initial injury was a fracture-dislocation. These lesions, if present, can be repaired through the tear in the rotator interval or arthroscopically prior to tuberosity fragment fixation. The tuberosity segment can then be shaped to match the donor site. Rigid fixation of the fragment to the shaft is the goal and can usually be achieved with one or two AO screws with washers. The screws should be angled inferomedially so that they engage the medial cortex of the humeral shaft, while remaining inferior to the articular surface of the humeral head **(Fig. 7–3B)**. Once fixation and ROM are assessed and found to be satisfactory, the rotator interval and deltoid are repaired.[6] Other treatment options include figure-eight tension-band constructs with nonabsorbable suture or wire. If the fragment is small, the rotator cuff may be detached and repaired primarily back to the bed with suture anchors following excision of the fragment.

Malunions resulting from three-part fractures, four-part fractures, and fracture-dislocations are extremely challenging reconstructions. If avascular necrosis is absent and the articular surface of the humeral head is preserved, osteotomies and internal fixation of the malunited segments, as described above, are indicated. In some cases, anatomic reconstruction may not be possible; however, satisfactory results are still obtained if the tuberosities are fixed about the head and shaft in such a way that motion is preserved without impingement.

In certain cases, the humeral head may have articular surface damage that involves <40% of the surface. In these cases, the head may be salvageable. The McLaughlin procedure, which involves transferring the subscapularis insertion, with or without the lesser tuberosity, into the defect may be indicated in situations such as these.

Humeral Head Sacrificing Techniques

Often the sequelae of three- and four-part fractures require prosthetic replacement. Appropriate soft tissue balancing is key to achieving a stable, well-functioning shoulder. Careful attention should be paid toward recreating humeral height, tuberosity alignment and fixation, and humeral head version. This is often best accomplished by osteotomizing the tuberosities to, in essence, *create* a four-part fracture, which is then reconstructed around the implant. A modular shoulder system, with different component sizes and eccentric humeral heads, allows for better soft tissue tensioning. It also allows intraoperative prosthetic trialing to improve stability and tuberosity position.[17] The decision to use a cemented versus noncemented humeral prosthesis should be made at the time of surgery and based on bone quality and component stability.

Humeral head prosthetic replacement is usually performed through an extended deltopectoral approach. Prior to addressing the bony pathology, the surgeon should deal with the associated soft tissue pathology. If external rotation contractures are present, a lesser tuberosity osteotomy or subscapularis lengthening should be performed. If the shoulder capsule is contracted, it should be released circumferentially at the glenoid edge. Subscapularis tendon adhesions require lysis, and the rotator cuff needs to be mobilized. At this point, the integrity of the cuff should be evaluated, as an irreparable tear is a relative contraindication to TSR.

Tuberosity position should be assessed to determine whether or not an osteotomy is necessary. If there is a block to external rotation at 20 degrees or less or elevation is <90 degrees, greater tuberosity osteotomy is indicated. If the tuberosity is malpositioned, but would lie below the level of the articular surface of the prosthesis, an osteotomy may not be necessary. However, in these cases, make sure that the position of the tuberosity does not block the appropriate insertion point for the stem.[18] If the lesser tuberosity is not replaced appropriately, the humeral head may subluxate posteriorly or coracoid impingement may occur with internal rotation. Although the osteotomy may sacrifice some bone, enough bone should remain attached to the rotator cuff to facilitate repair. There should also be a significant surface area of bony contact between the fragment and the humeral shaft.

The level of the humeral head osteotomy must account for any surgical neck malalignment and loss of height. As mentioned above, in severe cases, a scanogram can be helpful to elucidate the appropriate height. Once the humeral head osteotomy is completed, the head should be sized and the glenoid inspected. Glenoid erosion in the setting of an intact or repairable rotator cuff is an indication for TSR.

Shoulder stability, in large part, depends on proper height and version of the humeral component. The height must allow for repositioning of the tuberosities below the articular surface of the prosthesis and for appropriate soft tissue tensioning. Usually the prosthesis is retroverted 20 to 35 degrees; however, in the event of a chronic posterior dislocation, a posterior impression fracture, or recurrent instability, decreasing the amount of retroversion can improve stability.

Securing the tuberosities to the implant and humeral shaft can be done in a variety of ways. The senior author (DMD) uses five heavy, nonabsorbable sutures. Two of the sutures are placed through the tuberosity followed by insertion through the medial flange of the prosthesis. Two additional sutures are placed through each tuberosity and brought back to themselves. The fifth suture is placed through the shaft then brought up in a figure-eight fashion through the tuberosities. Appropriate drill holes are made in the humeral shaft, and the sutures are passed prior to implantation of the prosthesis. Shingling and bone grafting of the tuberosity are essential to ensure healing of the tuberosity back to the humeral shaft (see Chapter 6 for a more thorough description of the technique). An important point to be made is that in cases of type I and II malunions (as defined by Boileau et al), one can accept the stem being in varus and possibly perform a tuberosity osteotomy **(Fig. 7–4)**.

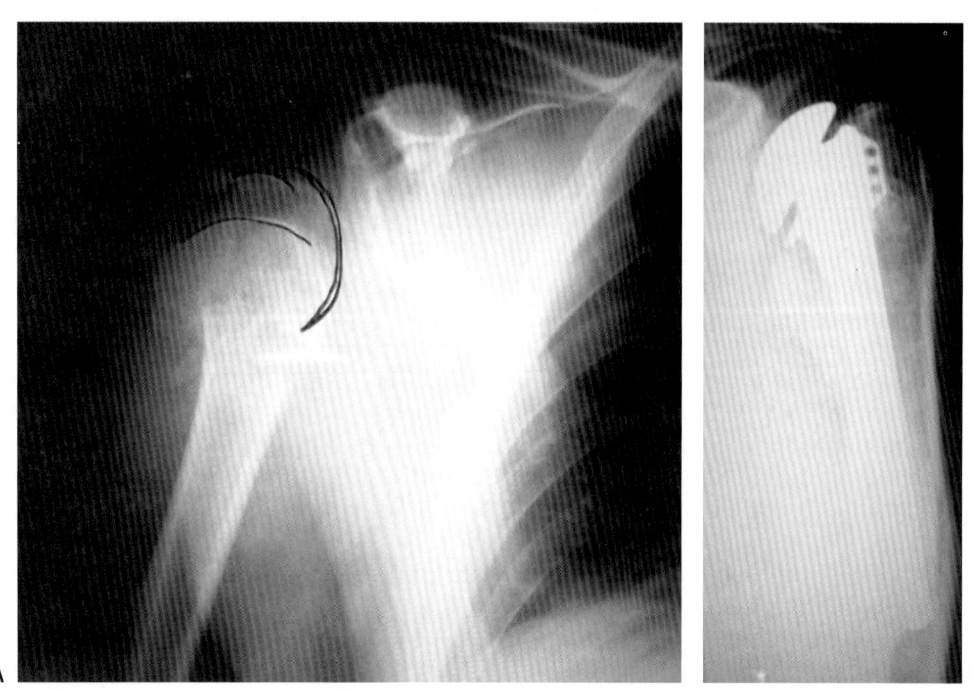

Figure 7–4 Preoperative radiograph **(A)** of a four-part malunion, and **(B)** postoperative radiograph of fracture treated with hemiarthroplasty, in which good results were achieved by placing stem in slight varus.

Prior to closure of the shoulder, stability should be assessed and the limits of passive ROM determined. It is important to document the intraoperative passive ROM that does not stress the repair of the tuberosities, as this will define the limits of ROM during the initial physical therapy phase. The rotator cuff and deltoid are repaired, and the wound is closed over a drain in layers.

Recently, in cases of severe tuberosity malunion (Boileau et al type III or IV), some surgeons have used the reverse-type shoulder prostheses because reported results for these patients are universally poor.

Postoperative Rehabilitation

If rigid internal fixation is achieved or if a prosthesis is used, passive ROM exercises are started on postoperative day 1. The limits of this motion are based on intraoperative stability. Gradually, assisted ROM exercises are instituted. Isometric exercises of the deltoid and rotator cuff are initiated once radiographic evidence of fragment union is visualized (usually about 6 weeks postoperatively). At 10 weeks, resistance exercises to strengthen the rotator cuff and deltoid can be started.

Results

There is a relative dearth of literature on results of operative treatment of proximal humerus malunions. Furthermore, the bulk of the literature that does exist addresses the entire spectrum of posttraumatic sequelae of proximal humerus fractures, not just malunions. This makes comparisons between different series complicated. Regarding two-part malunions of the surgical neck, one study exists.[16] Solonen and Vastamaki described the use of a valgus wedge derotational osteotomy secured with an AO T-plate in 7 patients. Preoperative varus angulation ranged from 40 to 60 degrees. Five of 7 achieved near-normal to normal results with much improved ROM. Two of the 7 had poor results, which the authors attributed to preoperative factors, such as associated soft tissue pathology and poor motivation for rehabilitation.

Few studies look solely at the results of reconstructive procedures for isolated tuberosity malunions. Morris et al reported on 3 of 6 patients with isolated greater tuberosity malunions treated by osteotomy and repositioning of the fragment. They concluded that such a procedure leads to a substantial increase in shoulder function.[11]

In Beredjiklian's study, 11 of the 39 reported cases involved isolated tuberosity malunion (type I malunion).[13] Eight of the 11 were treated with an osteotomy of the tuberosity and soft tissue reconstruction. Overall, 6 of 8 (75%) patients had a satisfactory result. Seven of the 8 had correction of the deformity to within 5 mm of the anatomic position. All patients reported lessening of their pain, and 7 of the 8 reported minimal to no pain. Functional capacity improved in 75% of the patients as well.

Results on prosthetic replacement for proximal humerus malunion are more prevalent. Tanner and Cofield[19] reported on 49 shoulders treated with arthroplasty for acute or chronic proximal humerus fractures. Sixteen of the 27 shoulders in the chronic fracture group were documented malunions with articular surface incongruities. Because this study was primarily a comparison of acute and chronic fracture treatments, the results as they pertain to malunions is limited. That being said, a few generalizations can be made. Mean age was 11 years younger in the chronic fracture group, and more careful attention was paid to postoperative immobilization and rehabilitation. To that end, ROM was better in the chronic group. Complications were more frequent in the chronic group and were attributed to the difficulty of the surgery, extensive scarring, and distorted anatomy.

Dines et al[17] reported on a series of 20 arthroplasties performed for chronic posttraumatic changes of the proximal humerus. This series included malunions, nonunions, avascular necrosis, and impression fractures. Preoperative malunion of the tuberosities or humeral head was present in 8 of 20 patients. Twelve of the 20 required an osteotomy based on external rotation <20 degrees and abduction <90 degrees. Overall, 90% of the patients had fair, good, or excellent results. When looking at the malunion group in isolation, The Hospital for Special Surgery Shoulder score improved from 27.4 preoperatively to 69.8 postoperatively. It was noted that patients younger than 70 and those that did not require a tuberosity osteotomy had better results. Furthermore, the authors found that using a modular-designed prosthesis facilitated soft tissue tensioning and tuberosity repair.

Norris et al[1] reviewed the results of 23 patients who failed the initial treatment for three- or four-part fractures and were subsequently revised to prosthetic arthroplasty. Initial treatment was operative for 13 of 23 and nonoperative for 10. Seventeen patients were classified as having malunions. Of note, all 10 three- or four-part fractures initially treated closed went on to develop malunions, and 7 of 13 (54%) treated operatively developed malunions. Norris' group agreed with previously published reports stating that tuberosity osteotomy is technically demanding. They did conclude that late arthroplasty following failed primary treatment of complex proximal humerus fractures improves pain, ROM, and function. However, the results are inferior to proximal humerus fractures treated acutely with prosthetic arthroplasty.

When looking solely at the patients in Beredjiklian's study who had proximal humerus malunions managed with prosthetic arthroplasty, 74% had satisfactory results. Twenty-three of the 39 patients in his study were treated in this manner. The authors defined satisfactory by the presence of at least 90 degrees of active forward flexion, at least 50% functional use of the arm compared with their normal side, and slight or no pain. The key to obtaining successful results rested on adequate treatment of all bony and soft tissue abnormalities. Of note, their complication rate was 30%, further testifying to the degree of difficulty associated with the management of proximal humerus malunions.

Boileau et al[12] retrospectively reviewed 71 shoulders treated with arthroplasty due to the posttraumatic sequelae of proximal humerus fractures. Of these 71, 16 were characterized as having severe malunions of the tuberosities. Overall results were good showing a significant reduction in pain, while increasing forward elevation and external rotation. However, when patients requiring tuberosity osteotomy were isolated, results were less encouraging. All patients requiring osteotomy had fair or poor results. The authors concluded that greater tuberosity osteotomy is the main cause of poor results following shoulder arthroplasty in the postfracture group. They recommended avoidance of osteotomy whenever possible. Again, the complication rate was high in this patient population (27%).

Antuna et al[20] assessed the long-term results of proximal humerus malunions treated with arthroplasty in 50 patients. Mean follow up was 9 years. They noted statistically significant improvements in pain and postoperative ROM. Again though, the complication rate was high (20%), and 25 of 50 patients had unsatisfactory results based on the Neer rating system. Echoing previous studies, patients who required a tuberosity osteotomy and those who had undergone previous operative treatment of their initial fracture had less postoperative ROM.

Recently, Mansat's group evaluated the results of shoulder arthroplasty for late sequelae of proximal humerus fractures.[21] Of these patients, 8 were classified as malunions. When compared with other etiologies, including avascular necrosis and posttraumatic arthritis without distortion, malunions and nonunions had the least favorable results. Again, the need for greater tuberosity osteotomy worsened the result. In their series, prognosis was positively influenced by the integrity of the rotator cuff at surgery. The authors suggest tolerating a malunion of the greater tuberosity if it does not compromise acceptable positioning of the humeral prosthesis (i.e., the surgery is made easier if one is able to seat the stem appropriately without performing an osteotomy).

Summary

Proximal humerus malunions are potentially painful, debilitating injuries that are difficult to correct surgically. An accurate history and thorough physical exam are necessary to fully appreciate the involved bony and soft tissue pathology. Imaging studies, such as plain films, CT scans, and MRIs, help assess the injury, but a basic understanding of the deforming forces involved is also necessary to understand the nature of the malunion.

The best treatment for a malunion is prevention. Appropriate diagnosis and treatment of the initial injury provide the patient with the best chance of an excellent result. When malunions do develop, treatment options must be tailored to each individual case. If patients cannot or do not want to undergo surgery, conservative treatment with nonsteroidal antiinflammatory drugs (NSAIDs) and physical therapy is appropriate. Operative management is technically demanding and fraught with a relatively high complication rate. The integrity of the articular surface of the humeral head and its blood supply determine whether or not a head sparing procedure can be performed. In cases of avascular necrosis or extensive articular damage, prosthetic replacement is necessary. Reports of malunion managed with osteotomy and realignment are limited, but encouraging. Pain and function typically both improve. Prosthetic arthroplasty also provides reliable pain relief and improvement of function, but the results are less favorable than those achieved with prosthetic replacement for acute fractures. It is essential to address all bony and soft tissue pathology to optimize the chances for a successful outcome. Cases of prosthetic replacement requiring tuberosity osteotomy routinely exhibit the worst results and highest complication rates. It can be argued that the poor results are probably because these cases are often the most difficult fracture deformities, and osteotomies are frequently needed for exposure. When an osteotomy is performed, secure fixation is critical to avoid healing problems; and when possible, such osteotomies should be avoided. The high incidence of complications reported in most series attests to the difficulty in managing this problem.

References

1. Norris TR, Green A, McGuigan FX. Late prosthetic arthroplasty for displaced proximal humerus fractures. J Shoulder Elbow Surg 1995;4:271–280
2. Neer CS II. Displaced proximal humerus fractures: part I. Classification and evaluation. J Bone Joint Surg Am 1970; 52:1077–1089
3. Keene JS, Huizenga RE, Engher WD, et al. Proximal humerus fractures: a correlation of residual deformity with long term function. Orthopedics 1983;6:173–178
4. Siegel JA, Dines DM. Techniques in managing proximal humerus malunions. Orthop Clin North Am 2000;31(1): 35–49

5. Mclaughlin H. Common shoulder injuries. Am J Surg 1947; 3:282–295
6. Craig EV. Open Reduction and Internal Fixation of Greater Tuberosity Fractures Malunions, and Nonunions. In: Craig EV, ed. Master Techniques in Orthopaedic Surgery: The Shoulder. New York: Raven Press; 2004
7. Wirth MA, Rockwood CA Jr. Complications of Treatments of Injuries to the Shoulder. In: Epps CH Jr, ed. Complications in Orthopaedic Surgery. 3rd ed. Philadelphia: JB Lippincott; 1994:174–193
8. Dines DM, Warren RF, Inglis AE, et al. The Coracoid Impingement Syndrome. J Bone Joint Surg Br 1990;72: 314–316
9. Bigliani LU, Flatow EL, Pollock RG. Fractures of the Proximal Humerus. In: Rockwood CA Jr, Green DP, Bucholz RW et al, eds. Rockwood and Green's Fractures in Adults. 5th ed. Philadelphia: Lippincott-Raven; 2002:997–1041
10. Kilcoyne RF, Shuman W. The Neer classification of displaced proximal humerus fractures: spectrum of findings on plain radiographs and CT scans. AJR Am J Roentgenol 1990;154:1029–1033
11. Morris M, Kilcoyne R, Shuman W, Matsen F. Humeral tuberosity fractures: evaluation by CT scan and management of malunion. Orthop Trans 1987;11:242
12. Boileau P, Trojani C, Walch G. Shoulder arthroplasty for the treatment of sequelae of fractures of the proximal humerus. J Shoulder Elbow Surg 2001;10:299–304
13. Beredjiklian PK, Iannotti JP, Norris TR, et al. Operative treatment of malunion of a fracture of the proximal aspect of the humerus. J Bone Joint Surg Am 1998;80: 1484–1497
14. Holloway GB, Schenk T, Williams GR, et al. Arthroscopic capsular release for the treatment of refractory postoperative or post-fracture shoulder stiffness. J Bone Joint Surg Am 2001;83:1682–1687
15. Cuomo F, Goss TP. Shoulder Trauma: Bone. In: Kasser JR, ed. Orthopaedic Knowledge Update 5. Rosemont, IL: American Academy of Orthopaedic Surgeons, 1996:267–283
16. Solonen KA, Vastamaki M. Osteotomy of the neck of the humerus for traumatic varus deformity. Acta Orthop Scand 1985;56:79–80
17. Dines DM, Warren RF, Altchek DW, et al. Posttraumatic changes of the proximal humerus: malunion, nonunion, and osteonecrosis: treatment with modular hemiarthroplasty or total shoulder arthroplasty. J Shoulder Elbow Surg 1993;2:11–21
18. Beredjiklian PK, Ianotti JP. Treatment of proximal humerus fracture malunion with prosthetic arthroplasty. Instr Course Lect 1998;47:135–140
19. Tanner MW, Cofield R. Prosthetic arthroplasty for fractures and fracture-dislocations of the proximal humerus. Clin Orthop Relat Res 1983;179:116–128
20. Antuna SA, Sperling JW, Sanchez-Sotelo J, et al. Shoulder arthroplasty for proximal humerus malunions: long term results. J Shoulder Elbow Surg 2002;11:122–129
21. Mansat P, Guity MR, Bellumore Y, et al. Shoulder arthroplasty for late sequelae of proximal humerus fractures. J Shoulder Elbow Surg 2004;13:305–312

8 Operative Treatment of Proximal Humeral Nonunions

René K. Marti and Christian van der Werken

In general, surgical neck fractures of the proximal humerus heal with nonoperative treatment. Good and excellent results can be expected after anatomic reduction and stable internal fixation of fractures of the proximal humerus.[1] Therefore, the prevalence of delayed union and nonunions after conservative and operative treatment is low. The etiology of nonunions following conservative treatment is severe displacement or interposition of soft tissue. Failed internal fixations are based on excessive soft tissue dissection, neglect of the basic principles of internal fixation, and finally vascular disturbance of the fracture area itself. For both treatment modalities, aggressive physiotherapy and poor patient compliance might be reasons for the nonunion as well.[2]

Established nonunions of the surgical neck pose a significant disability to the patient, causing pain, instability, and limitation of motion of the shoulder joint. In general, the patients are elderly and often have associated medical problems, posing a treatment challenge to the surgeon. Despite these obstacles, we believe that a joint-preserving approach is indicated because the functional outcome of hemiarthroplasty is questionable.[3]

Classification

In comparison with femoral neck fractures, a proximal humeral fracture should unite within 4 months, otherwise we consider it a nonunion. These nonunions are usually atrophic as a consequence of motion in the nonunion, leading to bone resorption with cavitation of the humeral head and producing a true pseudarthrosis. The combination of nonunion and humeral head necrosis is theoretically possible, but not seen in our series because most proximal humeral nonunions develop after two-part fractures of the surgical neck. Nonunions after three- and four-part fractures are rare.[4]

We might classify the proximal humeral nonunions in two specific types: Type A are nonunions with a rather big, well-vascularized head-metaphyseal fragment; type B are nonunions of the surgical neck leading to resorption with excavation of the humeral head.

Patient Assessment

History

Previous operation reports and analysis of the available x-rays will give the necessary information concerning the quality of the bone and rotator cuff.

Physical Examination

Range of motion (ROM) and neurovascular examination should be assessed before the operative intervention. A detailed examination of the axillary nerve function is critically important as well. Most or all of the shoulder motion results generally from motion at the false joint rather than at the glenohumeral joint **(Fig. 8–1)**. In those hypermobile nonunions, forward elevation is impossible or at least modest. Severe muscle atrophy is present and the rotator cuff function is difficult to assess.

Radiologic Evaluation

Standard anteroposterior and axillary radiographic examination is generally sufficient. Computed tomography (CT) or magnetic resonance imaging (MRI) has no influence on the indication for operative treatment. Fluoroscopy allows the evaluation of the ROM in the glenohumeral joint and in the nonunion. Stiffness occurs only when the tuberosities are involved. The goal of the preoperative evaluation is to decide which technique is most suitable and if bone grafting is indicated.

Laboratory Studies

Infection can be excluded by clinical examination and appropriate blood studies including complete blood count (CBC), erythrocyte sedimentation rate (ESR), C-reactive protein screening, and radionuclear scanning. All concomitant comorbid medical conditions need optimal treatment before the intervention.

A

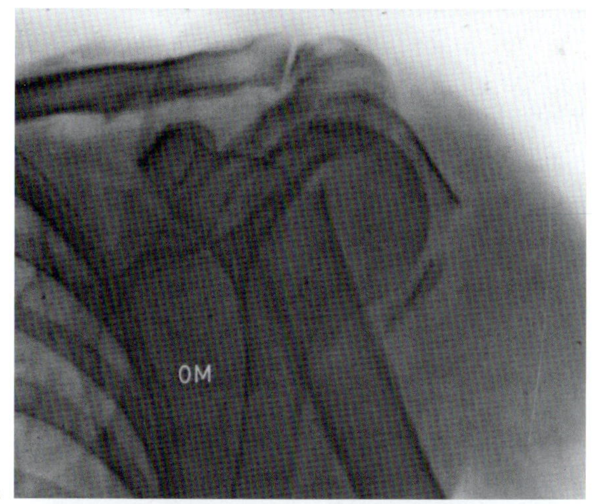

B

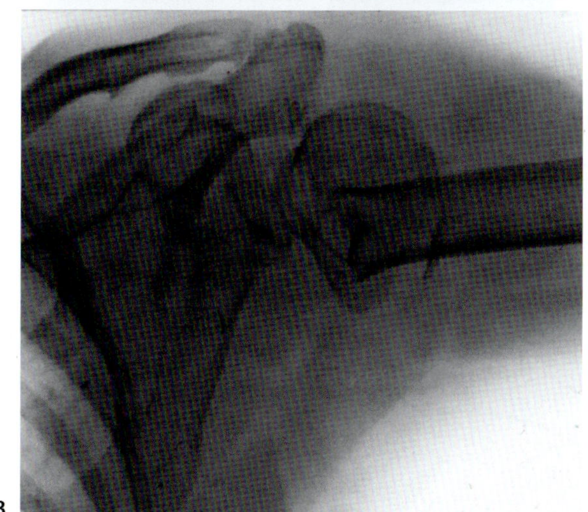

Figure 8–1 Type B nonunion – technique II (see Fig. 8–6).

Treatment

Nonsurgical Treatment

Not every nonunion needs surgical treatment: Operative interventions are indicated in patients whose nonunions cause relevant pain and result in a nonfunctional shoulder.

Surgical Treatment

Different stabilization techniques are used–intramedullary rods (Rush, Ender, etc.), intramedullary cortical bone grafts, open reduction, and internal fixation with tension-band techniques and plates.[2–10] Recently, the use of proximal humeral locking plate fixation techniques has been advocated for these nonunions. Those techniques are described in Chapter 4.

Fixation problems that one encounters in the treatment of acute proximal humeral fractures are often magnified in the setting of a nonunion. Nevertheless, the same principles, techniques, and implants are used to create the optimal stability that is necessary for any nonunion treatment. Approach and implant should not compromise the vascularity of the nonunion and the humeral head. Extra stability and biological stimulation by autologous bone grafting are often required, especially in atrophic nonunions of the resorption type.

Analyzing the literature and our own experience with referred patients, we conclude that the overall results of surgical treatments with nails of any type have not been satisfactory. Open reduction and internal fixation is the method of choice in the treatment of proximal humeral nonunions.

The principles of internal fixation are the same as in the primary fracture treatment.[1] Simple tension-band techniques may be sufficient if impaction of the shaft into the head of the humerus leads to intrinsic stability.[1,7]

Concerning surgical approaches, the use of blade plates is less invasive than those of T-plates, but for both similar results have been reported.[1,5,6] Double plating in combination with bone grafting using semi- or third-tubular plates is a valid alternative when there is cavitation of the humeral head (**Fig. 8–2**). In all these techniques, the purchase of the screws in the head of the humerus is compromised. Therefore, these have to be combined with impaction and tension bands that—if correctly applied—rely on the soft tissue attachments of the rotator cuff. Even in severe osteoporosis, the tendons and their attachment to the bone are able to withstand forces elicited by the wires. The new angle-stable plates provide a better fixation in the head of the humerus, but they will not eliminate the tension forces of the rotator cuff and will also rely on additional tension bands. The use of locking plate technology described in previous chapters can be helpful in some cases of difficult proximal fragment bone insufficiency.

Endoprosthetic replacement is only indicated in the presence of a split or necrotic humeral head and in preexistent glenohumeral arthrosis in the elderly patient. For the younger patient group, shoulder arthrodesis is still a valid option especially in case of associated infection.

Authors' Recommended Treatment

The surgical approach is classical and the same for all three techniques we will describe. Beach-chair position, shoulder, and ipsi- or contralateral iliac crest are draped freely. Full motion of the arm during the operation is a must.

A standard deltopectoral approach is used, respecting scars of earlier interventions. The placement of a Blount retractor under the deltoid allows visualization of the proximal humerus and the rotator cuff (**Fig. 8–3**). Release

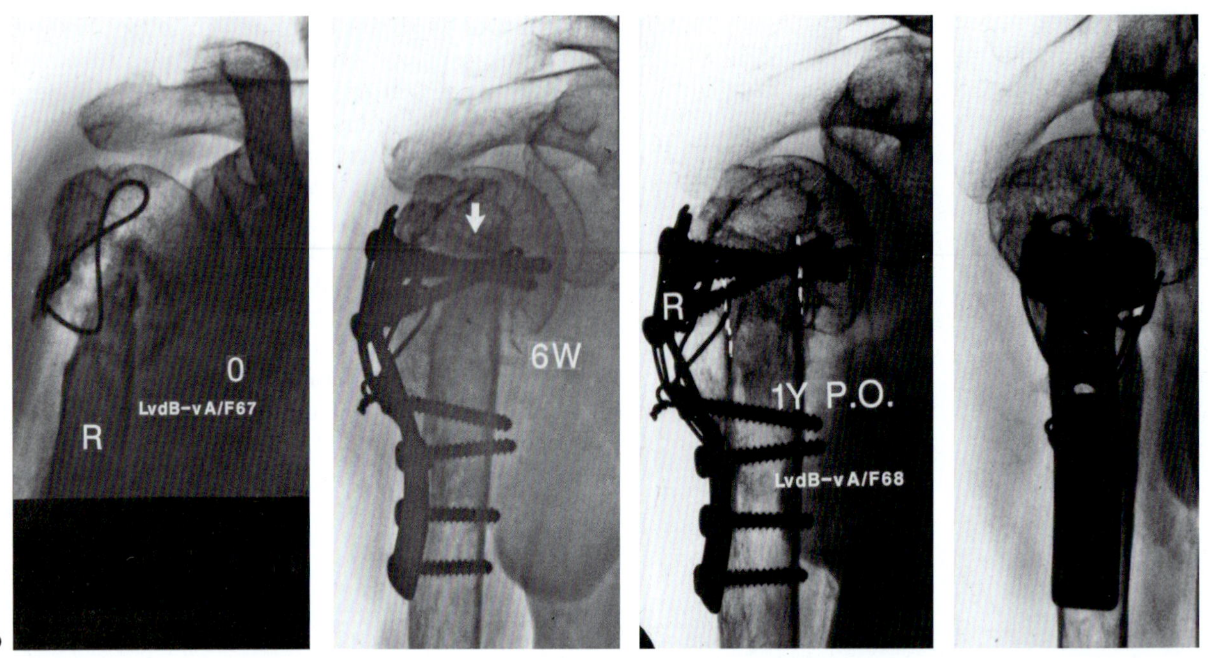

Figure 8–2 (A–D) Type B nonunion – technique IV. Severe excavation after primary tension-band internal fixation. Impaction and medialization of the shaft, lateral waved T-plate and iliac grafts, double tension band fixed below the plate around the first distal screw. There was uneventful healing and excellent functional results.

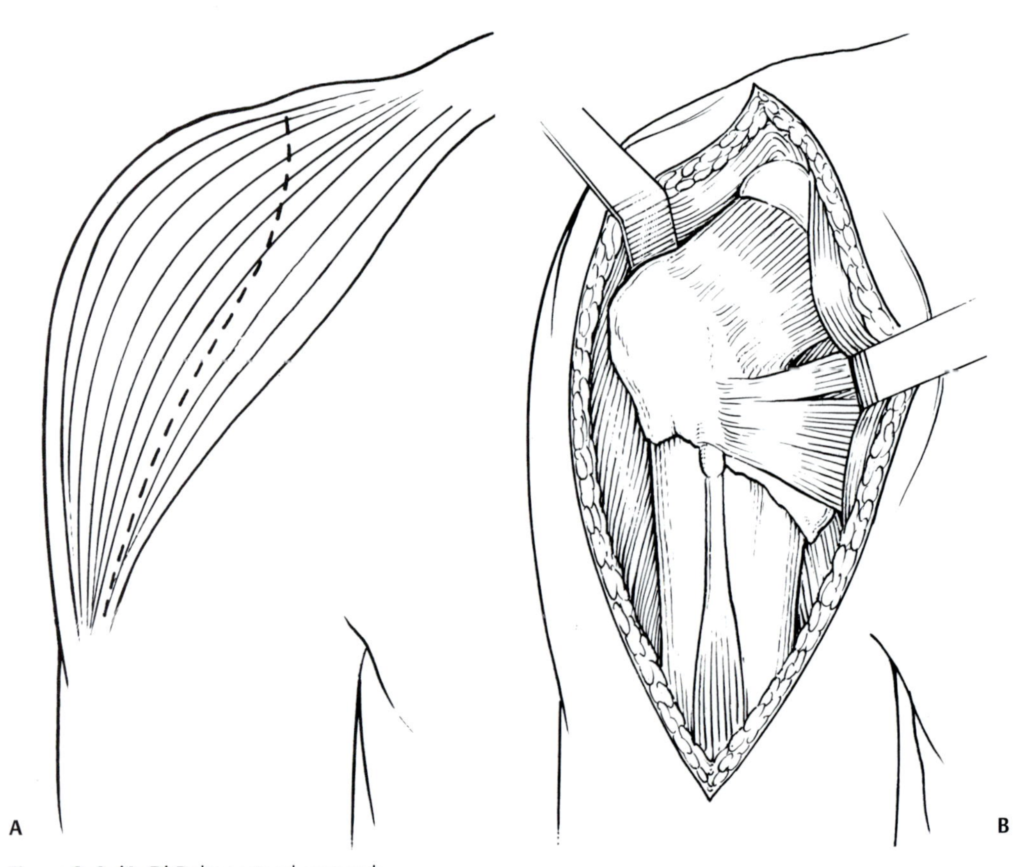

Figure 8–3 (A–D) Deltopectoral approach.

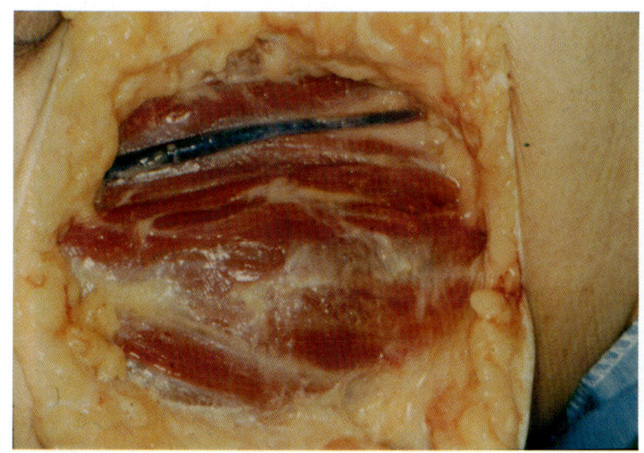
C

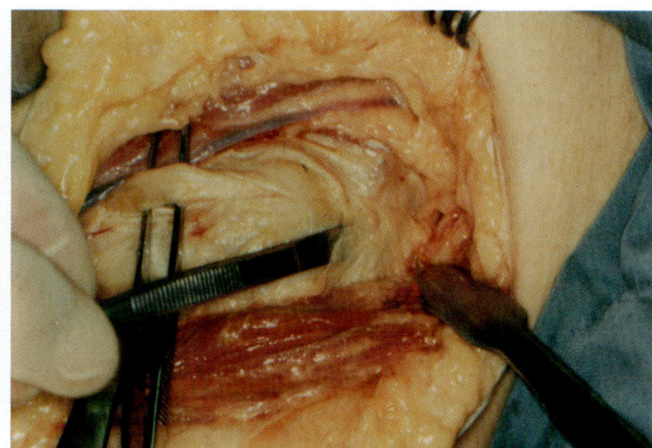
D

Figure 8–3 *(Continued)*

of the deltoid or pectoralis insertion is almost never necessary. To prevent injuries to the neurovascular structures, extended medial dissection should be avoided; the landmark to use is the biceps tendon.

Technique I

The treatment of type A proximal humeral nonunions below the surgical neck is similar to any other metaphyseal nonunion. Plate fixation in the big, well-vascularized head fragment is no problem. If both fragments are sclerotic, then impaction is not possible. The interposed fibrous tissue has to be removed, callus is decorticated, and both ends of the nonunion are débrided until bleeding bone is encountered. Now that the two fragments are adapted and compressed, a bridging graft may be necessary **(Fig. 8–4)**. All available implants can be used, angle blade plates, T-plates, the new angle stable plates (locking plates), and in delayed unions even a proximal humeral nail.

The challenge is the type B nonunion: the very proximal surgical neck nonunion. Analyzing our more than 30 years' experience, we developed a certain algorithm leading to three different techniques (II, III, and IV).

Technique II

The first step is, independent of the amount of bone resorption, the impaction of the shaft into the excavated head of the humerus. If the realized intrinsic stability is adequate, a pure, single or double tension-band technique can be applied **(Figs. 8–5** and **8–6)**.[1,7]

Technique III

If the intrinsic stability created by impaction is insufficient, the plate tension-band technique is our method of choice **(Fig. 8–7)**. The first step is the optimal placement of one or two tension-band wires under the insertion of the supraspinatus tendon to avoid secondary varisation. The second step is the impaction of the nonunion in a slight valgus overcorrection followed by the plate fixation, in former times with a T-plate, nowadays with angular stable plates (and/or locking plates). Important are the basic principles, independent of the chosen implant. Full compression using pointed reduction forceps must be applied before the eccentric distal holes are used for the final compression. The tension-band wire is placed beyond the plate around a screw and is tightened in a figure eight around the plate. The cerclage wire will not only eliminate the bending forces, but also avoid a breakout of a nonangle stable plate. Additional stability can be achieved by crossing the screws in the humeral head.

Technique IV

The described technique will not function in the presence of a severely excavated humeral head. Autogenous bone grafts are necessary to add extra stability and promote biology. Reduction and tension-band principles are the same as in technique III; the plate internal fixation is different. Either a T-plate or two flattened semitubular plates are waved laterally. The shaft fragment is displaced medially and the defect lateral in the humeral head and shaft is filled and bridged with solid corticocancellous grafts and free cancellous bone under the wave of the plates **(Fig. 8–2)**. By placement of the grafts laterally any neurovascular damage is avoided. One or two tension bands around the supraspinatus insertion eliminate the tension forces. A tension band around the subscapularis insertion is only indicated if the medial translation of the humeral shaft and the lateral grafts do not provide sufficient stability. Then we prefer the less

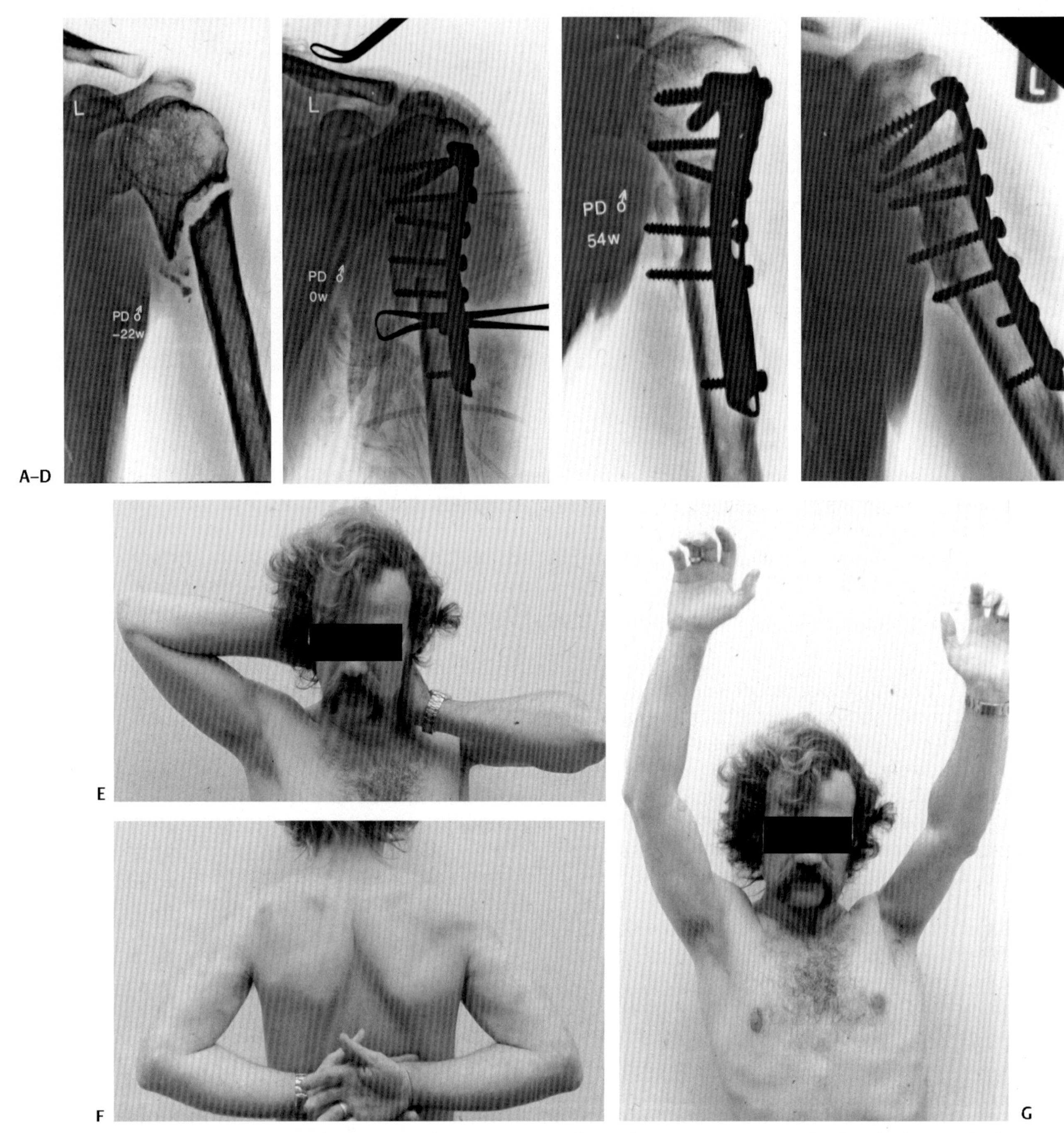

Figure 8–4 (A–G) Type A nonunion – technique I. Atrophic-interposition subcapital nonunion. Compressed T-plate, bridging graft. There were excellent results and graft resorption followed Wolff's law.

invasive application also used for primary fracture treatment **(Fig. 8–5B)**. The cerclage wire is placed under the biceps tendon and anchored in the same drill holes as the supraspinatus tension band. Drilling holes medial/inferior, as described by Kloen et al[7] are difficult to apply, require soft tissue stripping, and are a risk for the axillary nerve.

In all four techniques the glenohumeral joint is not opened. Subacromial débridement is rarely necessary and in a rare situation of a nonunion after three- or four-part

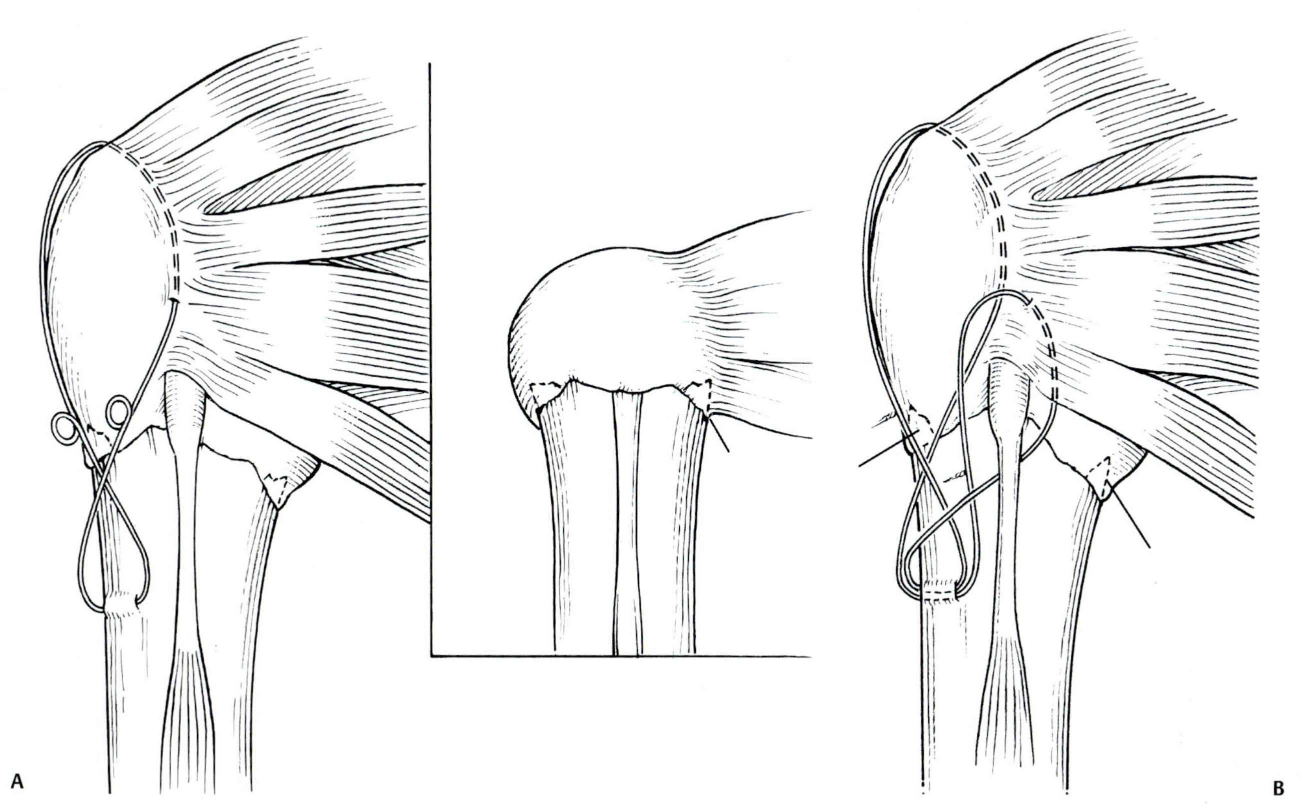

Figure 8–5 **(A)** Simple supraspinatus tension band. Tension is applied on both sides with a small pointed retractor. **(B)** Double tension band.

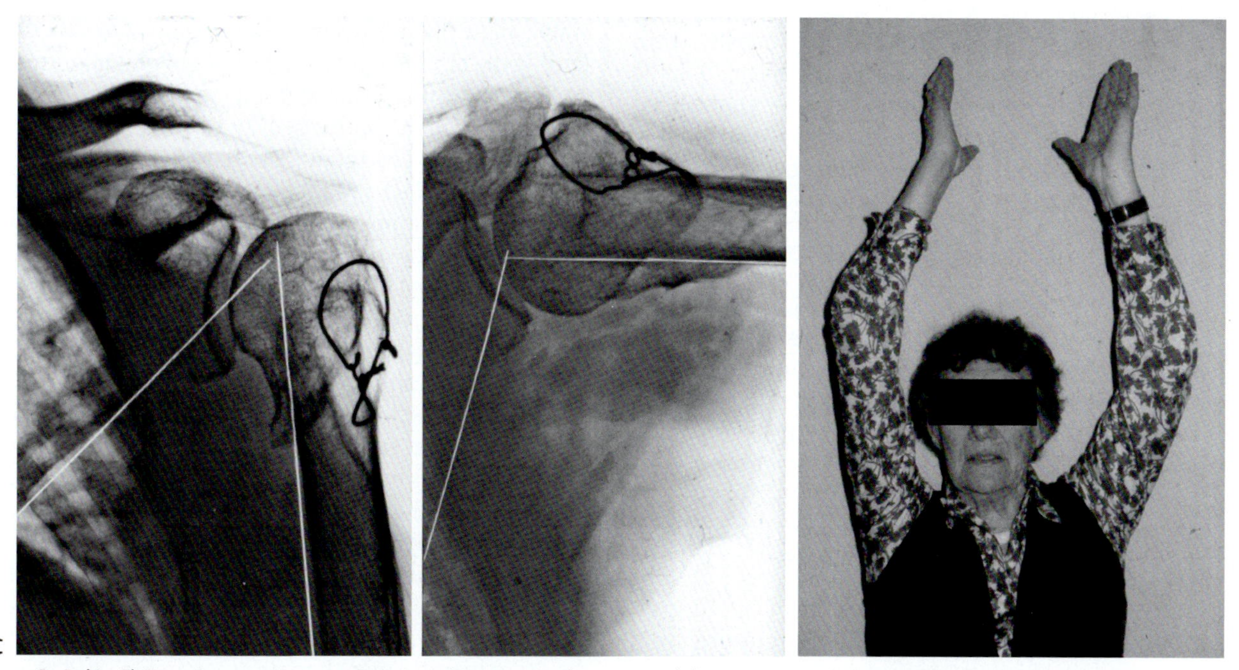

Figure 8–6 **(A–C)** Type B nonunion – technique II (see Fig. 8–1). Hypermobile nonunion. Impaction, optimal intrinsic stability, secured by supraspinatus tension band. There were excellent functional results. Technique III would be the additional plate fixation.

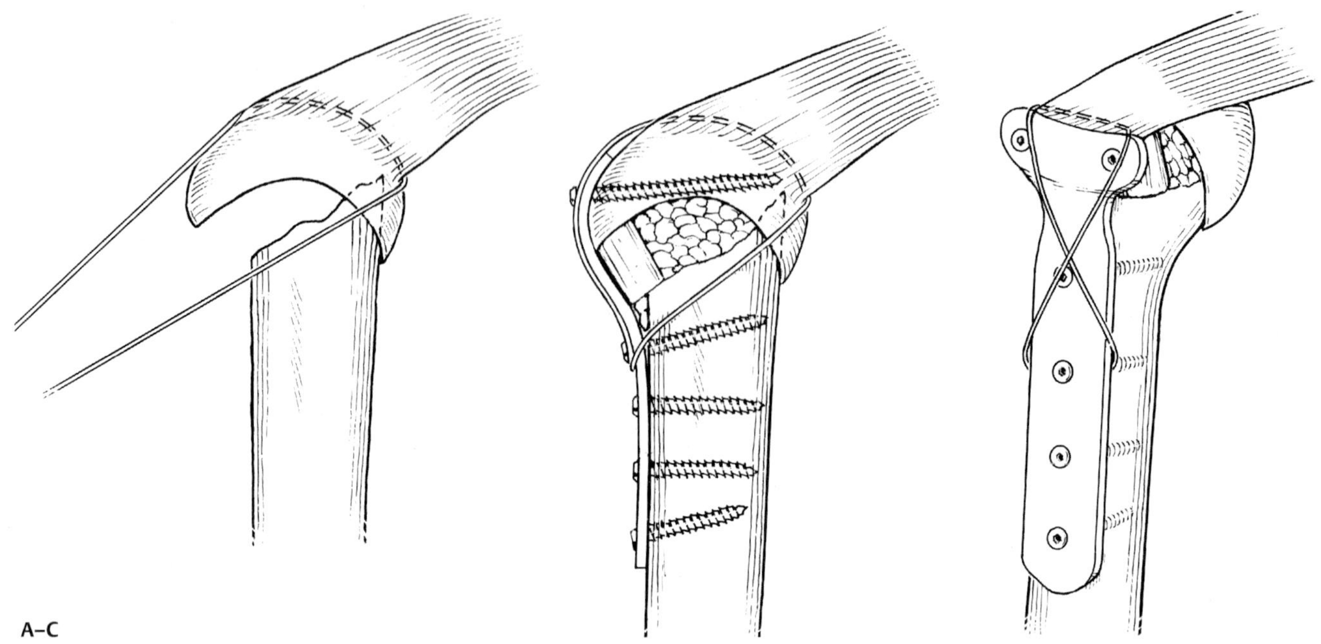

A–C

Figure 8–7 (A–C) Impaction, tension band around the plate.

fractures, the tuberosities have to be osteotomized and fixed by the already described tension-band technique.[10]

Complications

Neurovascular complications are possible, but not reported in the literature and not seen in our series. A temporary shoulder subluxation may be the consequence of an overlooked axillary nerve palsy or rotator cuff atrophy. The shoulder function restores after the healing of the nonunion and remaining stiffness is well tolerated and does not need manipulation under anesthesia. An eventual open arthrolysis could be combined with the hardware removal.

Postoperative Rehabilitation

Gentle pendulum exercises start on the first postoperative day, followed by passive shoulder mobilization up to 90 degrees elevation. Active motions in the same range are allowed after 4 weeks, full range after 6 weeks. Radiographs are obtained at 6 and 12 weeks to evaluate consolidation and a final control after 1 year.

Results

The best results of treatment of nonunions of the surgical neck of the proximal humerus in the literature are those reported using blade plate fixation. Ring et al[5] documented healing in 23 of 25 patients. Similar results were reported by Galatz et al[6] using internal fixation with blade plate or T-plate and autogenous bone graft in 13 patients.

The cases presented in those two articles do not show severe excavation of the humeral head (type B), compromising the anchorage of the blade plate. The impaction of the shaft into the excavated head does not allow the insertion of a seating chisel without destroying the achieved intrinsic stability. A valid alternative is certainly the new stable angle plates (locking compression plates [LCPs]) as long as the described basic principles of nonunion surgery are respected. Impaction and solid grafts create the necessary stability in the presence of an excavated head, secured by plate fixation and rotator cuff tension bands.

The relative lack of large numbers of patients and the multitude of fixation techniques make it difficult to compare the different studies and outline a standard protocol. We conclude that the best results of treatment of type II nonunions occurred after open reduction and internal fixation combined with autogenous grafting.

All our cases are well documented with a follow-up to 32 years. The described techniques led to union in all cases, even after several earlier interventions **(Fig. 8–8)**. The functional result was excellent in the type A nonunions (technique I) and acceptable for the mostly elderly patients group in the type B nonunions (techniques II to IV).

In recent years, LCP largely replaced the angled blade plate, especially in type B nonunions. The LCP proved its versatility with a simple and smooth insertion technique resulting in outcomes that are comparable with those of the other described methods. All nonunions that were treated with a LCP finally healed despite considerable

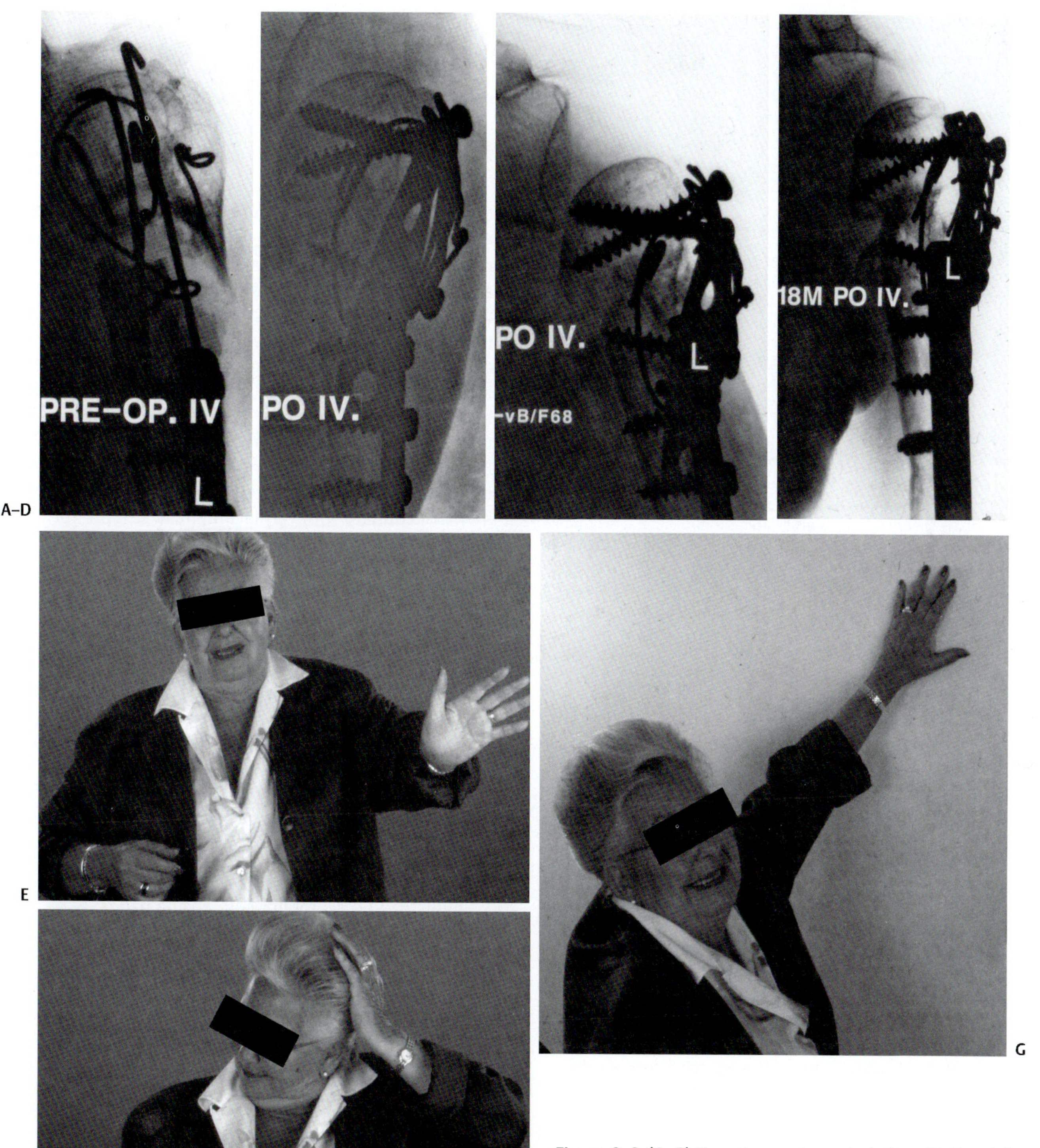

Figure 8–8 (A–G) Type B nonunion – technique IV. Remaining nonunion after three interventions and earlier plate fixation of a humerus shaft fracture. Mistake: no impaction, cerclage wires do not act as tension bands. Impaction-medialization of the shaft, two lateral, waved semitubular plates, iliac grafts. There was postoperative temporary subluxation because of the rotator cuff atrophy. Healing was uneventful; the patient had limited function, but was happy with her outcome.

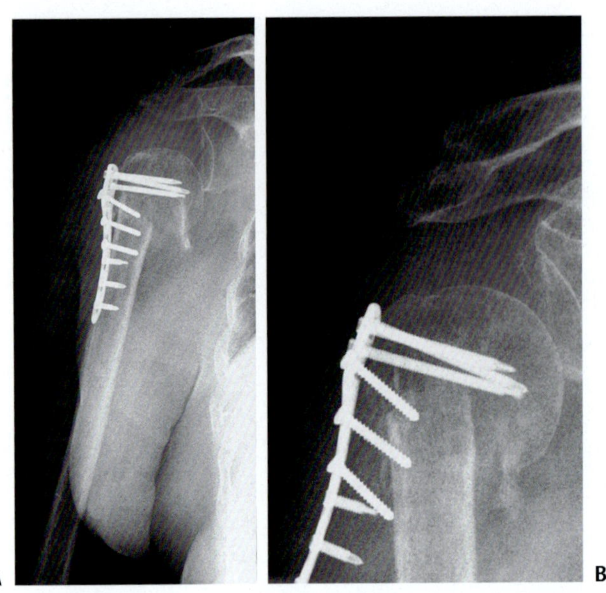

Figure 8–9 (A,B) Fixation of a type B nonunion with a compressed locking proximal humerus (LPH) plate. Insufficient impaction. Lateralization of the shaft. No bone graft. Within 3 months, the screws broke out of the shaft, but the screws in the excavated head were still stable.

complications rates if the described basic principles, impaction grafts, and tension band were not applied. The big advantage of the new plate is the safe anchorage of the screws even in an excavated head **(Fig. 8–9)**.

Summary

Concerning treatment modalities the classification in type A and B nonunions is useful. Type A, the real subcapital nonunion, can be treated as a fresh subcapital fracture and as any other metaphyseal nonunion. In type B, the treatment depends on the amount of bone resorption of the head. If there is no excavation, impaction and a simple cerclage tension band around the supraspinatus allow a limited invasive technique.[11] In the case of severe bone resorption impaction, corticocancellous bone grafting, plates, and tension bands produce the necessary stability. Following this algorithm, nonunions will heal, with functional results that mainly depend on the primary treatment. Secondary joint replacement is still an option as long as the rotator cuff is preserved.

References

1. Wijgman AJ, Roolker W, Patt TW, Raaymakers EL, Marti RK. Open reduction and internal fixation of three and four-part fractures of the proximal part of the humerus. J Bone Joint Surg Am 2002;84: 1919–1925
2. Healy WL, Jupiter JB, Kristiansen TK, et al. Nonunion of the proximal humerus: a review of 25 cases. J Orthop Trauma 1990;4:424–431
3. Marti RK, Lim TE, Jolles CW. On the treatment of comminuted fracture-dislocations of the proximal humerus: internal fixation or prosthetic replacement. In: Koibel R, Helbig B, Blauth W, eds; Telger TC, trans. Shoulder Replacement. New York: Springer; 1987:135–148
4. Neer CS. Displaced humeral fractures. Part II. The treatment of three-part and four-part displacement. J Bone Joint Surg Am 1970;52:1090–1103
5. Ring D, McKee MD, Perey BH, et al. The use of a blade plate and autogenous cancellous bone graft in the treatment of ununited fractures of the proximal humerus. J Shoulder Elbow Surg 2001;10:501–507
6. Galatz LM, Williams GR, Fenlin JM, et al. Outcome of open reduction and internal fixation of surgical neck nonunions of the humerus. J Orthop Trauma 2004; 18:63–68
7. Kloen P, Rubel IF, Helfet D. A two-tension-band technique for treatment of nonunions of the surgical neck of the humerus. Tech Shoulder Elbow Surg 2001;2(3):187–193
8. Nayak NK, Schickendantz MS, Reagan WD, et al. Operative treatment of nonunion of surgical neck fractures of the humerus. Clin Orthop Relat Res 1995;313:200–205
9. Walch G, Badet R, Nové-Josserand L, et al. Nonunions of the surgical neck of the humerus: surgical treatment with an intramedullry bone peg, internal fixation and cancellous bone grafting. J Shoulder Elbow Surg 1996; 5:161–168
10. Jupiter JB, Mullaji AB. Blade plate fixation of proximal humeral nonunions. Injury 1994;25:301–303
11. Marti RK, Besselaar PP, Raaymakers EL. In: Ruedi TP, Murphy WM, eds. AO Principles of Fracture Management. Stuttgart/New York: Thieme Medical Publishing; 2000:782–783

9 Arthroplasty for Proximal Humeral Fractures

David M. Dines and Russell F. Warren

Epidemiology and Mechanism of Injury

Complex fractures of the proximal humerus include three- and four-part fractures and fracture dislocations, intraarticular head splitting fractures, and chronic impression fractures. These injuries, which are historically quite rare, have become more common as the population ages and remains physiologically active. These injuries are generally the sequelae of low impact falls in elderly patients or high velocity trauma in younger patients, and are particularly disabling when they involve the dominant arm.[1-3]

Treatment

Severe complications in these fractures are the result of associated vascular compromise, which occurs because of interruption of the ascending branch of the anterior humeral circumflex artery as it courses around the proximal humerus and enters at the tuberosities around the bicipital groove.[4] These endosteal vessels are at risk in fractures that involve one or both tuberosities. Disruption of this major blood supply leaves the proximal humerus susceptible to avascular necrosis (AVN). Four-part fractures are particularly susceptible because they include disruption of both tuberosities and are associated with a high incidence of AVN ranging from 34 to 85%.[5-8]

In addition to vascular compromise, these fractures are often associated with significant comminution, which makes stable open reduction/internal fixation extremely difficult. Because of these factors, many surgeons have opted for a "wait-and-see" approach to treatment in some patients. The other treatment options have included closed reduction, open reduction with fixation, and hemiarthroplasty.[2,6,7,9-12]

Schai et al,[6] in comparing the results of these treatments in a group of patients who had sustained four-part proximal humeral fractures, noted that hemiarthroplasty gave statistically significant better results than both open reductions and internal fixation or conservative care. In other series, conservative treatment had only a 5% successful outcome.[7] Some authors have noted that four-part fractures treated acutely by hemiarthroplasty had significantly better results than those chronic four-part malunions treated later by arthroplasty.[13-15] With all these factors considered, hemiarthroplasty is, in the acute setting, the procedure of choice for most displaced proximal humeral fractures at risk for malunion or vascular compromise.[3,8,16-19]

Surgical Treatment

Indications for Surgery

Hemiarthroplasty is indicated in many patients who are medically suitable for such extensive surgery and are able to carry out the long rehabilitation process that is mandatory for a successful outcome. In rare cases of very young patients with displaced proximal humeral fractures and in a small subset of patients who have impacted four-part valgus fractures, attempts at open reduction/internal fixation with minimal hardware are indicated.[5,7,19,20] Minimal hardware is recommended so that if arthroplasty is necessary later the remaining soft tissue sleeve and vascularity to the humeral head will be preserved.[5,14,21]

Hemiarthroplasty is contraindicated in patients with medical frailty precluding surgery and those patients whose physical or mental condition makes them unable to comply with the required postoperative rehabilitation program.

In the older patient group, indications for arthroplasty are not based on chronological age, but are based on the patient's physiologic age, hand dominance, and activity requirements. In the younger patients an attempted open reduction/internal fixation is warranted to avoid prosthetic replacement and its associated complications. In these cases if AVN does occur, the tuberosities will be in a better anatomic position to facilitate conversion to a prosthesis.

Patient Assessment

As with all traumatic injuries, a careful history and physical exam and appropriate radiologic studies are mandatory. A careful history and physical exam is performed to determine

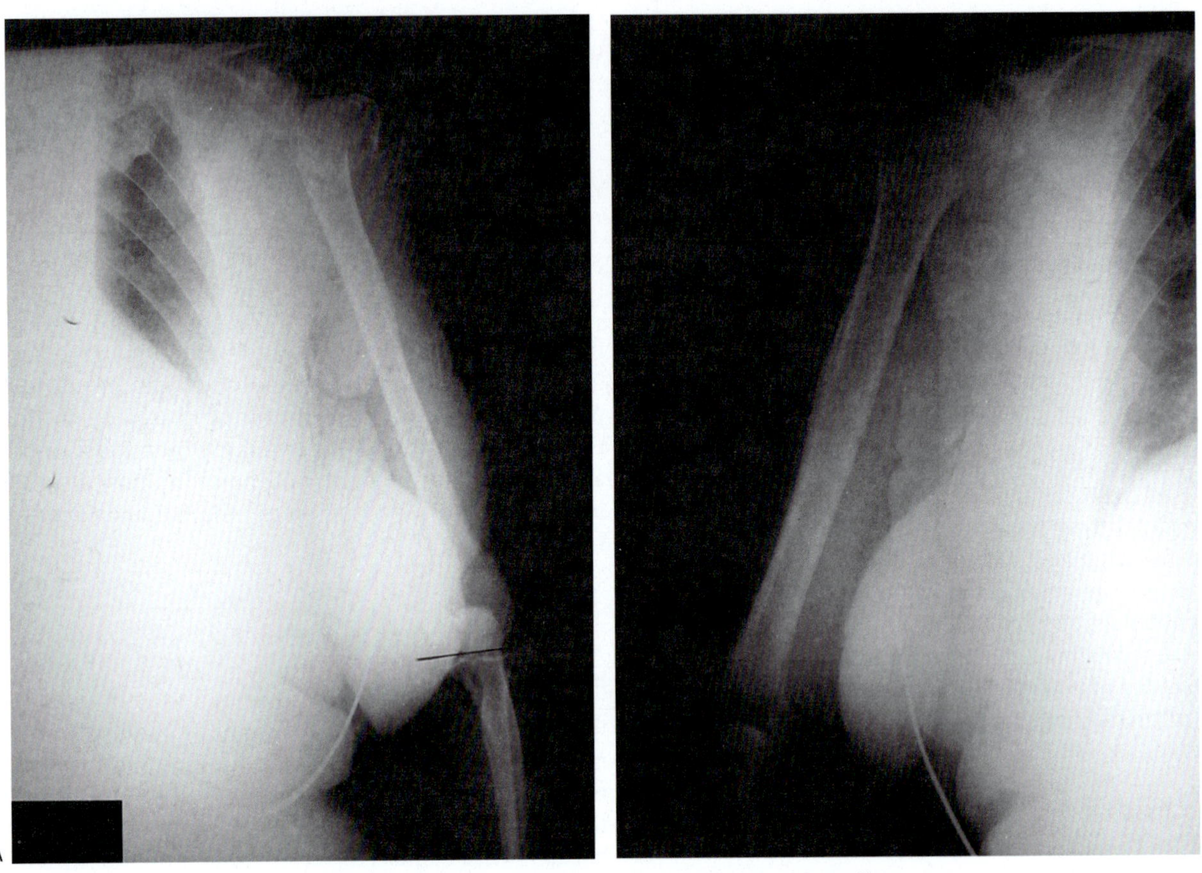

Figure 9–1 **(A)** Scaled x-ray of fractured proximal humerus. **(B)** Scaled x-ray of contralateral normal humerus.

any comorbid factors that might affect the surgical procedure and/or the postoperative rehabilitation process.

A thorough clinical examination of the shoulder is performed to determine the obvious deformity and neurovascular function. Special attention to the axillary nerve function and vascular compromise is important because many patients with complex proximal humeral fractures will have such injuries. Many patients with vascular injuries may have intact pulses distally due to the extensive collateral circulation around the proximal humerus. Deltoid contraction and sensory distribution may be tested and any vascular deficiency should be aggressively evaluated.

Radiologic Assessment

Standard x-rays should include a trauma series, which includes a true antereroposterior view of the scapula, a transcapular "Y" view, and an axillary view. In most cases, these views will supply the necessary information about the fracture complex to determine configuration; however, in some cases where displacement remains uncertain, computed tomography (CT) scans can be helpful, especially in distinguishing three- and four-part fractures. CT scans may also be helpful in detecting any head splitting or articular component of the fracture.

In an effort to reestablish proper height and length of the proximal humerus after hemiarthroplasty, we now routinely utilize full-length x-rays of both humeri to determine humeral length and properly use this measurement to help us later in recreating normal anatomy **(Fig. 9–1)**.

Treatment

Surgical Treatment

Techniques

Anesthesia

We utilize interscalene block anesthesia with supplemental general anesthesia when necessary. This allows for decreased use of anesthetic agents, especially in the older population. It also allows for significant pain relief postoperatively so that the patient may begin early physical therapy routines. A general anesthesia component is necessary for proximal muscle relaxation and eliminates discomfort of the patient lying in one position for extensive periods.

Patient Positioning

The patients are placed in a modified beach-chair position with the back elevated between 30 and 40 degrees. The head is well supported in a headrest or in a commercially available shoulder table. The patient is placed at the lateral edge of the table to allow free mobility of the operative arm, allowing unrestricted humeral extension, adduction, and rotation to facilitate the intramedullary reaming and allow for proper prosthetic component placement. The arm is appropriately prepped and draped free.

Surgical Exposure

We utilize a long deltopectoral incision, which is performed from the anterior portion of the acromioclavicular (AC) joint along the coracoid process and following the anterior deltoid distally. The surgeon develops a deltopectoral interval preserving the cephalic vein. Appropriate deltoid retractors are utilized between the deltoid and the conjoined tendon. Care should be taken to avoid injury to the musculocutaneous nerve, which crosses inferior to the coracoid. This can be done by partially tenotomizing the conjoint tendon.

The subacromial space is then cleared bluntly with gentle use of digital pressure or periosteal elevators. Proximal and distal deltoid insertion and origin are left intact and the pectoralis muscle tendon is retracted medially. The sternal head insertion may be partially released to decrease medial pull on the proximal shaft of the humerus and allow for better exposure. The fracture figuration is now exposed after hemorrhagic bursa and fracture hematoma is carefully excised.

Identification and Mobilization of Fracture Fragments

The biceps tendon is isolated and identified. This is a key surgical landmark that helps locate the tuberosity fragments because the fracture configuration is medial or deep to the exposure. The fracture line is found between the tuberosities slightly posterior to the bicipital groove. The intertubercular fracture line is followed proximally to the rotator interval, which is opened to allow better access to the tuberosities that can then be identified. The lesser tuberosity will be displaced medially and the greater tuberosity will be displaced posterior superiorly. In many cases, there are soft tissue attachments that must be gently freed utilizing periosteal elevators or osteotomes; however, care should be taken to avoid injury to the periosteal attachments.

The cancellous portion of the isolated tuberosity fragments are often oversized and may need to be trimmed for reduction and repair later. The bone that is removed can be saved and used later as bone graft during tuberosity reconstruction. At this point three #5 nonabsorbable or fiber-wire sutures are placed at the bone tendon interface between the cuff and the bony surface of the greater tuberosity from proximally to distally. One traction suture is also placed at the bone tendon interface of the lesser tuberosity as well. Once control of the tuberosities has been achieved the humeral head is teased out of the glenohumeral joint. Sometimes this requires the use of osteotomes or periosteal elevators to release it from its soft tissue or bony attachments.

The head fragment will then be measured using calipers or sizing guides to select the proper head size for later reconstruction. At this point with adequate exposure, the glenoid is evaluated for concomitant fracture or damage. In cases of severe damage, bone loss or even concomitant arthritis glenoid replacement might be considered.

The long head of the biceps insertion into the glenoid is resected and the remaining stump removed. The remaining tendon will later be tenodesed to the soft tissue reconstruction.

Prosthetic Insertion

With the tuberosities retracted and the humeral head removed, the intramedullary canal is now exposed. The first critical step in prosthetic replacement is placement of the humeral component at the appropriate height (length) and version. This is a critical step in the operative process, which actually begins preoperatively. In some cases the humeral head will fracture at the articular surface making replacement at the appropriate height relatively easy. In other cases where there is significant proximal comminution, the surgeon must recognize the bone loss based on the findings of the preoperative x-rays, the intraoperative findings, and the evaluation of full-length scaled x-rays of the injured and contralateral humerus with a ruler of defined length. This information utilized in conjunction with either an external or intramedullary fracture sizing guide will ensure proper humeral length reconstruction. Many commercially available fracture arthroplasty systems will have associated extramedullary or intramedullary fracture placement guides, which will ensure proper height and fixation.

Preoperative assessment of the proximal humeral comminution is also critical to allow the surgeon to place the humeral component at the proper height. Comminution of the medial humeral neck should be assessed and pieces measured to help identify the position in which the humeral component must be placed. The arm is extended and adducted to deliver the shaft anteriorly. The canal is now prepared with progressive hand-held sequential reamers.

The stem size can be predetermined on preoperative radiographs using appropriate templates. Appropriate reamers are used to "sound" the canal to its largest diameter. At this point, an intramedullary or extramedullary fracture device is utilized.

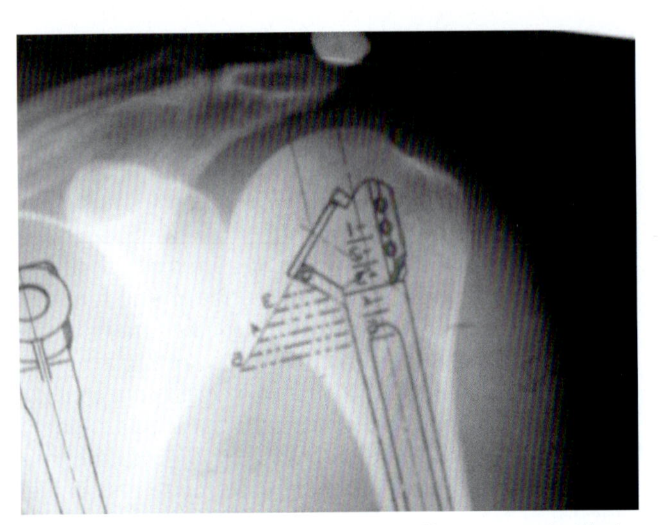

Figure 9–2 Templating the normal proximal humerus to decide the appropriate "hash mark" for proper height placement of prosthesis on the affected side.

The intramedullary fracture-positioning sleeve device is utilized at our institution (Biomet, Warsaw, IN). This device will place and maintain the humeral stem component at the appropriate height that had been calculated from operative x-rays, preoperative scanograms, and intraoperative observation of medial proximal humeral bone loss. Once the appropriate height has been calculated, the depth of the position of the fracture sleeve can be determined. Utilizing templates over x-rays of the contralateral normal proximal humerus, the appropriate "hash mark" depth for the intramedullary fracture sleeve is chosen **(Fig. 9–2)**. The amount of proximal bone loss, if present, is calculated based on preoperative x-rays and intraoperative measurements and added to the chosen hash mark depth to insure proper placement.

Once the appropriate hash mark has been identified the canal is reamed to size. Next, the appropriate diameter tap is used to the depth chosen by the "hash mark (±bone loss)" for proper positioning of the intramedullary fracture sleeve. Finally, the fracture sleeve is inserted to that depth to maintain the appropriate height for the humeral component **(Fig. 9–3)**.

The intramedullary fracture-positioning sleeve does not regulate version. This must be done by flexing the elbow to 90 degrees and the transverse epicondylar access of the elbow to zero degrees. The arm is externally rotated to the desired degree of retroversion between 20 and 30 degrees. Excessive version in either direction

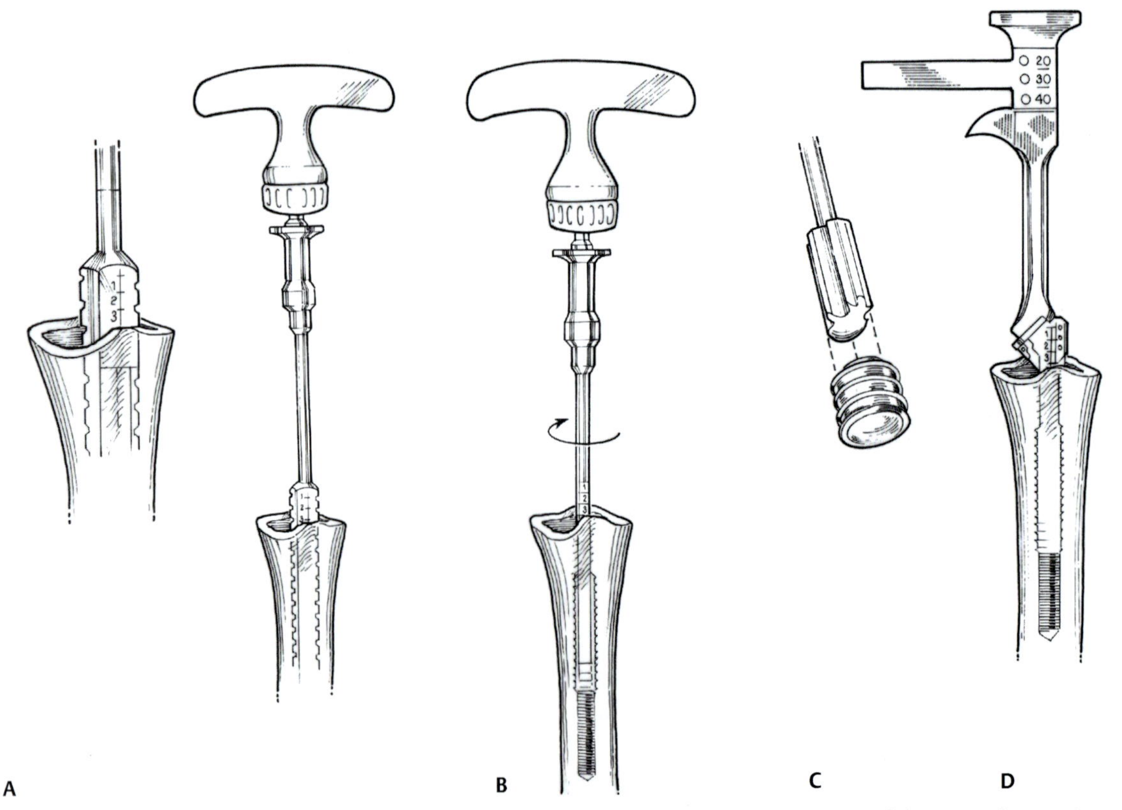

Figure 9–3 Use of the intramedullary fracture-positioning sleeve device. **(A)** Ream the humeral canal to the chosen hash mark. **(B)** Use the cutting reamer to the chosen hash mark to prepare the canal for placement of the sleeve in proper position. **(C)** Fracture sleeve on inserter/holder. **(D)** Figure of fracture sleeve and humeral fracture stem placed to the chosen position utilizing the fracture sleeve.

can lead to problems of stability of the implant and/or compromise of the greater tuberosity fixation. In cases with excess retroversion the greater tuberosity is placed under greater stress during internal rotation leading to nonunion or failure.

Once the fracture sleeve has been placed a trial reduction can be performed in the following manner. A trial prosthesis of the appropriate diameter to match the fracture sleeve is inserted in the appropriate version determined by external rotation. Next, a trial humeral head component chosen by direct measurement of the removed fracture fragment of the humeral head is placed on the trial stem. At this point, the arm is reduced and the humeral component should point directly at the glenoid. There should be 50% override anteriorly or posteriorly and inferiorly with traction on the arm. The humeral component should clear the acromion at 90 degrees of abduction with good rotation. Recreation of the appropriate height of the component is critical to recreate adequate tension in the deltoid myofascial sleeve. If the implant is placed in a position that is too proud, impingement and loss of motion will occur. If the implant is placed in a position that is too short, the effective length of the deltoid will be diminished and this will cause a loss of power and instability.

Once the appropriate components have been chosen based on these trial reductions and intraoperative measurements, as well as intraoperative x-rays if necessary, then cementing of the chosen humeral component may commence. As with any prosthesis, cement technique is critical. We avoid the use of pressurized cement and cement restrictors because this can cause increased pressure with the humeral canal and may allow cement to protrude through the thin posterior cortex and into the soft tissue space possibly compromising the radial nerve.

Prior to cementing, two drill holes are placed in the humeral shaft ~1.5 cm distal to the fracture line of the humerus at the bicipital groove and posterior to the bicipital groove by ~1.5 cm. These drill holes are then utilized to place a #5 nonabsorbable suture from front to back and a #5 nonabsorbable suture posteriorly through the posterior hole for later tuberosity reconstruction, which will be defined in the next section. These sutures must be placed prior to cementing the component, as there will be no possible way to place them after the cement has hardened.

The humeral component is cemented utilizing the appropriate technique; excess cement is removed and the component is maintained in the proper position until the cement has hardened.

Once the stem component has been securely cemented in the correct position, the proper sized humeral head component is now firmly impacted in place after thorough drying of the Morse taper to avoid head instability. Fixation of the head component can be assessed by trying to rotate the head component on the stem. It should not be movable.

Tuberosity Reconstruction and Rotator Cuff Repair

In addition to proper component placement, the success of the operation is directly dependent on the appropriate tuberosity reconstruction with eventual complete healing of the tuberosities to the humeral shaft and to each other in the proper position below the top of the prosthesis. The #5 sutures previously placed at the superior, middle, and inferior supraspinatus tendon insertion of the greater tuberosity will now be utilized to secure the tuberosities around the humeral component, both utilizing the medial fixation slot in the humeral component and utilizing the posterior longitudinal suture for two-point fixation of the greater tuberosity to the shaft. This is followed by transverse fixation to the lesser tuberosity and completed with a figure-eight tension band of the tuberosity construct.

It is critical to remember that the tuberosity placement must be secure enough to allow for early range of motion (ROM) and must be in contact with the humeral shaft to ensure healing. It is critical not only for the tuberosities to heal, but for them to be placed in a position where they can recreate normal rotator cuff function. To achieve this, the top of the tuberosity must lie between 5 and 10 mm below an imaginary line over the highest point of the humeral head. There are many different techniques for tuberosity fixation and some are dependent upon the prosthetic system that is being utilized.

We utilize the following technique in tuberosity reconstruction:

1. The greater tuberosity is first fixed to the shaft and around the implant utilizing the top and bottom suture (#1 and #3) and the posterior longitudinal suture (B) through the shaft. The top and bottom suture through the greater tuberosity are placed through the medial fixation slot in the implant and then brought around and tied to themselves with the sutures holding the greater tuberosity in the correct position below the humeral head and against the anterior fin of the component and impacted over the posterior fin for enhanced fixation. The anterior fin represents placement to the “natural bicipital groove” for anatomic reconstruction. The posterior longitudinal suture (suture B), which was placed inside out around the superior portion of greater tuberosity, is now tied to insure rigid fixation. Prior to tying these sutures the other transverse suture (#2) through the greater tuberosity is placed to fix the lesser tuberosity either transversely around the implant or through the lateral fin. Prior to securing the

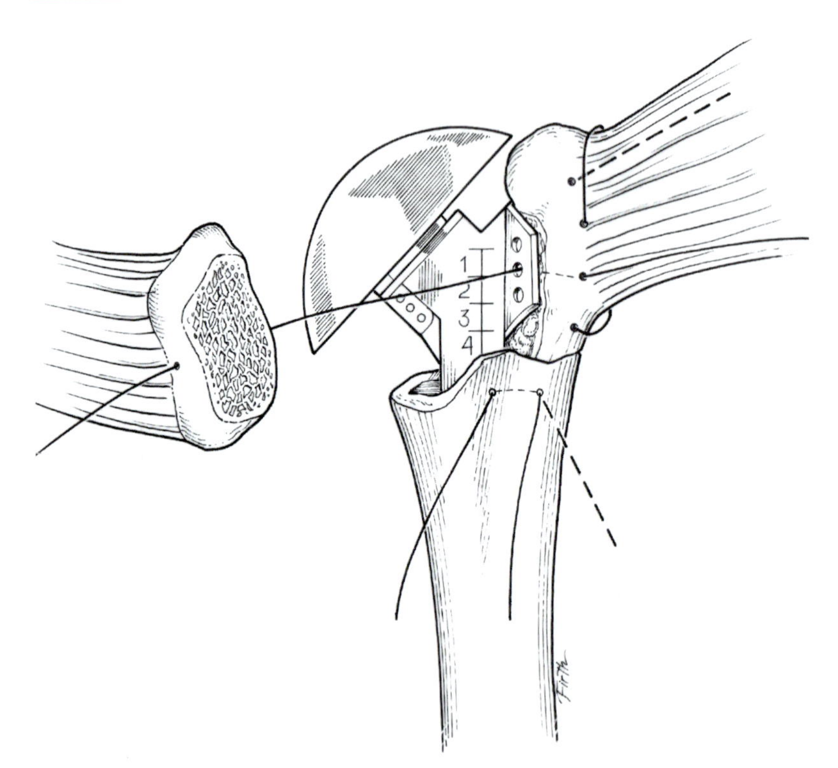

Figure 9–4 Appropriate sutures placed through the tuberosities and the humeral shaft as noted in the text for fixation of the tuberosities to the humeral shaft.

tuberosities, the cancellous bone graft harvested from the removed humeral head and tuberosities is packed about the stem and fin **(Fig. 9–4)**.

2. Utilizing the transverse suture #2 (one strand as seen here or with two strands depending upon the size of the tuberosity) which has been passed through the greater tuberosity, the lesser tuberosity is brought similarly against the fin of the prosthesis and the greater tuberosity. It is also placed below the top of humeral head component and may be held by a towel clamp while the suture(s) are tied in sequence **(Fig. 9–5)**.

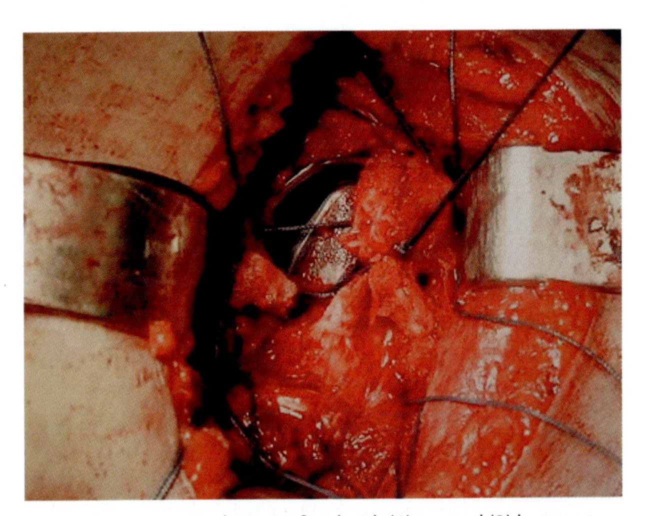

Figure 9–5 Greater tuberosity fixed with (1) top and (3) bottom transverse sutures and the posterior longitudinal suture (B) as described in the text. Transverse suture 2 to be used to fix the lesser tuberosity.

3. With the tuberosities now secured to the shaft and to the fin of the prosthesis, the front to back strand previously placed through the proximal humeral shaft **(Fig. 9–6A)** is now utilized and placed in a figure-eight fashion through the soft tissue above the tuberosities to create a tension-band effect through the tuberosities on the shaft. The tuberosities should overlap the humeral shaft slightly to ensure healing **(Fig. 9–6)**.
4. Finally, the stump of the biceps tendon which remains is fixed by soft tissue repair to the tuberosity reconstruction in effect tenodesing the long head of the biceps tendon. Although some surgeons advocate saving the biceps tendon within the groove, we have recently studied problems in hemiarthroplasty and have found a biceps tenodesis effect can occur in some cases where the tendon is saved, creating stiffness and restricted motion. For this reason, we now routinely excise the intraarticular portion of the long head of the biceps tendon and create a soft tissue tenodesis of the tendon to tuberosity repair as described above.

Next, the rotator interval is closed using #1 nonabsorbable sutures while placing the arm in external rotation to avoid contracture. The tuberosity reconstruction is inspected to make sure it moves as a solid unit and to determine the parameters of a safe range in the early postoperative period. These ranges of motion should allow clearance of the acromion in abduction at 90 degrees and allow for at least 45 degrees of external rotation. Forward elevation should be well above shoulder height; generally

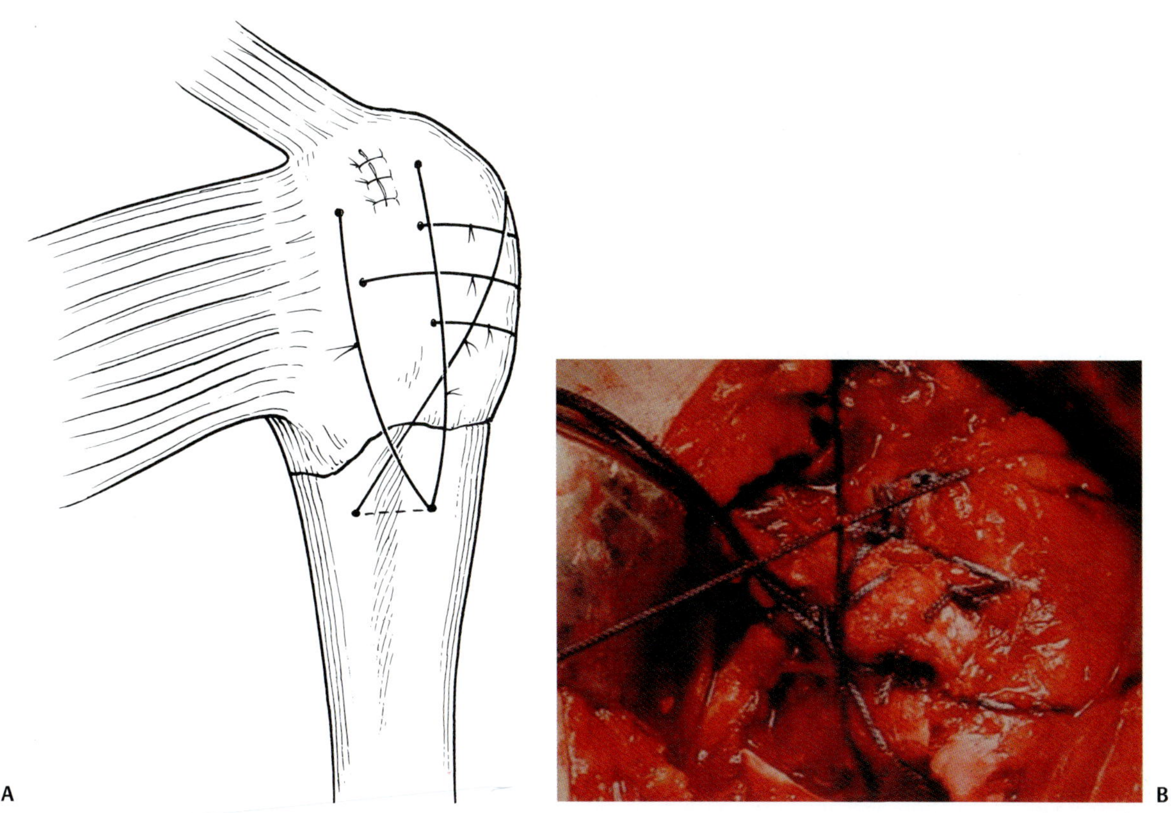

Figure 9–6 (A) Greater and lesser tuberosities fixed with sutures tied around the implant as described in the text. **(B)** Operative picture of completed tuberosity reconstruction.

~150 degrees. Noting this ROM enables the surgeon to plan the postoperative rehabilitation program properly with the physical therapist in the postoperative period.

Tuberosity position is also critical. The tuberosity must be placed below the top of the head of the prosthesis and should be placed in a position that creates normal humeral offset as described by Rietveldt et al to ensure proper deltoid function after arthroplasty.[22] Recent studies by Cuomo et al and others confirm that the tuberosities must be placed below the top of the humeral head component 0.5 to 1.0 cm for best results **(Fig. 9–7)**.[16,23–25]

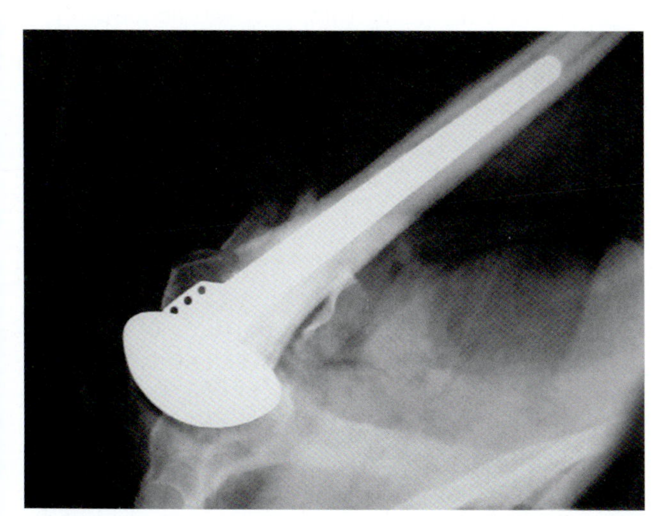

Figure 9–7 X-ray of hemiarthroplasty of the proximal humerus after displaced comminuted fracture demonstrating proper component placement and fixation of the tuberosities in proper position.

Postoperative Rehabilitation

Successful hemiarthroplasty for four-part fractures depends upon a proper rehabilitation program.[8,11,17] A physician-directed program that begins immediately after surgery and addresses the importance of early passive mobility to prevent adhesions is necessary. A sling is used for 4 to 6 weeks except during exercises. During the first 6 weeks, only passive exercises are allowed. Passive ROM exercises in the supine position and gravity-assisted pendulum exercises are instituted initially. The goal during this time is to achieve 140 degrees of elevation in a scapular plane and 30 to 35 degrees of external rotation. In cases of severe comminution, osteoporosis, or in cases where the tuberosity reconstruction is not as secure a longer period of immobilization with limited passive motion may be considered.

The passive ROM phase continues until there is clinical and roentgenographic evidence of tuberosity healing. At this point, isometric rotator cuff and deltoid exercises and active assisted elevation are initiated. At 8 weeks, once tuberosity healing is achieved, active elevation and gradual stretching to regain full ROM are encouraged. Early strength training against gravity and activities of daily living are started at this time. By 3 months, strength training is fully initiated. This includes resistance strengthening of the rotator cuff utilizing rubber tubing, light weights, and isometrics. Strengthening exercise should include scapular rotation exercises and deltoid strengthening exercises. These should be continued for up to 1 year. ROM exercises and stretching should also continue for up to 1 year as functional improvement can be expected during this time.

Complications

There are several reported complications that can occur after hemiarthroplasty for proximal humeral fractures.[1,3,8,13,17–19] The overall rate of complications has been reported as high as 35%.[1,19] Although infection or neurovascular complications have rarely been reported, technique-related complications are the most common causes of a poor result. These technique-related complications include tuberosity nonunion and/or failure, instability due to component malposition, and rotator cuff insufficiency due to failure of the tuberosity reconstruction. Scarring of the long head of the biceps tendon has been reported as a cause of restricted motion and stiffness.[26]

Instability

Placement of the humeral component in a position that is either too high or too low will lead to various forms of instability. Implants that are placed too high will lead to superior instability, leading to secondary impingement and further tuberosity failure.[18,27,28] Implants which are implanted too low will lead to poor tension in the myofascial sleeve, leading secondarily to inferior subluxation and loss of function of the rotator cuff even in the face of a good tuberosity reconstruction.

Tuberosity Reconstruction Failure

To regain proper rotator cuff function, the tuberosities must heal to the shaft of the humerus as well as themselves and around the prosthesis in the right position. Tuberosity position is also critical. The tuberosity must be placed below the top of the head of the prosthesis and should be placed in a position which creates normal humeral offset as described by Rietveldt et al[22] to ensure proper deltoid function after arthroplasty. Recent studies by Cuomo et al[23] confirm that the tuberosities must be placed below the top of the humeral head component 0.5 to 1.0 cm. In their series, those tuberosity reconstructions that were placed in this position below the top of the humeral head component had statistically significant better results than those tuberosities placed immediately below the humeral head or those that were placed above the humeral head. Placement of the tuberosities above the humeral head leads to impingement.[8,16,24,25,28–30]

Excessive humeral component retroversion or even anteversion can also lead to instability. In addition, excessive retroversion may put undue stress on the greater tuberosity reconstruction during internal rotation leading to failure of fixation or nonunion.[16,24,28] Failure of healing, or malposition of either or both tuberosities will lead to rotator cuff insufficiency and clinical failure. There are many causes for tuberosity failure, mostly related to technique. The tuberosities must be fixed to themselves and the shaft utilizing proper suture technique, bone graft, and proper postoperative rehabilitation to avoid active motion before healing has occurred. Tuberosity failure is a preventable severely disabling complication that restricts ROM, stability, and function.

Results

The results of hemiarthroplasty treatment for complex fractures including four-part fractures have been mixed.[1,3,6,8,9,11,17–19] Few authors have reported results similar to those reported in Neer's original article.[11] Others have reported more disappointing results in terms of return to function.[1,6,8,18] Most authors report minimal pain, but varying results with regard to function, motion, and strength.

Factors affecting outcomes include problems with greater tuberosity healing, patient age, the timing of surgery, and component position.[16,17,23–25,29,30] In our own earlier series, we had 85% good to excellent results utilizing sound surgical techniques and appropriate physiotherapy.[9,17] In this series and another on malunions, we found the results were better in patients younger than 70, as well as in those cases in which the hemiarthroplasty was performed less than 4 weeks from the time of injury.[9,14,17] These findings have been confirmed by others.[15,16] Utilizing the fracture sleeve described in this article, we now are able to reproduce the premorbid humeral anatomy in 90% of cases utilizing the fracture sleeve to ensure proper humeral height.

Summary

Hemiarthroplasty for complex fractures of proximal humerus is standard of care in most elderly patients who are medically stable and are able to undergo extensive physical therapy that is required. Hemiarthroplasty in this difficult set of patients is technically demanding and requires meticulous attention to surgical detail. Proper component positioning, proper tuberosity reconstruction, and appropriate physician-directed physiotherapy are mandatory for successful results.

References

1. Bigliani LU, Flatow EL, McClusky GN, Fisher RA. Failed prosthetic replacement for displaced proximal humeral fractures. Orthop Trans 1991;15:744–748
2. Biglianai LU. Fractures of the proximal humerus. In: Rockwood CA, Matsen FA, eds. The Shoulder. Philadelphia: W.B. Saunders; 1990:278–334
3. Bigliani LU, McClusky GN. Prosthetic replacement in acute fractures of the proximal humerus. Semin Arthroplasty 1990;1:129–137
4. Laing PG. The anterior blood supply of the adult humerus. J Bone Joint Surg Am 1956;38:1105–1116
5. Knight RA, Mayne JA. Comminuted fractures and fracture dislocations involving the articular surface of the humeral head. J Bone Joint Surg Am 1957;39:1343–1355
6. Schai P, Imhoff A, Preiss S. Comminuted humeral head fractures: a multicenter analysis. J Shoulder Elbow Surg 1995;4(5):319–330
7. Young TB, Wallace A. Conservative treatment of fractures and fracture dislocations of the upper end of the humerus. J Bone Joint Surg Br 1985;67:373–377
8. Zuckerman JD, Cuomo F, Koval KJ. Proximal humeral replacement for complex fractures: indications and surgical technique. In: Springfield DS, ed. Instructional Course Lectures. Vol 46. St. Louis, MO: American Academy of Orthopaedic Surgeons; 1997:7–14
9. Moeckel BH, Dines DJ, Warren RF, Altchek DW. Modular hemiarthroplasty for fractures of the proximal part of the humerus. J Bone Joint Surg Am 1992;74:884–889
10. Neer CS II. Displaced proximal humerus fractures. Part I. Classification and evaluation. J Bone Joint Surg Am 1970;52:1077–1089
11. Neer CS II. Displaced proximal humerus fractures. Part 2. Treatment of 3-part and 4-part fracture displacement. J Bone Joint Surg Am 1970;52:1090–1103
12. Neer CS II, Rockwood CA. Fractures and dislocations of the shoulder. In: Rockwood CA, Green DP, eds. Fractures. 2nd ed. Philadelphia: J.B. Lippincott; 1984:675–707
13. Bosch U, Skutek M, Frenerey W, Tsecherne H. Outcome after primary and secondary arthroplasty in elderly patients with fractures of the proximal humerus. J Shoulder Elbow Surg 1998;7:479–484
14. Dines DM, Coleman S, Warren RF. Arthroplasty for acute and chronic fractures of the proximal humerus. Orthopaedics Spec Ed 2000;1(4):25–34
15. Norris TR, Green A, McGuigan FX. Late prosthetic shoulder arthroplasty for displaced proximal humerus fractures. J Shoulder Elbow Surg 1995;4:271–280
16. Boileau P, Walch G, Krishnan S. Tuberosity osteosynthesis and hemiarthroplasty for four-part fractures of the proximal humerus. Tech Shoulder Elbow Surg 2000;1(2): 96–109
17. Dines DM, Warren RF. Modular shoulder hemiarthroplasty for acute fractures. Clin Orthop Relat Res 1994;307:18–26
18. Goldman RT, Koval KJ, Cuomo F, et al. Functional outcome after humeral head replacement for acute 3 and 4 proximal humeral fractures. J Shoulder Elbow Surg 1995;4:81–86
19. Tanner MW, Cofield RH. Prosthetic arthroplasty for fractures and fracture dislocations of the proximal humerus. Clin Orthop Relat Res 1983;179:116–128
20. Compito CA, Self EB, Bigliani LU. Arthroplasty in acute shoulder trauma. Clin Orthop Relat Res 1994;307:27–36
21. Jakob RP, Miniaci A, Anson PS, et al. Four part valgus impacted fractures of the proximal humerus. J Bone Joint Surg Br 1991;73:295–298
22. Rietveld ABN, Dannen HAM, Rozing PM, et al. The lever arm in glenohumeral abduction after hemiarthroplasty. J Bone Joint Surg Br 1988;70:561–565
23. Cuomo F, Zuckerman JD, et al. The effect of tuberosity placement on results of hemiarthroplasty for fractures of the proximal humerus. Paper presented at: open and closed meetings of the American Shoulder and Elbow Society; October 4th, 1999; Philadelphia, PA, and March 18th, 2000; Orlando, FL
24. Mighell MA, Kolm GP, Collinge CA, et al. Outcomes of hemiarthroplasty for failures of the proximal humerus. J Shoulder Elbow Surg 2003;12:569–577
25. Frankle MA, Greenwald DP, Markel BA, Ondrovic LE, Lee WE III. Biomechanical effects of malposition of tuberosity fragments on the humeral prosthetic reconstruction for four-part proximal humerus fractures. J Shoulder Elbow Surg 2001;10(4):321–326
26. Hirsch JC, Dines DM. Arthroscopy for failed shoulder arthroplasty. J Arthroscopy Related Surg. 2000;16(6):1–5
27. Dines DM, Warren RF, Altchek DW, et al. Post traumatic changes of the proximal humerus: malunion, nonunion and osteonecrosis: treatment with modular hemiarthroplasty or total shoulder arthroplasty. J Shoulder Elbow Surg 1993;2:11–21
28. Krishnan SG, Pennington SD, Burkhead WZ, Boileau P. Shoulder arthopasty for fracture: restoration of the "gothic arch." Tech Shoulder Elbow Surg 2005;6(2): 57–66
29. Green A, Barnard WL, Limbard RS. Humeral head replacementfor acute, four-part proximal humerus fractures. J Shoulder Elbow Surg 1993;2:249–254
30. Demirhan M, Kilicoglu O, Altinel L, Eralp L, Akalin Y. Prognostic factors in prosthetic replacement for acute proximal humerus fractures. J Orthop Trauma 2003;17:181–189

10 Nonunions of the Humeral Shaft

Paul S. Issack, Margaret H. Lauerman, and David L. Helfet

The humeral shaft consists of the region between the superior border of the insertion of the pectoralis major to a location just above the supracondylar ridge.[1] Fractures of this region account for 3 to 5% of all fractures; most can be managed nonoperatively with good to excellent results.[1–4] In a study of 620 patients with humeral shaft fractures treated in a functional brace, nonunion rates were 2% for closed fractures and 6% for open fractures. Varus-valgus and anteroposterior angulation were maintained within 5 degrees.[2] Perfect alignment is not essential; 20 to 30 degrees of angulation and up to 3 cm of shortening can be tolerated in the upper extremity without significant functional impairment.[1] Angulation can be compensated for functionally by motion at the shoulder and elbow and aesthetically by the musculature and subcutaneous tissues of the arm.

A nonunion of the humeral shaft is said to be present when the healing process, which should be completed by 4 months, fails to progress.[1] If union is not observed by 24 to 32 weeks after injury, the fracture is unlikely to heal and is considered a nonunion.[1,3] Humeral shaft nonunions occur in up to 10% of fractures treated nonoperatively and in up to 15% of fractures treated surgically.[1–4] As a nonunion develops, fracture lines will become wider and the edges will become sclerotic. With persistent motion at the fracture site, a synovial pseudoarthrosis or "false joint" may form with a synovium-like cavity and fluid.[5] The type of nonunion that develops depends on the blood supply to the fracture. If there is good vascularity, periosteal cartilaginous callus will form. With continued motion, endosteal callus will accumulate and seal off the medullary canal. This hypertrophic nonunion has biological healing potential, but lacks mechanical stability. Hypertrophic nonunions should be treated with rigid stabilization to provide mechanical stability; supplemental bone grafting is unnecessary. If there is poor vascularity at the fracture edges, such as after excessive surgical periosteal stripping, little callus will form and an atrophic nonunion results. In addition to providing mechanical stability, these nonunions require bone grafting to provide biological healing potential.

Etiology

Several factors contribute to the development of a humeral shaft nonunion. These can be broadly grouped into factors related to the personality of the fracture, patient characteristics, and the type of treatment rendered. Factors related to the personality of the fracture include pattern, location, and soft tissue disruption. Certain fracture patterns, such as the transverse, short oblique, or comminuted fractures, are probably more difficult to heal and are likely to go on to nonunion. There is less surface area for healing in these fractures and increased strain, with greater likelihood for displacement and granulation tissue formation.[1,3] Recently, a long lateral butterfly fragment of the humeral shaft was been described as a fracture pattern associated with nonunion.[6] The fracture originated at the junction of the proximal and middle third of the diaphysis as a hemitransverse medial fracture, which extended with a large, lateral butterfly third fragment. Eight of nine of these fractures progressed to nonunion after nonsurgical management. The healing pattern was identical in all eight: The proximal humeral fragment healed with the proximal portion of the butterfly fragment, but a nonunion between the proximal humeral fragment, the distal humeral fragment, and the distal portion of the third fragment developed.[6] Location of the fracture may also predispose to delayed union or nonunion. Fractures at the junction of the middle and distal thirds of the humeral diaphysis may disrupt the primary nutrient artery to the humerus, which may result in problems with fracture healing.[3] Blood vessels, nerves, and soft tissue can be interposed at the fracture site, resulting in nonunion and neurovascular compromise.[1,3,4] Open fractures of the humeral diaphysis are more likely to go onto nonunion than closed fractures. This is likely due to the soft tissue disruption and periosteal stripping, which occur with the open injury. These types of injuries also predispose to infections that can result in sequestrum formation, osteolysis, implant loosening, and impaired fracture healing.[1,3–5,7]

Patient factors may also predispose to the development of nonunion. Obesity may predispose a patient to development of nonunion because of difficulty immobilizing the obese arm.[3,8] Alcoholism, malnutrition, and smoking may contribute to poor healing potential.[1,3,4] Stiffness or ankylosis at the shoulder or elbow can result in increased motion at the fracture site, thus inhibiting union.[4] Finally, the type of treatment the patient receives, operative or nonoperative, may determine the healing potential of the humeral shaft fracture. Closed reduction with soft tissue interposition or overdistraction with a hanging arm cast may predispose patients to develop nonunion.[1] However, nonunions of the humeral shaft are more likely to occur after operative treatment, with rates varying according to the specific surgical intervention. Excessive surgical exposures with periosteal stripping will disrupt the vascularity and biological healing potential of fractures.[5] Treatment of humeral shaft fractures with intramedullary nailing has been reported to result in nonunion rates of 0 to 23%. Risk of nonunion remains significant following plating ranging from zero to 13%.[9–14] Irrespective of the type of implant, fixation with inadequate stabilization results in persistent motion at the fracture site. Mechanical instability will result in implant failure before fracture union.[1,3,5,7,13,15] Poor quality bone, such as in osteoporosis or pathologic fractures, may make it difficult to achieve rigid stability with internal fixation necessitating alternative techniques to achieve stability and eventually union.[4,16]

Treatment

Nonsurgical Treatment

Patients with a humeral shaft nonunion may present with limitations in function and pain that prevent them from performing activities of daily living. In general, this problem should be treated operatively. There are, however, limited indications for the nonoperative treatment of humeral shaft nonunions. If patients have little pain and functional disability or have medical comorbidities that may place them at unacceptable risk for surgical intervention, they may be managed nonsurgically in a functional brace.[2,4] Patients with a painless synovial pseudoarthrosis may require the motion at this site to compensate for stiffness at the shoulder and elbow; hence, correcting the pseudoarthrosis in these patients may result in significant loss of function of the extremity.[5,7]

Electrical stimulation of humeral shaft nonunion has a success rate of 40 to 50% and is therefore not indicated.[17] Low-intensity pulsed ultrasound and extracorporeal shock wave therapy have been reported to have inconsistent results on the healing of a nonunion.[18,19] Furthermore, these treatments cannot correct deformity; thus, they may not be able to address the functional impairment associated with nonunion.

Surgical Treatment

The goals of surgical treatment include correction of deformity and achieving union to relieve pain and restore function of the upper extremity. There are several different surgical techniques that have been described to treat humeral nonunions, including plating, intramedullary nailing, and external fixation. Generally, plating techniques are preferred to treat humeral shaft nonunions. The need for débridement of the nonunion site, bone grafting, and additional techniques to improve vascularization is determined by the biological healing potential of the nonunion (i.e., atrophic versus hypertrophic). Special techniques and implants that do not depend on screw purchase into host bone for stability may be required to treat nonunions in osteoporotic bone.

Techniques

Plating Techniques

Compression plating, with or without bone grafting, is widely considered the gold standard for treatment of humeral shaft nonunions. The humeral shaft may be approached through several exposures. The anterolateral (Henry) approach may be used to expose the proximal aspect of the shaft.[20] A posterior triceps-splitting approach may be used to expose the middle and distal aspects of the humeral shaft.[20] A modified posterior approach to the humeral shaft has been described in which the medial and lateral heads of the triceps muscle are subperiosteally elevated and retracted medially with the radial nerve.[21] With the standard posterior triceps-splitting approach without mobilization of the radial nerve, the proximal dissection can expose the distal 55% of the humerus. With the modified posterior approach, the distal 94% of the humerus can be exposed. In addition to the greater visualization of the posterior aspect of the humerus, this approach reflects the medial head of the triceps as a unit, thus maintaining continuity of the fibers and preserving triceps function. In a series of 7 patients who underwent treatment of acute humeral shaft fractures or nonunion using this approach, none had evidence of radial nerve dysfunction or triceps weakness at follow-up.[21] A medial approach, though rarely used, may reduce potential injury to the radial nerve in patients who have had previous postero-or anterolateral exposures with associated scarring. If a microvascular bone transfer is required, this approach allows access to the brachial artery and its vena comitantes.[8]

Humeral shaft nonunions treated with rigid 4.5-mm compression plating, lag screw fixation when possible, débridement of the fracture edges, and supplemental autogenous bone grafting have been demonstrated to achieve high union rates (**Fig. 10–1**).[9,15,22–25] A minimum of eight cortices of fixation proximal and distal to the fracture site should be obtained. Union rates after compression plating and bone grafting have been reported to be as high as 100%.[8,16,23,24,26] In 10 patients with humeral shaft nonunions, Foster and colleagues observed an 80% union rate with compression plating. A 73% union rate was seen in 11 humeral shaft unions treated with a

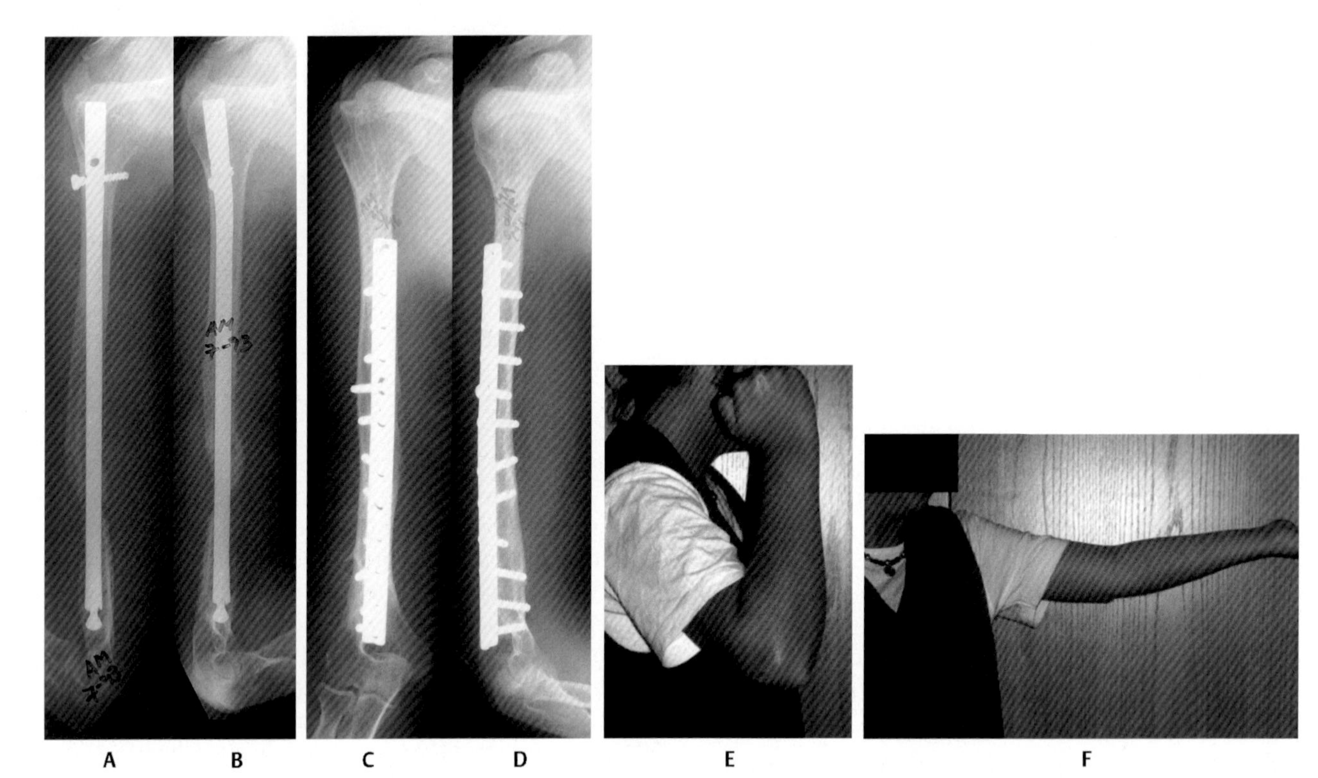

Figure 10–1 (A) Anteroposterior and **(B)** lateral radiographs of a nonunion of the humerus. The fracture was previously treated with a retrograde intramedullary device. The patient underwent an antegrade exchange nailing, but failed to heal and an atrophic nonunion developed. **(C)** Anteroposterior and **(D)** lateral radiographs of the humerus taken 3 years after treatment with a single posterior plate. **(E,F)** The nonunion healed completely with an excellent functional result. (From Rubel IF, Kloen P, Campbell D, et al. Open reduction and internal fixation of humeral nonunions: a biomechanical and clinical study. J Bone Joint Surg Am 2002; 84:1315-1322. Reprinted by permission.)

Kuntscher nail. Subacromial impingement and decreased shoulder motion were seen in the majority of patients who underwent nailing.[9]

For humeral shaft nonunions, double plating may be indicated in cases of poor bone quality, persistent micromotion after application of one plate, and to counteract significant deformity. In biomechanical studies, the combination of a posterior limited-contact dynamic compression plate and a lateral 3.5-mm reconstruction plate with or without an interfragmentary screw demonstrated greater axial and rotational stiffness than a posterior limited-contact dynamic compression plate alone.[23] In a clinical study of 37 patients plated for humeral shaft nonunions, 18 cases were double plated because of concerns about the adequacy of the stability after application of the single plate construct. No significant differences in healing rate were noted between single- and double-plating techniques; the overall union rate was 92% at an average of 4.8 months postoperatively **(Fig. 10–2)**.[23] Thus, the use of a two-plate construct may be helpful when bone quality is poor, or when micromotion is still evident at the nonunion site after application of the first plate. Although excessive soft tissue stripping is a potential concern with double plating, the dissection needed to correct deformity and debride the fibrous tissue allowed application of the second plate without additional exposure. Furthermore, the addition of the second plate did not decrease healing rates.[23]

The locking compression plate (LCP; Synthes, Paoli, PA) incorporates the option of threaded screw holes into a standard bone plate. The previous standard dynamic compression-unit plate hole has been replaced by a figure-eight screw hole with a threaded hole on one end and an oval dynamic compression plate on the other end. If osteoporosis sufficient to compromise screw purchase is encountered, the surgeon can switch to a locking screw. A screw locked to the plate functions as a fixed-angle device and does not depend on purchase between screws and host bone for stability. In addition, as locked screws do not bring the plate to the bone, there is limited contact between the plate and the bone thus preserving the blood supply to the fracture and enhancing healing. Ring and colleagues reported on 24 patients (9 delayed unions and 15 nonunions of the humeral shaft) with an average age of 72 years, who underwent fixation with a LCP with either autograft or demineralized bone matrix. All healed with 22 of 24 reporting good to excellent results.[16]

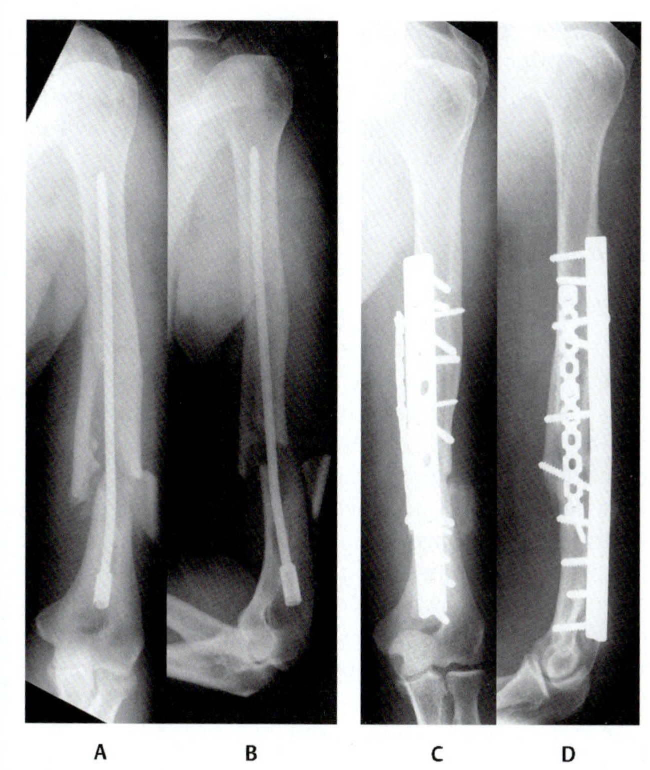

Figure 10–2 **(A)** Anteroposterior and **(B)** lateral radiographs of a nonunion of the humerus. The fracture was originally treated with a retrograde intramedullary device. **(C)** Anteroposterior and **(D)** lateral radiographs taken 8 months after open reduction and internal fixation with dual plates and an interfragmentary screw. Solid bridging callus is seen. (From Rubel IF, Kloen P, Campbell D, et al. Open reduction and internal fixation of humeral nonunions: a biomechanical and clinical study. J Bone Joint Surg Am 2002; 84-A:1315-1322. Reprinted by permission.)

For nonunions of the proximal humeral shaft, a dynamic compression plate may be contoured in a spiral fashion to preserve the insertion of the deltoid, the so-called spiral compression plate. The plate fixes the proximal humerus laterally over the greater tuberosity and anteriorly over the midhumeral shaft.[27]

Disadvantages of plating include having to open the fracture site, thus potentially devitalizing the periosteum and providing an increased risk of infection, especially in grade III open humeral shaft fractures.

Intramedullary Nailing

Intramedullary nailing, either antegrade or retrograde, may be used to treat humeral nonunions. Intramedullary nailing of humeral shaft nonunions has several disadvantages. The nail, if unlocked, does not provide rotational stability. Shoulder pain predominates secondary to injury at the rotator cuff insertion site with nail entry and subacromial impingement. Incidence of elbow pain is high following retrograde nailing. In addition, the nail may migrate out the entry site.[10,28] Union rates following intramedullary nailing are lower than that seen after plating.[10,15] Higher union rates have been described with open nailing techniques and bone grafting. Lin and colleagues[29] reported on 26 of 28 patients with a humeral shaft nonunion who achieved union following this technique. Similarly, Martinez and colleagues[30] reported on 21 of 21 patients with a humeral shaft nonunion, who achieved union following open nailing and bone grafting.

Nonunion of the humerus following failed intramedullary nailing can be difficult to manage. Removal of the previous nail can create further injury to the rotator cuff insertion resulting in shoulder pain.[10,15] These cases should be plated.[10,13,15] McKee and colleagues reported on 9 of 9 patients who achieved union following conversion to plate fixation with autogenous bone grafting. In contrast, only 4 of 10 patients achieved union following exchange nailing.[15] Robinson and associates similarly reported poor results following exchange nailing with only 2 of 5 achieving union.[10] In addition, a humerus that had failed locked nailing often demonstrated bone loss severe enough that in some cases, the cortical integrity of the bone itself was disrupted. Such bone loss cannot be reliably managed with exchange nailing.[15]

External Fixation/Ilizarov Techniques

Several authors have reported successful treatment of a humeral nonunion with the Ilizarov method.[6,31–35] Patel and colleagues reported on 16 patients with a humeral shaft nonunion following previous surgical treatment. In 10 of these cases, nonunion followed intramedullary nailing. All achieved union following application of an Ilizarov frame and compression. In the 10 patients previously treated with a nail, the nail was left in place, the locking screws were removed, and the frame was used to compress the nonunion over the nail.[35] In the remaining 6 cases, the nonunions were explored, prior hardware was removed, and fibrous tissue was débrided. Similarly, Lammens and colleagues reported on 28 of 30 patients with a humeral shaft nonunion who achieved union after application of an Ilizarov external fixator.[33] Complications include pin tract infections, shortening of up to 8 cm, refracture after frame removal, and nail protrusion. An apparent advantage of this technique is that bone graft is apparently not necessary to achieve union, even in cases of atrophic nonunion.[33–35]

After application of an Ilizarov frame, a technique termed *callus massage* has been described to stimulate healing. Short periods of progressive distraction are alternated with periods of compression (0.5 mm of distraction a day for 7 days, followed by 1 mm of compression a day for 7 days over a 4-week period). The result is net compression with union and slight, but acceptable, shortening.[34,35]

Techniques to Improve Biological Healing Potential

The biological healing capacity of the nonunion determines whether additional techniques to improve vascularization are necessary. For hypertrophic nonunions, providing mechanical stability through rigid plate fixation is sufficient to allow healing; supplemental bone grafting is not required. In an atrophic nonunion, the biological healing capacity of the fracture ends is diminished. In these nonunions, exposure and débridement of the fracture site is necessary to reestablish the medullary canal and allow for ingress of pluripotent mesenchymal cells. Bone grafting of the nonunion site is essential in an atrophic nonunion. The choice of bone graft, either autologous or allograft, is not as critical as the plating technique. Hierholzer and colleagues noted a 100% union rate in 46 humeral shaft nonunions treated with plating and iliac crest autograft and a 97% union rate in 34 humeral shaft nonunions treated with demineralized bone matrix. Time to union was similar in both groups with union at 4.5 months in the iliac crest autograft group and 4.1 months in the demineralized bone matrix group. Functional outcome did not differ between the two groups. However, because 37% of patients who underwent bone graft harvesting from the iliac crest demonstrated prolonged donor site pain,[36] demineralized bone matrix may become the standard choice of graft augmentation.

In atrophic nonunions, techniques to improve vascularity such as bridge plating, shingling, or petaling are recommended.[5,7,25] Bridge plating preserves the vascular envelope provided by the surrounding muscle. The plate is contoured so that a gap of 0.5 to 1 cm is left between the bone and the plate at the site of the nonunion minimizing devascularization in this region.[25] The gap, which extends from one screw hole proximal to one screw hole distal to the limits of the bone defect, allows circulation from the surrounding soft tissue envelope to supply the autograft. Ring and colleagues reported on 14 of 15 patients with atrophic nonunion who achieved union at a mean follow-up of 30 months with a bridge plate and cancellous autograft. All patients with healed fractures had no pain and good function.

Shingling and petaling may be used to revascularize the cortex around a nonunion. Shingling, or decortication, is the raising of thin osteoperiosteal flaps with a sharp osteotome from the outer cortex from both sides of the nonunion. Fragments ~2 to 3 mm thick and ~2 cm long are elevated on either side of the nonunion for approximately two thirds the circumference of the bone. The periosteum and muscle are attached to the elevated fragments preserving the vascularity of these fragments. Cancellous bone graft can be inserted into the space between the shingles and the decorticated cortex.[5] Gentler procedures such as petaling are recommended for osteoporotic bone. Petaling or fish-scaling can be performed with a gouge, elevating osteoperiosteal flakes. Alternatively, cortical bone flanking the nonunion can be drilled with a 2.7-mm drill bit. These procedures should be performed on the side of the bone not covered with the plate.[5]

Special Situations

Infection

The treatment of an infected nonunion requires solving two problems sequentially: (1) eradication of the infection, and (2) achievement of fracture union. The evaluation of an infected nonunion begins with a history to determine the length of time the infection and nonunion have been present and previous surgical and nonsurgical treatments. The longer an infection has been present, the more likely a chronic osteomyelitis has taken hold, which often requires bony débridement. Physical examination of the skin and previous surgical incisions as well as presence of sinus tracts should be noted. Preoperative laboratory studies, specifically a white blood count (CBC), C-reactive protein screening, and erythrocyte sedimentation rate (ESR), will allow for a diagnosis of infection to be made and will provide easily measured serum markers, which may be followed after surgical débridement to evaluate resolution of infection. Definitive treatment requires thorough débridement of the nonunion site, rigid internal fixation, and postoperative culture-specific antibiotics. These cultures should be deep cultures obtained from the bone intraoperatively to be reliable.[7]

Osteopenia

There are several modifications of standard internal fixation that may be used to enhance fixation in osteopenic bone. Loose 4.5-mm cortical screws may be replaced with 6.5-mm cancellous bone screws. Alternatively, polymethylmethacrylate cement can be placed into screw holes in a semiliquid state. Screws are placed in the holes and tightened when the cement has hardened.[5] Cortical allograft or fibular autograft struts can be placed medially, opposite the plate. A screw can be passed across both cortices of the humerus and both cortices of an allograft strut to gain quadricortical purchase.[37,38] Biomechanical studies have shown that quadricortical fixation is stronger than bicortical fixation.[39] Union rates of up to 100% within 4 months have been reported in humeral shaft nonunions treated with this technique.[37,38] Fibular allograft struts can also be placed in the medullary cavity with screws passing through the fibula and both humeral cortices. Eight of nine humeral shaft nonunions treated with this technique united at an average of 3.5 months.

With standard nonlocking plates, host bone quality determines screw purchase. The stability of the plate–bone construct results from friction between the undersurface of the plate and the bone and requires bicortical purchase to prevent toggling of the screws. Fixed angle implants such as the blade plate, the addition of spiked nuts (Schuli nuts; Synthes, Paoli, PA) that lock screws into the plate,[40] or locked compression plates in which the threads on the screw head lock into corresponding threads on the screw hole of the plate are helpful when bone quality is poor.[41] The screws cannot toggle in the plate. With locked plating, compression of the plate to the underlying bone is not required to achieve construct stability. It is therefore not essential to obtain bicortical purchase to achieve stability.[41] Ring and colleagues[16] obtained union in 24 osteoporotic delayed unions or nonunions of the humeral shaft using a single locked compression plate.

Segmental Bone Defects

Microvascular-free bone transfer is advantageous in treating humeral nonunion with local devascularization and infection. Its success does not depend on the surrounding soft tissue envelope, which may be ischemic from previous surgery, infection, or trauma. Vascularized fibular graft, corticoperiosteal graft from the medial supracondylar region of the femur and scapular grafts have been used as donors.[8,42] Jupiter reported on 4 patients with an atrophic nonunion of the humeral shaft treated with a medial approach, an anterior plate, and vascularized fibular graft. The graft was inserted into the medullary canal medially if the cortex was deficient or a trough was fashioned on the medial aspect of the humeral cortex to inlay the graft. The graft was fixed to the humerus with one screw on each end and peroneal anastomoses with the brachial artery and venae comitantes was performed. Three of four healed within 4 months with regained use of the injured limb. The fourth case required a longer plate and additional grafting to heal.[8] Muramatsu and colleagues reported on 21 of 23 humeral shaft nonunions, which healed with vascularized grafts from the fibula, femur, or scapula at an average time of 6, 4, and 7 months, respectively. Donor site complications were minimal.[42]

Bone transport with the Ilizarov technique has also been used to treat humeral shaft nonunion with significant bone loss and shortening. Sidor and colleagues reported on eight cases of humeral length deficits in which a 9.8 cm mean lengthening was achieved using the Ilizarov technique. All achieved over 80% of the desired length with six restored to full length. No permanent neurovascular or infectious complication occurred.[43] Pullen and colleagues[30] reported on 4 patients with humeral shaft nonunion and shortening treated with a hybrid Ilizarov frame. Three nonunions were atrophic and infected, and one was hypertrophic. All patients obtained union of the humeral fracture with resolution of infection. Length was restored to within 1 cm in 3 patients; the fourth patient had a residual limb length discrepancy of 3 cm, but began with 11 cm of shortening. Complications included pin tract infections and refracture after removal of the fixator.

Pathologic Bone

Humeral shaft fractures in patients with metabolic bone diseases such as osteoporosis, Paget's disease, and tumors, present two challenges for treatment: (1) poor quality bone that compromises the stability of internal fixation, and (2) diminished healing potential. In these patients, there is an uncoupling of bone formation and bone resorption, which diminishes the material and structural properties of bone and increases the likelihood of development of a humeral shaft nonunion.[44,45] Bisphosphonate drugs such as alendronate have been used to restore this balance by decreasing bone resorption; this improves bone density and strength.[45–47] In a patient with a fracture, however, these agents may inhibit healing. Remodeling is impaired and although increases in callus strength may be noted, the quality of bone formed is poor.[48,49] Clinical trials specifically addressing the effect of bisphosphonates on fracture healing will provide an optimal treatment algorithm for the use of these agents in the osteoporotic patient who has sustained a fracture.

Parathyroid hormone (PTH) is an agent that appears to have promise in the treatment of nonunions in pathologic bone. PTH is an anabolic agent that enhances osteoblastic bone formation. Teriparatide, the active N-terminal fragment of PTH (residues 1–34) has been approved by the U.S. Food and Drug Administration for the treatment of postmenopausal women with osteoporosis who are at high risk for fracture.[44] When administered in intermittent doses, PTH can increase bone density, bone quality, and accelerate healing in animal fracture models.[50–52] Caution must be exercised when using PTH when the underlying cause of the pathologic bone is a tumor; PTH may act as a growth factor and enhance the aggressiveness of the tumor. The potential role of PTH in treating nonunions must be further examined in animal models and clinical trials.

Bone morphogenetic proteins (BMPs) may play a role in the treatment of difficult humeral shaft nonunions in metabolic bone diseases. Recombinant forms of human BMPs have been used clinically to promote healing in tibial shaft nonunions and appear to have the ability to promote union at other sites.[53–57] As in the case of PTH, potential stimulation of an underlying malignancy is a concern with their use in pathologic bone. Further clinical trials are necessary to fully define the role of these agents in the treatment of humeral shaft nonunions.

Summary

Humeral shaft nonunions are a challenging problem and can result in significant pain and disability. Treatment requires identifying the potential mechanical and biological causes for the impaired healing. Although nonoperative treatment is indicated in limited instances, nonunion is essentially a problem that should be treated surgically. Mechanical stability can be most reliably achieved with open reduction and internal fixation with compression plating; the indications for intramedullary nailing and external fixation are more limited. A poor biological healing response can be augmented with several techniques to improve vascularity including bone grafting, shingling/petaling, and bridge plating. Special techniques such as cement augmentation, quadricortical fixation into allograft or autograft, and locked plating are used to address osteopenia. Microvascular free bone transfer and bone transport with the Ilizarov device are used to treat segmental bone defects. Finally, nonunions in patients with metabolic bone diseases may require newer pharmacotherapies to enhance osteogenesis. Addressing both the mechanical and biological causes of failed fracture healing should reliably improve union rates and function.

References

1. Zuckerman JD, Koval KJ. Fractures of the shaft of the humerus. In: CAJ Rockwood CAJ, Green DP, Bucholz RW, Heckman JD, eds. Rockwood and Green's Fractures in Adults. 4th ed. Philadelphia, PA: Lippincott-Raven; 1996:1025–1053
2. Sarmiento A, Zagorski JB, Zych GA, Latta LL, Capps CA. Functional bracing for the treatment of fractures of the humeral diaphysis. J Bone Joint Surg Am 2000;82:478–486
3. Jupiter JB, von Deck M. Ununited humeral diaphyses. J Shoulder Elbow Surg 1998;7:644–653
4. Pugh DM, McKee MD. Advances in the management of humeral nonunion. J Am Acad Orthop Surg 2003;11:48–59
5. Rosen H. Nonunion and malunion. In: Browner BD, Jupiter JB, Levine AM, Trafton PG, eds. Skeletal Trauma: Fractures, Dislocations, Ligamentous Injuries. 2nd ed. Philadephia, PA: W.B. Saunders; 1998:619–660
6. Castella FB, Garcia FB, Berry EM, et al. Nonunion of the humeral shaft: long lateral butterfly fracture–a nonunion predictive pattern? Clin Orthop Relat Res 2004;424: 227–230
7. Rosen H. The treatment of nonunions and pseudarthroses of the humeral shaft. Orthop Clin North Am 1990;21: 725–742
8. Jupiter JB. Complex non-union of the humeral diaphysis. Treatment with a medial approach, an anterior plate, and a vascularized fibular graft. J Bone Joint Surg Am 1990; 72:701–707
9. Foster RJ, Dixon GLJ, Bach AW, Appleyard RW, Green TM. Internal fixation of fractures and non-unions of the humeral shaft. Indications and results in a multi-center study. J Bone Joint Surg Am 1985;67:857–864
10. Robinson CM, Bell KM, Court-Brown CM, McQueen MM. Locked nailing of humeral shaft fractures. Experience in Edinburgh over a two-year period. J Bone Joint Surg Br 1992;74:558–562
11. Rommens PM, Verbruggen J, Broos PL. Retrograde locked nailing of humeral shaft fractures. A review of 39 patients. J Bone Joint Surg Br 1995;77:84–89
12. Crates J, Whittle AP. Antegrade interlocking nailing of acute humeral shaft fractures. Clin Orthop Relat Res 1998;350:40–50
13. Flinkkila T, Ristiniemi J, Hamalainen M. Nonunion after intramedullary nailing of humeral shaft fractures. J Trauma 2001;50:540–544
14. Chapman JR, Henley MB, Agel J, Benca PJ. Randomized prospective study of humeral shaft fracture fixation: intramedullary nails versus plates. J Orthop Trauma 2000; 14:162–166
15. McKee MD, Miranda MA, Riemer BL, et al. Management of humeral nonunion after the failure of locking intramedullary nails. J Orthop Trauma 1996;10:492–499
16. Ring D, Kloen P, Kadzielski J, Helfet D, Jupiter JB. Locking compression plates for osteoporotic nonunions of the diaphyseal humerus. Clin Orthop Relat Res 2004;425:50–54
17. Esterhai JLJ, Brighton CT, Heppenstall RB, Thrower A. Nonunion of the humerus. Clinical, roentgenographic, scintigraphic, and response characteristics to treatment with constant direct current stimulation of osteogenesis. Clin Orthop Relat Res 1986;211:228–234
18. Biedermann R, Martin A, Handle G, et al. Extracorporeal shock waves in the treatment of nonunions. J Trauma 2003;54:936–942
19. Nolte PA, van der Krans A, Patka P, et al. Low-intensity pulsed ultrasound in the treatment of nonunions. J Trauma 2001;51:693–702
20. Hoppenfeld S, deBoer P. Surgical Exposures in Orthopaedics: The Anatomic Approach. Philadelphia, PA: J.B. Lippincott; 1994
21. Gerwin M, Hotchkiss RN, Weiland AJ. Alternative operative exposures of the posterior aspect of the humeral diaphysis with reference to the radial nerve. J Bone Joint Surg Am 1996;78:1690–1695
22. Borus TA, Yian EH, Karunakar MA. A case series and review of salvage surgery for refractory humeral shaft nonunion following two or more prior surgical procedures. Iowa Orthop J 2005;25:194–199

23. Rubel IF, Kloen P, Campbell D, et al. Open reduction and internal fixation of humeral nonunions: a biomechanical and clinical study. J Bone Joint Surg Am 2002;84-A:1315–1322
24. Marti RK, Verheyen CC, Besselaar PP. Humeral shaft nonunion: evaluation of uniform surgical repair in fifty-one patients. J Orthop Trauma 2002;16:108–115
25. Ring D, Jupiter JB, Quintero J, Sanders RA, Marti RK. Atrophic ununited diaphyseal fractures of the humerus with a bony defect: treatment by wave-plate osteosynthesis. J Bone Joint Surg Br 2000;82:867–871
26. Otsuka NY, McKee MD, Liew A, et al. The effect of comorbidity and duration of nonunion on outcome after surgical treatment for nonunion of the humerus. J Shoulder Elbow Surg 1998;7:127–133
27. Gill DR, Torchia ME. The spiral compression plate for proximal humeral shaft nonunion: a case report and description of a new technique. J Orthop Trauma 1999;13:141–144
28. Lin J, Shen PW, Hou SM. Complications of locked nailing in humeral shaft fractures. J Trauma 2003;54:943–949
29. Lin J, Hou SM, Hang YS. Treatment of humeral shaft delayed unions and nonunions with humeral locked nails. J Trauma 2000;48:695–703
30. Martinez AA, Herrera A, Cnenca J. Good results with unreamed nail and bone grafting for humeral nonunion: a retrospective study of 21 patients. Acta Orthop Scand 2002;73:273–276
31. Pullen C, Manzotti A, Catagni MA, Guerreschi F. Treatment of post-traumatic humeral diaphyseal nonunion with bone loss. J Shoulder Elbow Surg 2003;12:436–441
32. Catagni MA, Guerreschi F, Probe RA. Treatment of humeral nonunions with the Ilizarov technique. Bull Hosp Jt Dis Orthop Inst 1991;51:74–83
33. Lammens J, Bauduin G, Driesen R, et al. Treatment of nonunion of the humerus using the Ilizarov external fixator. Clin Orthop Relat Res 1998;353:223–230
34. Raschke M, Khodadadyan C, Maitino PD, Hoffmann R, Sudkamp NP. Nonunion of the humerus following intramedullary nailing treated by Ilizarov hybrid fixation. J Orthop Trauma 1998;12:138–141
35. Patel VR, Menon DK, Pool RD, Simonis RB. Nonunion of the humerus after failure of surgical treatment. Management using the Ilizarov circular fixator. J Bone Joint Surg Br 2000;82:977–983
36. Hierholzer C, Sama D, Toro JB, Helfet DL. Plate ORIF of humeral shaft delayed unions and nonunions of the humeral shaft: is healing dependent on type of bone graft? J Bone Joint Surg Am 2006; 88:1442–1447
37. Hornicek FJ, Zych GA, Hutson JJ, Malinin TI. Salvage of humeral nonunions with onlay bone plate allograft augmentation. Clin Orthop Relat Res 2001;386:203–209
38. Van Houwelingen AP, McKee MD. Treatment of osteopenic humeral shaft nonunion with compression plating, humeral cortical allograft struts, and bone grafting. J Orthop Trauma 2005;19:36–42
39. Wright TW, Miller GJ, Vander Griend RA, Wheeler D, Dell PC. Reconstruction of the humerus with an intramedullary fibular graft. A clinical and biomechanical study. J Bone Joint Surg Br 1993;75:804–807
40. Ring D, Perey BH, Jupiter JB. The functional outcome of operative treatment of ununited fractures of the humeral diaphysis in older patients. J Bone Joint Surg Am 1999; 81:177–190
41. Haidukewych GJ. Innovations in locking plate technology. J Am Acad Orthop Surg 2004;12:205–212
42. Muramatsu K, Doi K, Ihara K, Shigetomi M, Kawai S. Recalcitrant posttraumatic nonunion of the humerus: 23 patients reconstructed with vascularized bone graft. Acta Orthop Scand 2003;74:95–97
43. Sidor ML, Golyakhovsky V, Frankel VH. Humeral lengthening and bone transport using the Ilizarov technique. Bull Hosp Joint Dis 1992;52:13–16
44. Madore GR, Sherman PJ, Lane JM. Parathyroid hormone. J Am Acad Orthop Surg 2004;12:67–71
45. Lin JT, Lane JM. Bisphosphonates. J Am Acad Orthop Surg 2003;11:1–4
46. Levis S, Quandt SA, Thompson D, et al. Alendronate reduces the risk of multiple symptomatic fractures: results from the fracture intervention trial. J Am Geriatr Soc 2002;50:409–415
47. Black DM, Cummings SR, Karpf DB, et al. Randomised trial of effect of alendronate on risk of fracture in women with existing vertebral fractures. Fracture Intervention Trial Research Group. Lancet 1996;348:1535–1541
48. Adolphson P, Abbaszadegan H, Boden H, Salemyr M, Henriques T. Clodronate increases mineralization of callus after Colles' fracture: a randomized, double-blind, placebo-controlled, prospective trial in 32 patients. Acta Orthop Scand 2000;71:195–200
49. Peter CP, Cook WO, Nunamaker DM, et al. Effect of alendronate on fracture healing and bone remodeling in dogs. J Orthop Res 1996;14:74–79
50. Alexander JM, Bab I, Fish S, et al. Human parathyroid hormone 1–34 reverses bone loss in ovariectomized mice. J Bone Miner Res 2001;16:1665–1673
51. Alkhiary YM, Gerstenfeld LC, Krall E, et al. Enhancement of experimental fracture-healing by systemic administration of recombinant human parathyroid hormone (PTH 1–34). J Bone Joint Surg Am 2005;87:731–741
52. Kim HW, Jahng J. Effect of intermittent administration of parathyroid hormone on fracture healing in ovariectomized rats. Iowa Orthop J 1999;19:71–77
53. Zlotolow DA, Vaccaro AR, Salamon ML, Albert TJ. The role of human bone morphogenetic proteins in spinal fusion. J Am Acad Orthop Surg 2000;8:3–9
54. Issack PS, DiCesare PE. Recent advances toward the clinical application of bone morphogenetins proteins in bone and cartilage repair. Am J Orthop 2003;32: 429–436
55. Makino T, Hak DJ, Hazelwood SJ, Curtiss S, Reddi AH. Prevention of atrophic nonunion development by recombinant human bone morphogenetic protein-7. J Orthop Res 2005;23:632–638
56. Friedlaender GE, Perry CR, Cole JD, et al. Osteogenic protein-1 (bone morphogenetic protein-7) in the treatment of tibial nonunions. J Bone Joint Surg Am 2001;83-A:S151–S158
57. Govender S, Csimma C, Genant HK, et al. Recombinant human bone morphogenetic protein-2 for treatment of open tibial fractures: a prospective, controlled, randomized study of four hundred and fifty patients. J Bone Joint Surg Am 2002;84-A:2123–2134

11 Complex Fractures of the Distal Humerus

Jesse B. Jupiter

Injuries involving the distal humerus comprise a constellation of complex articular injuries.[1-5] Although recommendations for treatment have varied,[6,7] there has now been general acceptance of the advantages of operative treatment.[8-28] Advances have been made in understanding the variety of fracture patterns, preoperative imaging, surgical exposures, and the techniques and technology for the internal fixation of these difficult fractures–yet several recognized difficulties and complications remain.[29-39] These include loss of elbow mobility, nonunion, malunion, posttraumatic arthritis, and ulnar nerve dysfunction.

In this chapter, I will concentrate on contemporary issues in the assessment and management of distal humeral fractures, as well as complex fracture patterns. These include multifragmentary articular fractures at or distal to the olecranon sulcus, chondral articular shearing fractures, fractures involving osteopenic bone, and the issues involved with the alternative of total elbow arthroplasty as definitive fracture management. Issues related to surgical exposures, new technologies for internal fixation, and postoperative rehabilitation will be highlighted. The assessment and management of complications postfracture will be addressed elsewhere in this text.

Anatomy

An understanding of the operative anatomy of the distal end of the humerus and its correlation to resultant fracture patterns and surgical fixation is essential.[40] The distal humerus is composed of two bony columns, one medial and one lateral, which flare out distally and are separated by the olecranon and coronoid fossa and, more distally, the trochlea.

The goal in the surgical reconstruction of the articular anatomy and bony support of the distal humerus is to reconstruct an equilateral triangle consisting of both columns and the intervening trochlea. Instability of the fixation of any one of these three limbs will dramatically weaken the entire surgical repair. Some of the contemporary issues regarding the type and location of plate fixation that will provide optimal skeletal repair will be discussed later.

What is important to understand is the relevant relationship of the ulnar and radial nerves to the posterior aspect of the distal humerus. Approximately 10 cm proximal to the medial epicondyle, the ulnar nerve traverses the medial intermuscular septum from the anterior to posterior compartments. The nerve passes distal and posterior to the medial epicondyle enclosed in a fibrous sheath, which is the top of the cubital tunnel. Upon exiting, it courses between the two heads of the flexor carpi ulnaris traveling distally through the anterior compartment of the forearm.

The radial nerve crosses the posterior aspect of the humerus ~20 cm proximal to the medial epicondyle. The nerve splits into a branch to the medial head of the triceps, the lower lateral brachial cutaneous nerve, and the posterior interosseous and superficial radial sensory nerves. The posterior interosseous nerve traverses through the lateral intermuscular septum ~10 cm proximal to the lateral epicondyle.

Patient Assessment

Radiologic Evaluation

With the exception of "simpler" fracture patterns such as the "T" or "Y" fractures, the more complex multifragmented or "smashed" fractures, or those featuring chondral shearing components are not readily appreciated from standard radiographs, even those obtained after traction applied to the arm.[41] The evolution of computed tomography (CT) scanning, especially three-dimensional (3D) reconstructions, have added immeasurably to more accurately assessing the fracture patterns preoperatively **(Fig. 11–1)**.[42]

The reliability and diagnostic accuracy of two-dimensional (2D) versus 3D CT in the classification and management of distal humeral intraarticular fractures was evaluated in our Hand and Upper Extremity Center. Five independent observers evaluated CT scans of 30 consecutive fractures for the presence of five fracture characteristics: a coronal plane fracture line, articular comminution, metaphyseal comminution, presence of separate entirely articular fragments, and articular surface impaction. The results showed that 3D CT reconstruction improved both the intra- and interobserver reliability for the AO/ASIF comprehensive classification and the Mehne/Malta classification systems when compared with 2D CT scans.

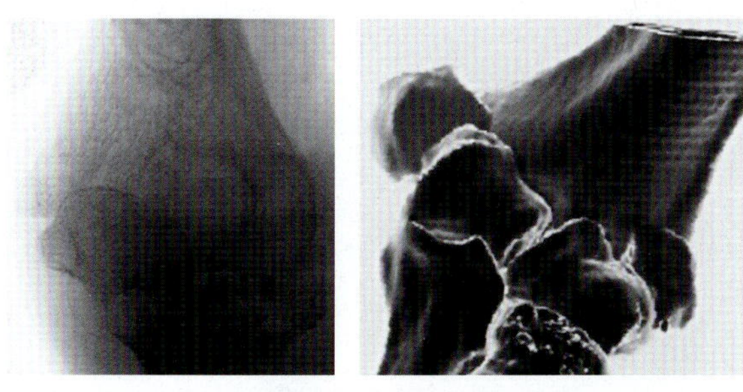

Figure 11–1 The development of three-dimensional computed tomography (CT) scanning has greatly enhanced the preoperative understanding of complex articular fractures. **(A)** This shearing articular fracture is poorly visualized in standard radiographs. **(B)** The three-dimensional CT more accurately depicts the fracture.

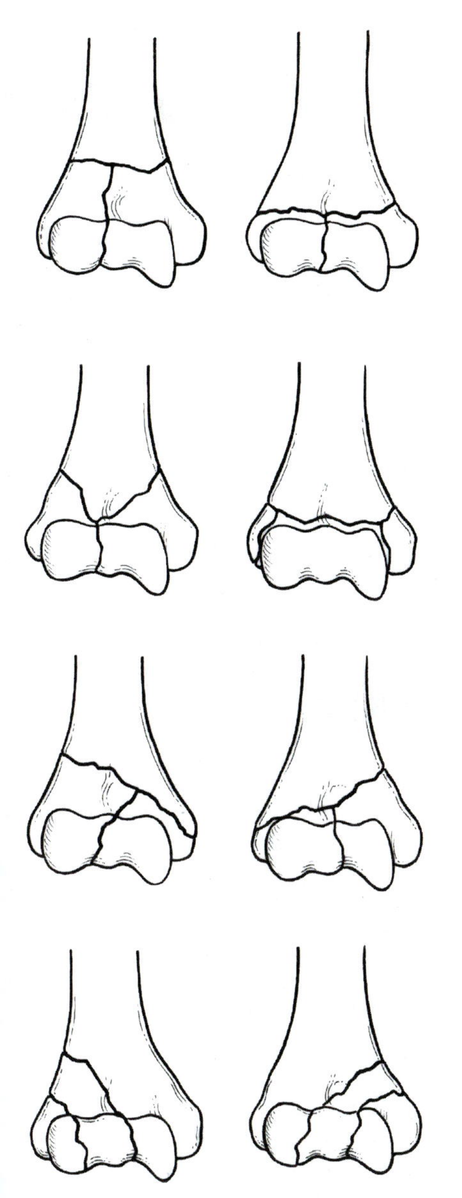

Figure 11–2 The Mehne and Matta classification is useful to appreciate variable patterns of bony column involvement.

Classification

The historical convention of describing intraarticular distal humeral fractures as "T" or "Y" fractures has been supplanted by more detailed attempts to define the specific features of each fracture.[43–46] Rather than describe the variety of classifications, I will concentrate on but a few contemporary useful classifications.

Mehne and Malta based their classification on the surgical anatomy as well as the involvement of the distal humeral bony columns **(Fig. 11–2)**.[37,47] Four basic categories were identified–intraarticular, extraarticular, intracapsular, and extracapsular. The intraarticular fractures are divided into single or bicolumnar injuries, and capitellar fractures or trochlea fractures. The bicolumnar fractures can be viewed both by the slope as well as location of the fracture lines and the orientation of the intraarticular components(s). The "H" type would represent the more complex intraarticular patterns with articular fragments separated with adequate bony support.

The comprehensive classification (AO/ASIF) system represents an alphanumeric system with three major types including extraarticular (type A), partial articular (type B), and complete articular (type C).[48,49] Within each type are three groups and three subgroups, extending from simple to more complex fracture patterns involving both articular and metaphyseal involvement (see Chapter 13, Fig. 13–1).

There continues to be an evolution in recognition and classification of the articular injuries of the distal humerus.[50] A constellation of patterns of articular shearing fractures has been identified with their basic feature being little or no supporting metaphyseal subchondral bone.[51–53] Understanding the specific features of the fracture patterns will play an important role in decision-making and operative tactics. Although some patterns have been identified within the comprehensive classification B3 group, the full extent of the variation and complexity has only recently been described. With the advent of 3D CT reconstruction, a more accurate representation of the fracture pattern preoperatively will permit more accurate preoperative planning of both the surgical approach as well as method of internal fixation **(Fig. 11–3)**. The specific fracture types reflect a progression of injury severity extending from an isolated capitellum (B3.1), trochlea fracture (B3.2), or combined capitellar-trochlea (coronal shear) displaced in the frontal plane to combinations of shearing and impaction injury of both articular surface and distal metaphyseal bone.[19, 54] Those injuries associated with impaction may prove to be the most difficult to reduce anatomically unless the metaphyseal bony impaction is recognized and elevated.

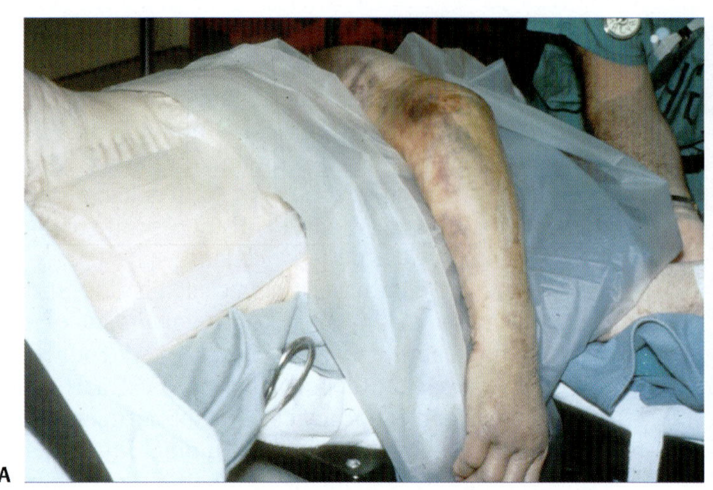

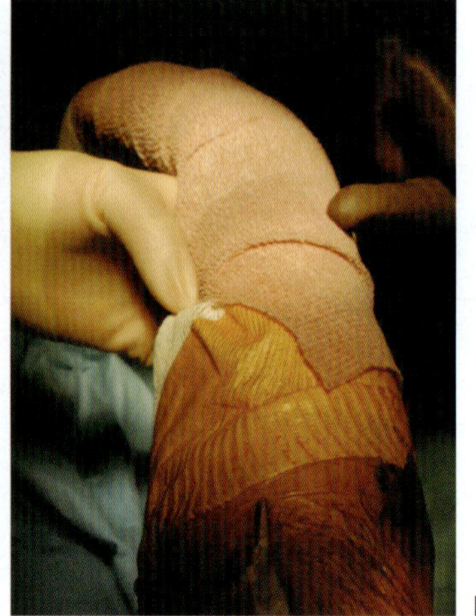

Figure 11–3 The lateral decubitus position permits excellent access to the injured limb as well as to the ipsilateral iliac crest. **(A)** The patient is placed in the lateral position with surgical preparation of the ipsilateral iliac crest. **(B)** Dependent edema of the hand and forearm is prevented by wrapping the distal limb in elastic wrap. (Case courtesy of Dr. David King.)

Treatment

Surgical Treatment

For the more complex distal humeral fractures, patient positioning and surgical exposure is crucial to achieving a successful result.[55] The patient's position will depend, in part, upon the surgeon's preference as well as the nature of fracture and/or associated injuries. With the exception of some chondral shearing fractures, which may be approached through a lateral incision with the patient supine and arm extended on a hand table, the preferred position would be in the lateral decubitus or prone position **(Fig. 11–3)**. The ipsilateral iliac crest can be prepared and draped in the event that autogenous bone graft will be required. As the repair of these fractures may prove technically difficult and lengthy, general anesthesia and the use of a sterile tourniquet are preferred.

Under sterile tourniquet control, a straight dorsal incision is made elevating the medial and lateral skin flaps.[56] The traditional approach is to curve the incision slightly around the tip of the olecranon to avoid hypersensitivity upon contact; however, I have never found this to be necessary.

How to approach and protect the ulnar nerve is a subject of continued discussion. Although it is very reasonable to expose the nerve and perhaps protect it with a nerve loop, continued traction on the nerve during the procedure will risk a traction neuritis.[28, 57] By the same token, will mobilization of the nerve proximally up to the medial intermuscular septum and distally through the two heads of the flexor carpi ulnaris to end up in a subcutaneous position really prevent postsurgical nerve dysfunction **(Fig. 11–4)**? In a preliminary study in our service comparing a cohort of patients in whom the ulnar nerve was identified at the onset of the procedure but not mobilized with a similar group of patients in whom the nerve was extensively mobilized and moved into a subcutaneous position, there was no statistically significant difference in postoperative ulnar nerve dysfunction.

Although the more commonly used approaches have been both through an olecranon osteotomy or triceps splitting exposure, several additional options exist and may prove useful for specific fracture problems.

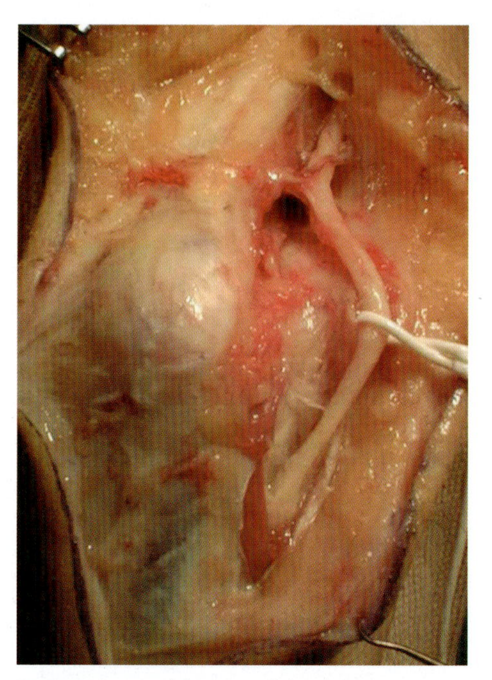

Figure 11–4 Mobilization of the ulnar nerve 6 cm proximal and distal to the cubital tunnel will permit the nerve to lie in a subcutaneous position at the conclusion of the surgery.

The transolecranon approach will provide excellent exposure,[58] but enthusiasm for this technique has been tempered by reports identifying associated complications including nonunion, hardware prominence, or proximal migration of longitudinal Kirschner wires, which may inhibit elbow extension.[59,60] In addition, when faced with multifragmented fractures in the older patient where total elbow arthroplasty would be an option, an alternative exposure will be required.[61]

When performing the olecranon osteotomy, several technical features will help minimize potential complications **(Fig. 11–5)**.[62] The osteotomy is preferentially done in the middle of the olecranon, where there is the least amount of articular cartilage. By elevating part of the anconeus, this can be directly visualized. The creating of a "chevron" osteotomy with the apex pointed distally will enhance later realignment and fixation. I have found that placing two Kirschner wires obliquely from the dorsal aspect of the proximal ulna to exit just medial to the ventral ridge of the ulna will avoid the wires "backing out" as well as impinging upon the radius during forearm rotation. For the tension band, I use two smaller gauge stainless steel wires (20- or 22-gauge) spaced several centimeters apart in the proximal ulna. These wires are brought under the attachment of the triceps against the very tip of the proximal olecranon. Lastly, to help prevent the Kirschner wires from migrating proximally, these are bent into two 90-degree bends and hammered into the proximal olecranon. There has been some concern regarding the stability of such fixation and whether or not early mobilization is advisable. I

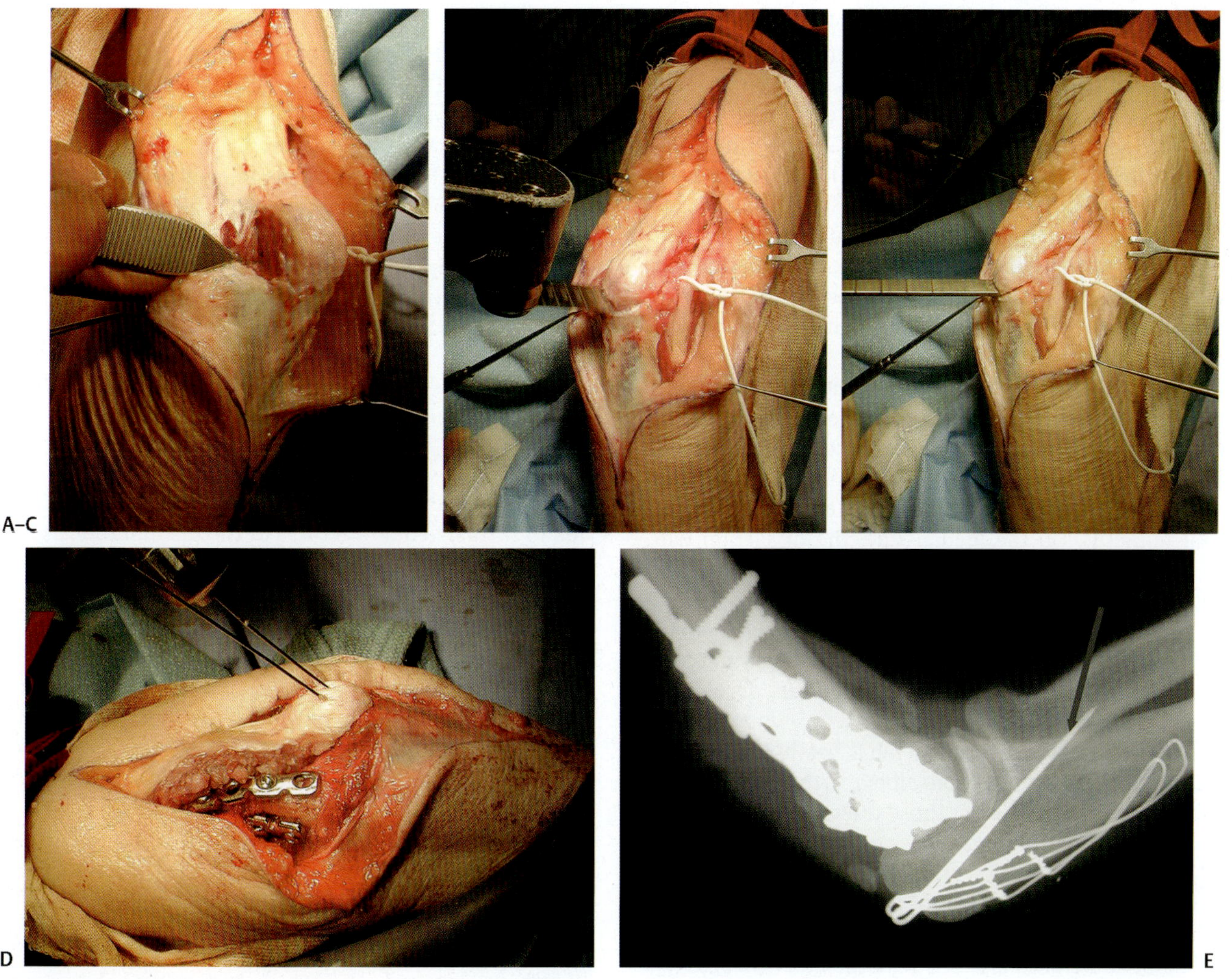

Figure 11–5 The technical points of performing an olecranon osteotomy. **(A)** By elevation of a small portion of the anconeus, direct exposure of the olecranon articular surface permits a more accurate placement of the osteotomy in the center where there is a minimal amount of articular cartilage. **(B)** Using a thin blade, a cut is created in a chevron pattern, stopping just at the opposite cortex. **(C)** The osteotomy is completed using a thin blade osteotomy. **(D)** Fixation of the osteotomy begins with two smooth 0.45-inch Kirschner wires, directed toward the anterior cortex of the proximal ulna and away from the proximal radius to avoid impingement. **(E)** Two tension wire loops enhance fixation and the proximal Kirschner wires are bent in a 90-degree fashion and impacted into the proximal olecranon.

have not found this to be the case at all. In a consecutive series of 44 olecranon osteotomies that I performed, there were no nonunions with requirement for second procedure to gain union.[63] Only 13% of patients required a second procedure to remove symptomatic wires.

Alternative surgical exposures include the paratricipital posterior approach, triceps split exposure, triceps-reflecting anconeus pedicle (TRAP), triceps sparing elevation, and/or extended lateral exposure.[64] The paratricipital posterior approach involves mobilization of the triceps from the medial and lateral intermuscular septa, as well as posterior aspect of the humerus.[65,66] This exposure may be more applicable for these fractures at the supracondylar level or simple articular injuries or those complex fractures in which arthroplasty is to be performed. The paratricipital approach will be less optimal for more complex articular injuries especially those at or distal to the olecranon sulcus.

The triceps-splitting approach involves splitting the triceps in the midline from the distal third of the humerus to the proximal one fourth of the length of the ulna.[67] This approach may prove advantageous in open fractures in which the distal tip of the humeral shaft penetrates the triceps aponecrosis. It is critical to repair the triceps back to the proximal ulna with transosseous suture, as an inadequate repair can adversely affect elbow extension and may inhibit postoperative rehabilitation. When performed carefully, McKee and colleagues[68] found no difference in the strength of elbow extension when compared with patients treated with an olecranon osteotomy.

The TRAP exposure preserves the neurovascular supply to the anconeus muscle and provides an extensile exposure of the distal humerus.[69] The dissection begins distally, elevating the anconeus from the ulna extending proximally toward the lateral epicondyle and the lateral column of the distal humerus. On the medial side, the dissection will extend distally to merge with the distal extent of the lateral exposure followed by sharp elevation of the triceps insertion from the ulna. The entire flap can be mobilized proximally to expose the distal humerus and articular fracture including these complex multifragmented very distal fracture patterns.

The triceps elevation approach has been traditionally used when performing total elbow arthroplasty (**Fig. 11–6**).[70,71] It may be used in those fractures in which internal fixation may not prove possible and arthroplasty is to be considered. The dissection of the triceps starts medially off the ulna as an osteoperiosteal flap and continues until the anconeus and triceps can be retracted over the lateral humeral condyle. As with the other triceps elevation procedures, a meticulous repair of the triceps mechanism with transosseous sutures is mandatory.

The final alternative surgical exposure is that of the lateral approach.[72,73] This exposure is most useful for lateral column fractures as well as articular shearing chondral fractures. For simpler capitellar or unicondylar fractures the lateral collateral ligament complex can be spared or elevated with an osteotomy of the lateral epicondyle extending the dissection to elevate the lateral triceps insertion from the proximal ulna. The elbow can be "hinged open" supported only on the medial soft tissues and affording excellent exposure of the entire anterior surface of the capitellum and trochlea (**Fig. 11–7**). At the conclusion of the procedure, the lateral soft tissues and/or epicondyle must be carefully repaired with transosseous sutures.

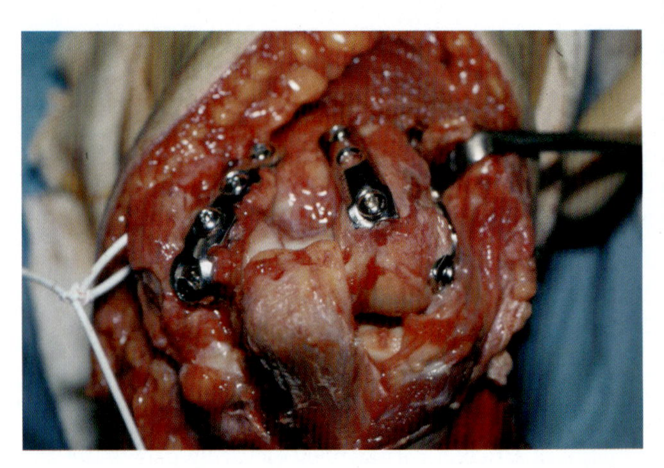

Figure 11–6 The triceps elevation exposure is to be considered when the possibility of elbow arthroplasty exists.

Techniques

Internal Fixation Techniques

Although the general principles of definitive internal fixation of intraarticular fractures of the distal humerus are well recognized, the task becomes substantially more

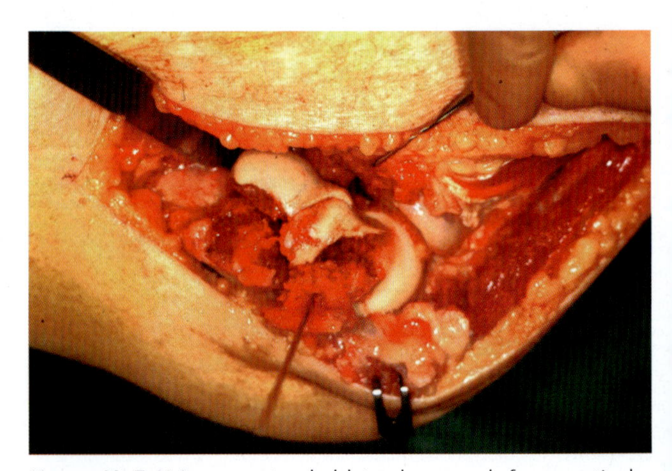

Figure 11–7 Using an extended lateral approach for an articular shearing fracture, the elbow can be "hinged open" to expose the entire articular surface.

complex when faced with multifragmented articular fractures at or distal to the olecranon sulcus. Irrespective of the fracture pattern(s), the basic goal revolves around realignment of the trochlea as close as possible to its original width. By doing so, the inherent stability of the elbow is enhanced.

Several technical points will facilitate the internal fixation of the more complex articular fractures. With the very comminuted articular fractures, it may prove beneficial to provisionally reassemble the larger articular fragment onto one of the bony columns using smooth 0.062-inch Kirschner wires. The use of an oscillating drill is very helpful when applying the Kirschner wires, as it will negate the risk of injury to the nearby ulnar nerve.

When the articular injury involves a fracture plane not only in the sagittal plane, but also in the coronal plane, definitive fixation may require the use of headless screws and/or small threaded Kirschner wires, which can be buried beneath the articular surface, although the latter are subject to migration **(Fig. 11–8)**.[50,74]

Some complex injuries exist in which the trochlea is not only fragmented, but also has a structural defect due to impaction. The goal must be to preserve the anatomic width of the trochlea using a compact cancellous graft to preserve elbow stability **(Fig. 11–9)**. When using screw fixation to stabilize the trochlea, interfragmentary compression is to be avoided to maintain the trochlea width.

To establish the mechanical stability of the fixation of the articular reconstruction onto the bony columns, the placement of two plates 90 degrees to each other is required.[75,76] This concept has recently been challenged with the development of contoured humeral plates shaped to sit on the lateral and medial columns 180 degrees to each other **(Fig. 11–10)**.[77,78]

Although technologic advances have produced precontoured implants for distal humeral fractures, many fractures – even very complex patterns – can be adequately stabilized using standard reconstruction-type implants. One special tactic is based upon contouring the medial plate to bend around and "cradle" the medial epicondyle **(Fig. 11–11)**. The most distal two screws are placed at 90 degrees to each other, enhancing their stability. An alternative technique, in particular when the medial epicondyle is fragmented, is to direct a long screw from the "cradle" to extend proximally to engage in the lateral bony column.

On the lateral side with the complex articular fractures located at and/or below the olecranon sulcus, two options exist for lateral plate fixation. One option involves placement of a plate on the dorsal surface to extend distally to the posterior limit of the articular surface of the capitellum **(Fig. 11–12)**. The most distal screw should be directed proximally and laterally to engage the more secure cortical bone of the lateral ridge of the bony column. A second option, which can be used either as the sole lateral column fixation or in addition to the posterior lateral plate, involves the placement of a plate along the very lateral column with the most distal screw directed across the

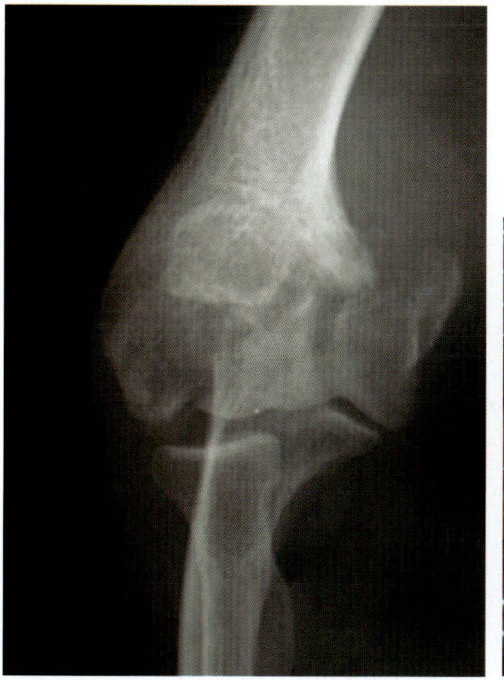

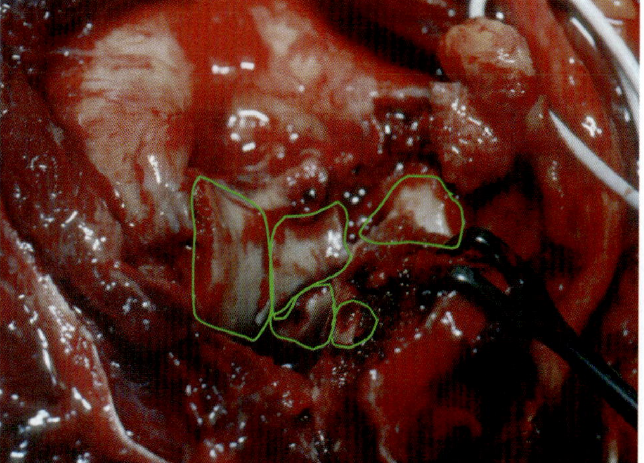

Figure 11–8 A very comminuted fracture in a 70-year-old woman, distal to the olecranon sulcus involving sagittal and coronal fracture lines. **(A)** The preoperative radiograph. **(B)** Intraoperative appearance of articular injury.

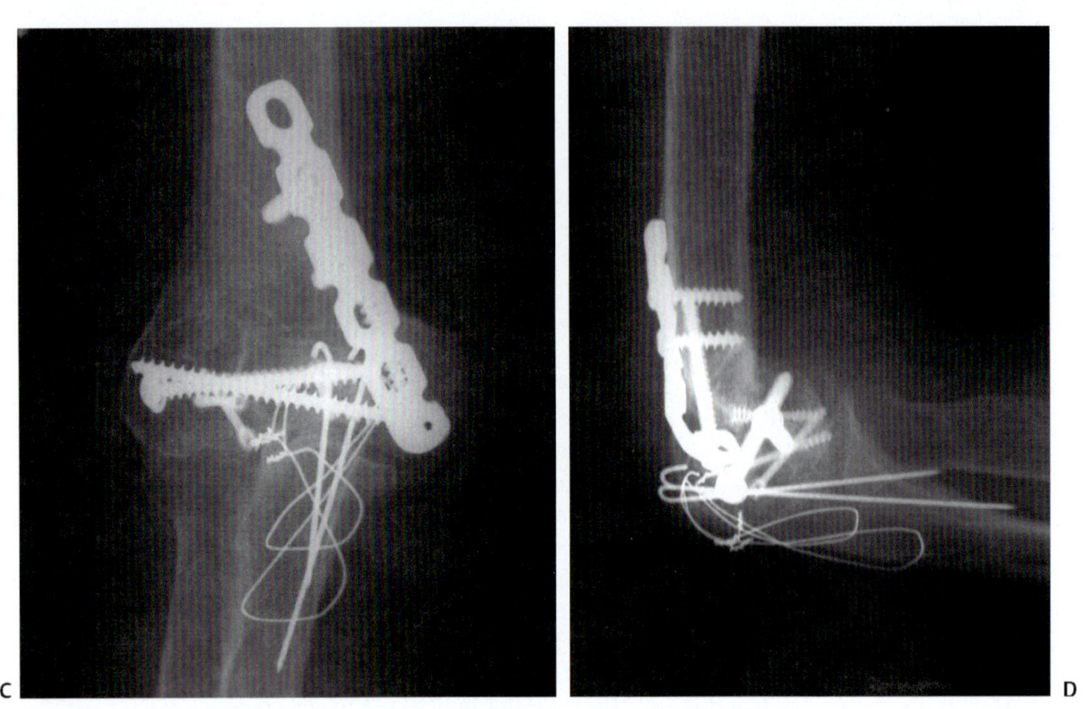

Figure 11–8 (*Continued*) **(C,D)** Fixation of the coronal fracture lines required headless screws.

trochlea reconstruction into the firm subchondral cancellous bone **(Fig. 11–13)**.

In an effort to enhance the stability of the plate fixation for the more difficult comminuted fractures, especially when associated with osteoporosis, custom precontoured implants have been developed. These include plates specific to the unique anatomy of the distal humerus, placing contoured plates on the medial and lateral bony ridges to face each other, and the development of angular stable locked screws to enhance the stability of the plate fixation **(Fig. 11–14)**.

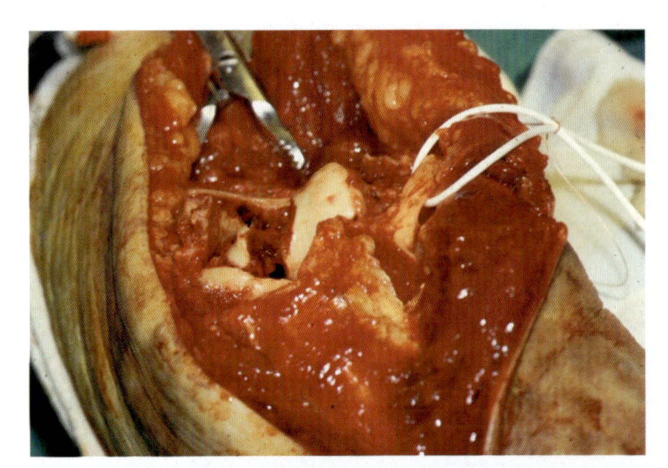

Figure 11–9 A critical component of articular reconstruction is to maintain the anatomic width of the trochlea even if it requires autogenous bone graft.

One approach advocated by O'Driscoll and colleagues is based not only on preshaped implants, but also on a principle-based fixation.[77,79] This includes:

1. Every screw should pass through a plate.
2. Each screw should engage a fragment on the opposite side that is also fixed to a plate.
3. As many screws as possible should be placed into the distal fragments.
4. Each screw should be as long as possible.
5. Each screw should engage as many articular fragments as possible.
6. Plates should be applied such that compression is achieved at the supracondylar level for both bony columns.
7. Plates should be strong and stiff enough to resist bending or breaking at the supracondylar level.

There are several other precontoured implants now available for the fixation of the more complex articular fractures. Angular stable screws, which lock into the plate, offer additional fixation advantages.

Several other technical "pearls" should be recognized. Avoid having both plates end proximally at the same level, as this presents a potential risk for fracture **(Fig. 11–15)**.

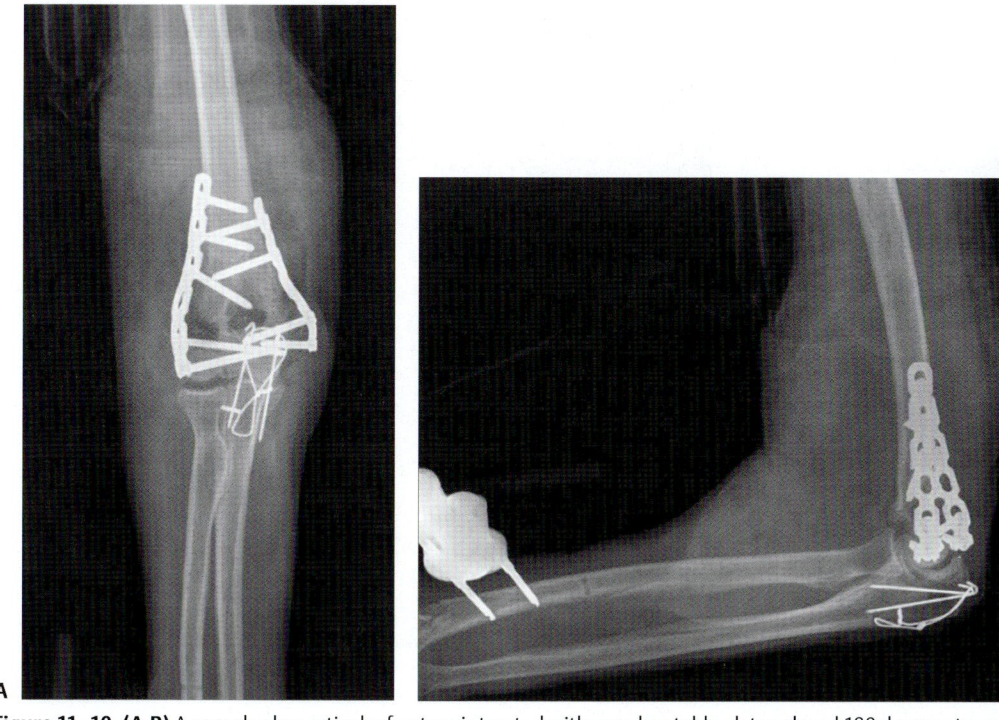

Figure 11–10 (A,B) A complex low articular fracture is treated with angular stable plates placed 180 degrees to each other on the medial and lateral columns.

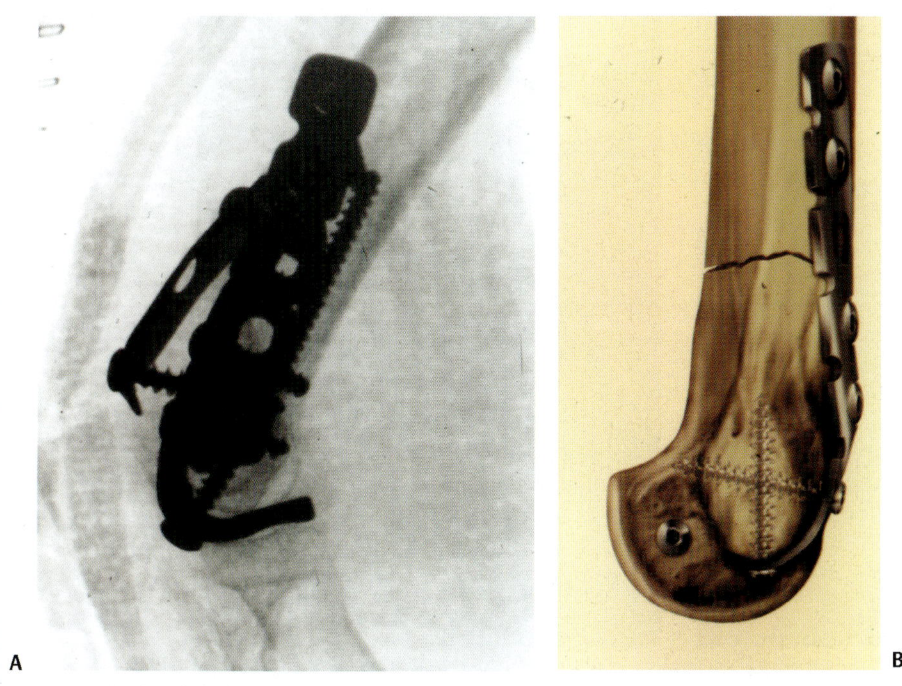

Figure 11–11 (A,B) A schematic of a reconstruction plate placed along the medial column and contoured distally to cradle the medial epicondyle.

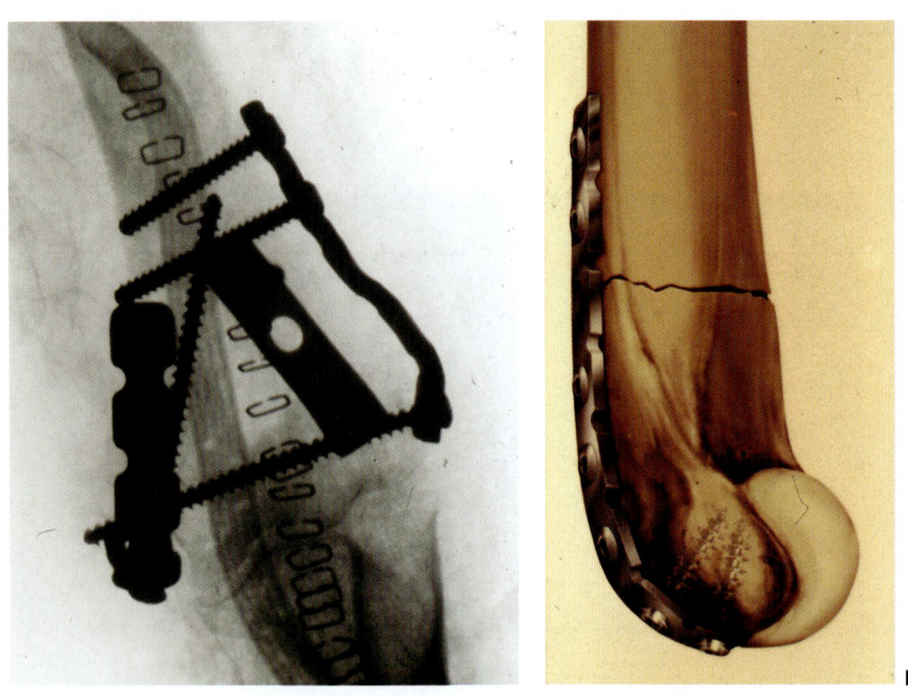

Figure 11–12 (A,B) A lateral plate can be placed posteriorly on the lateral column extending to the proximal aspect of the capitellar cartilage with the distal screws directed proximally and laterally.

A second "pearl" applies to fractures, which include extensive metaphyseal comminution. The fracture can be shortened to enhance bony contact and the stability of the plate fixation. This will result in little if no functional deficits.[80]

Chondral Shearing Fractures

With the exception of those shearing fractures, which extend across the articular surface to also involve the medial epicondyle, most chondral shearing fractures are effectively approached using an extended lateral exposure.[81–84] Those

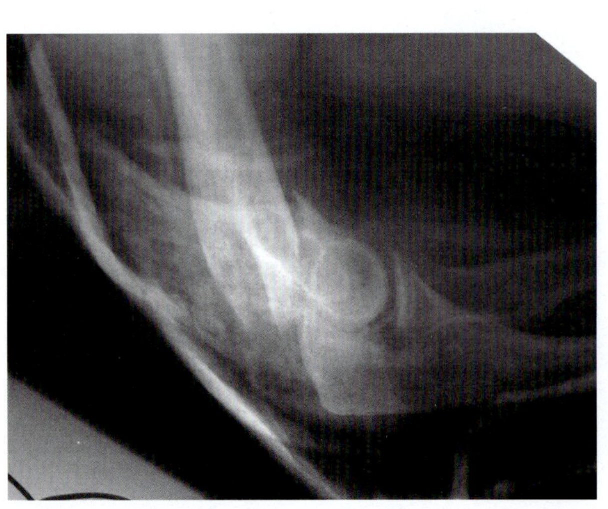

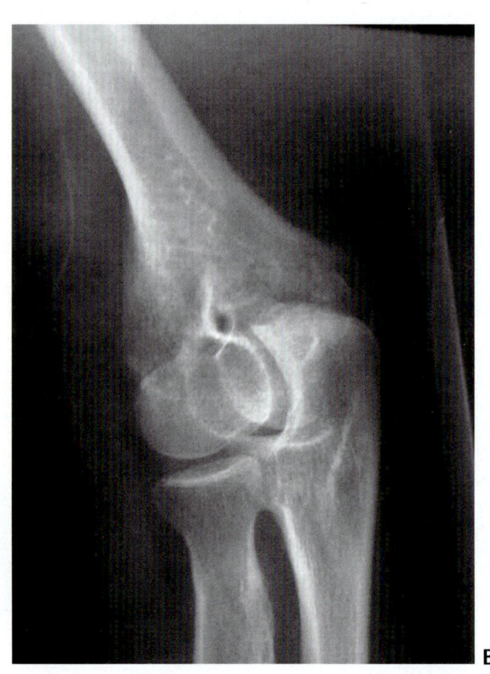

Figure 11–13 A low distal humerus articular fracture in a 62-year-old woman, treated with three strategically placed plates. **(A,B)** The preoperative anteroposterior and lateral x-rays.

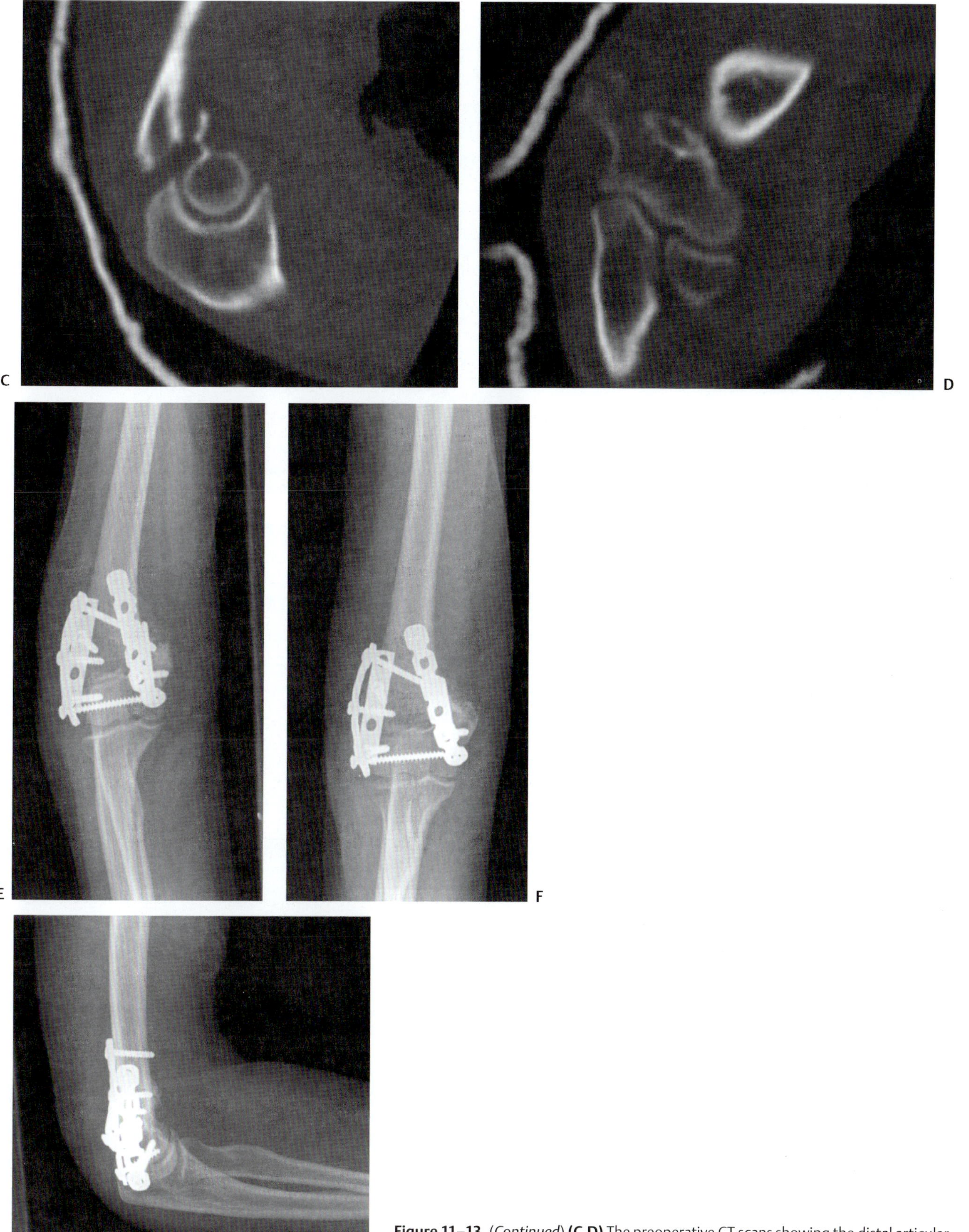

Figure 11–13 (*Continued*) **(C,D)** The preoperative CT scans showing the distal articular monoblock fragment. **(E–G)** The internal fixation with three standard plates.

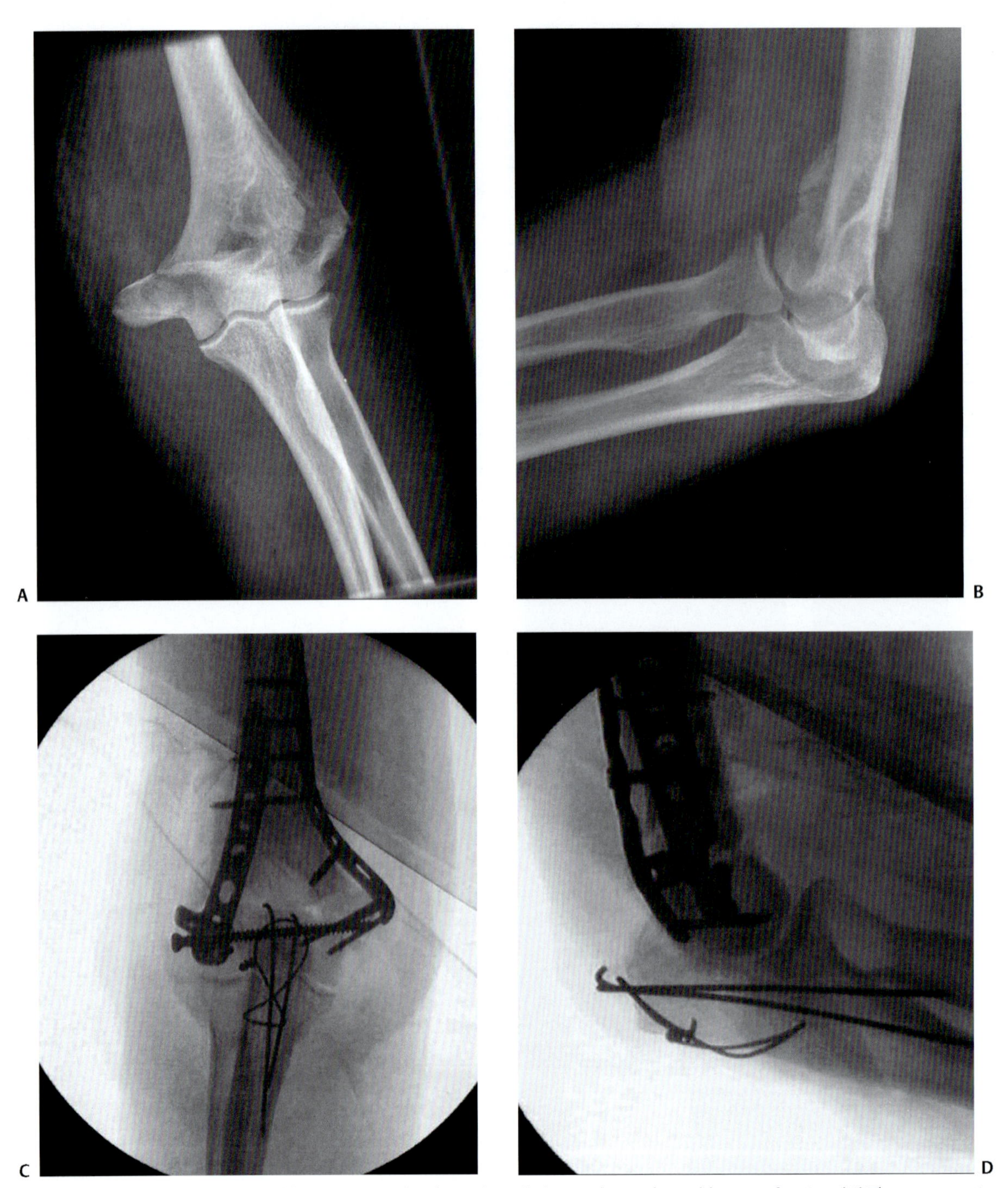

Figure 11–14 A low distal humeral fracture treated with preshaped plate with angular stable screw fixation. **(A)** The preoperative anteroposterior (AP) and **(B)** lateral radiographs. Fixation with angular stable plates and screws. **(C)** The postoperative AP and **(D)** lateral radiographs.

involving the medial epicondyle are best approached through an olecranon osteotomy **(Fig. 11–16)**.

When the fracture involves the lateral epicondyle, lateral exposure is facilitated by elevating the epicondyle with its attached soft tissues, which include the wrist and digital extensors and lateral collateral ligament complex. Alternatively, an osteotomy of the lateral epicondyle can be performed **(Fig. 11–17)**.

Typically, the fracture fragment(s) are found displaced medially and proximally with little or no soft tissue attachments.[85] Once realigned, temporary fixation is done using 0.045- or 0.062-inch smooth Kirschner wires. An important caveat to bear in mind, when anatomic reduction is not achievable, is the fact that this may be the result of impaction of the posterior aspect of the lateral bony column and/or impaction of part or all of the posterior trochlea.

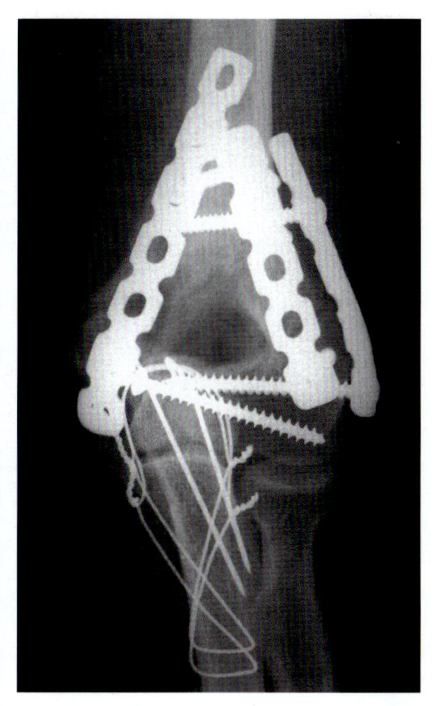

Figure 11–15 Care is always taken to avoid plates ending at the same level proximally.

Definitive fixation is achievable in most cases using headless screws placed through the cartilage from anterior to posterior. A large lateral epicondylar fragment can be screwed with a contoured small plate and screws or a tension band wire technique.[46, 86]

Timing of Surgery

With the exception of open distal humerus fractures, a few conditions require immediate operative treatment. The combination of the complexities of the injury and operative fixation, the need for specific equipment and implants, the potential for overlying soft tissue trauma, and the importance of adequate imaging and preoperative planning would all suggest that the surgery be delayed and performed electively. In addition, in the older patient, comorbidities must be evaluated and the decision regarding the role of total elbow arthroplasty discussed.

Open fractures require emergent care **(Fig. 11–18)**. In addition to irrigation and débridement of the open fracture, questions remain regarding the timing of internal fixation. Some recommend delaying fixation until the wound is defined and free of contamination; however, my preference is to consider fixation of at least the articular fracture fragments except when the wound is highly contaminated. In one study of open articular fractures, the authors recorded infection in 3 of 26 open fractures treated with immediate definitive fixation with only 1 patient ultimately developing deep sepsis.[87] On rare occasions with massive bone loss in younger patients, an elbow allograft has been used.[88]

Total Elbow Arthroplasty

The issues related to the indications, techniques, and outcomes of total elbow arthroplasty are addressed in another chapter. From my perspective, a word of caution must be expressed regarding too much enthusiasm for this approach, given the exceptional difficulties inherent in the salvage of a failed elbow arthroplasty. At the same time, those fractures made more complex by underlying arthrosis, extreme fragmentation in osteoporotic bone, or combinations of these in a patient who has relatively low functional demand – all represent appropriate indicators for total elbow arthroplasty.[61,89–96]

Postoperative Care and Rehabilitation

Optimally, sufficient stability can be achieved with internal fixation to permit early postoperative mobilization of the

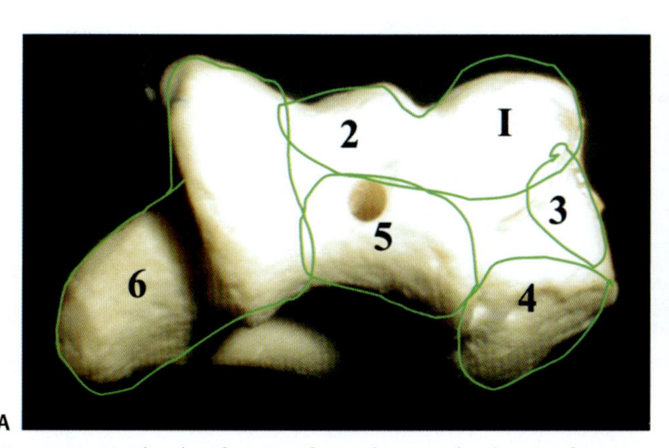

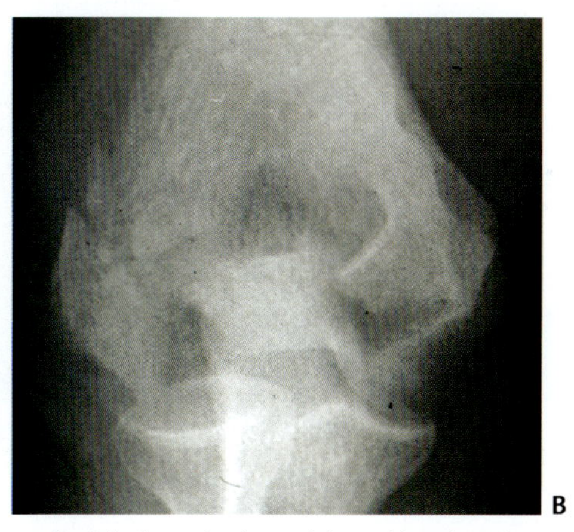

Figure 11–16 The classification of complex articular shearing fractures. (1) Capitellum. (2) Coronal shear fracture. (3) Shear fracture including lateral epicondyle. (4) Shear fracture involving parted of the posterior wall of the lateral column. (5) Trochlea shear fracture involving anterior and posterior articular fragments. (6) Shear fracture extending across the articular surface to involve the medial epicondyle.

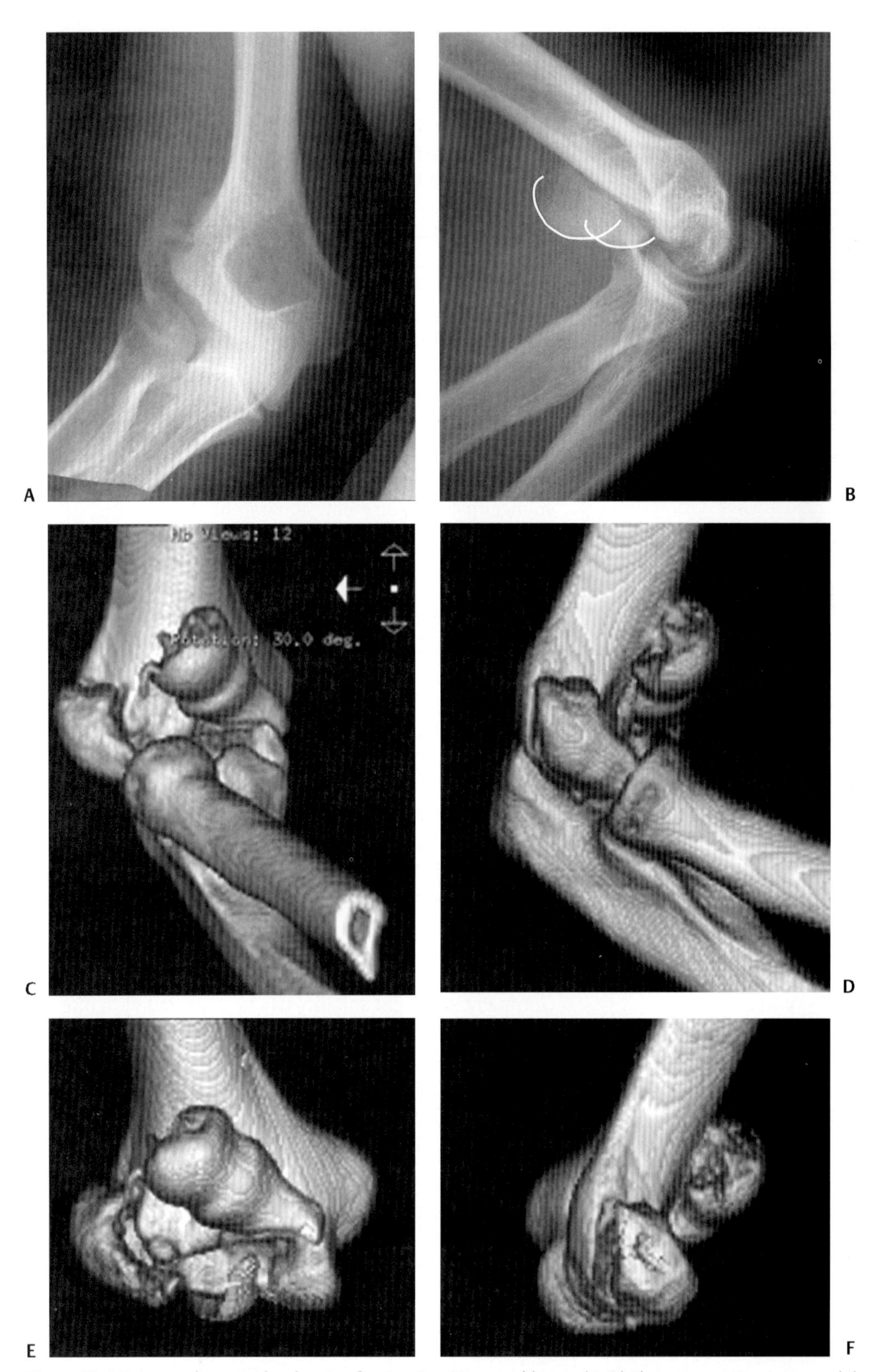

Figure 11–17 A complex articular shearing fracture in a 35-year-old man. **(A–F)** The preoperative x-rays and three-dimensional computed tomography scans.

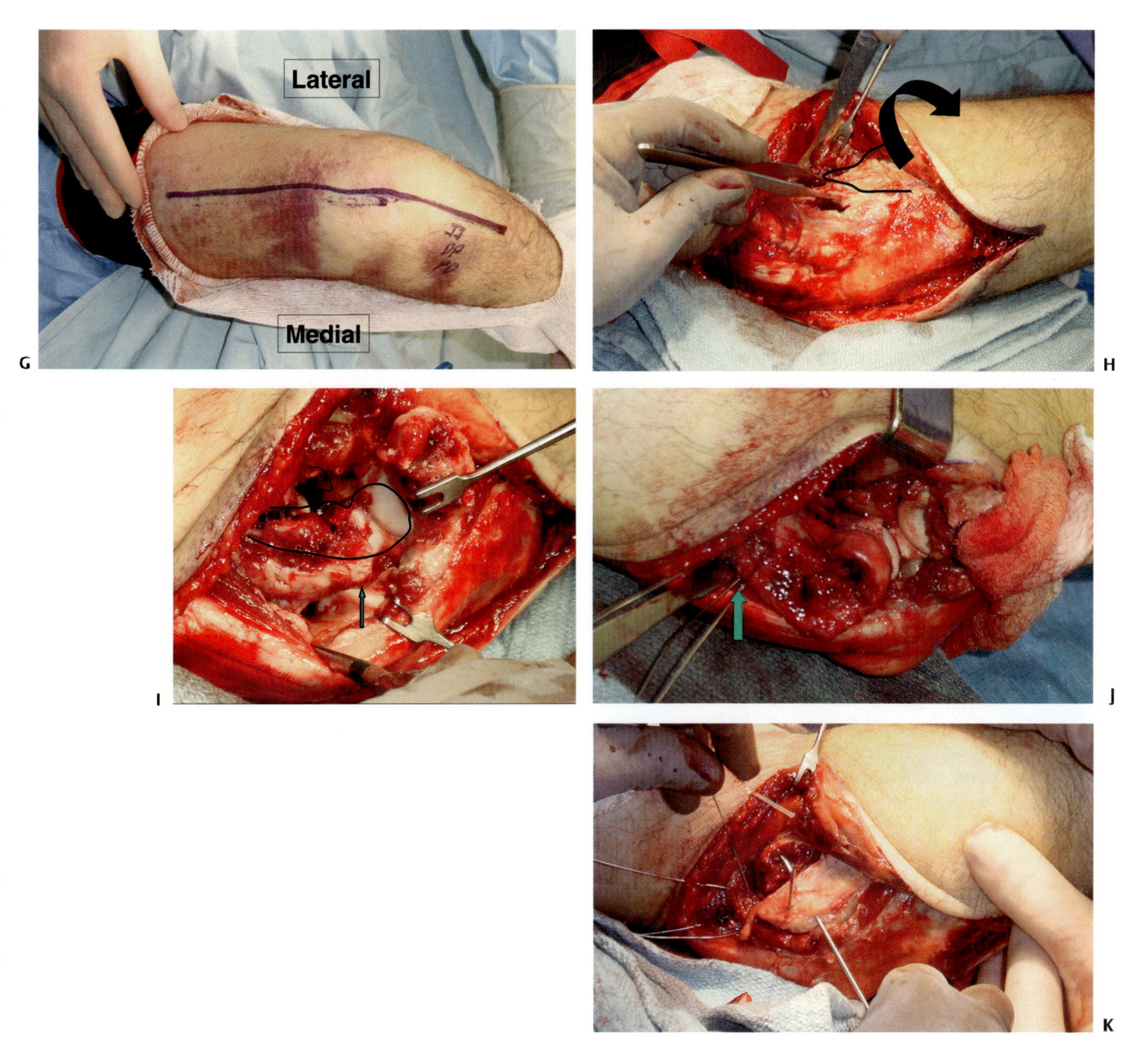

Figure 11–17 (*Continued*) **(G)** A straight posterior incision will allow exposure to the ulnar nerve as well as lateral column. **(H)** By elevating the fractured lateral epicondyle distally and the lateral triceps posteriorly, the elbow can be "hinged open," gaining access to the anterior elbow and the fracture fragments. **(I)** The impacted posterior wall of the lateral column is disimpacted (*arrow*) allowing anatomic reduction and internal fixation with headless compression screws. **(J,K)** The lateral epicondyle is repaired with tension wires.

surgically repaired elbow. Prolonged immobilization will risk permanent loss of motion. There will be some cases, as in complex chondral shearing fractures, which can be stabilized only by small threaded headless screws that may well benefit from immobilization for 14 to 21 days, accepting the possibility of some residual loss of motion.

I prefer to splint the elbow for the initial postoperative night in full extension and elevated on several pillows (**Fig. 11–19**). Active motion using gravity-assist maneuvers should be initiated within the first 48 hours postoperatively. Supervision with a physiotherapist is preferred; however, it is crucial that the patient understand the exercise protocol and perform the exercises independently of the therapist (**Fig. 11–20**). Once swelling has diminished over the succeeding 4 to 6 weeks, a gradual increase in the elbow range of motion is to be anticipated. When limitation of motion is appreciated, turnbuckle-type splints as well as extension splints to use at night should be initiated.

It has been our experience that the majority of patients should be expected to achieve a functional range of elbow motion of approximately a 100-degree combined arc of

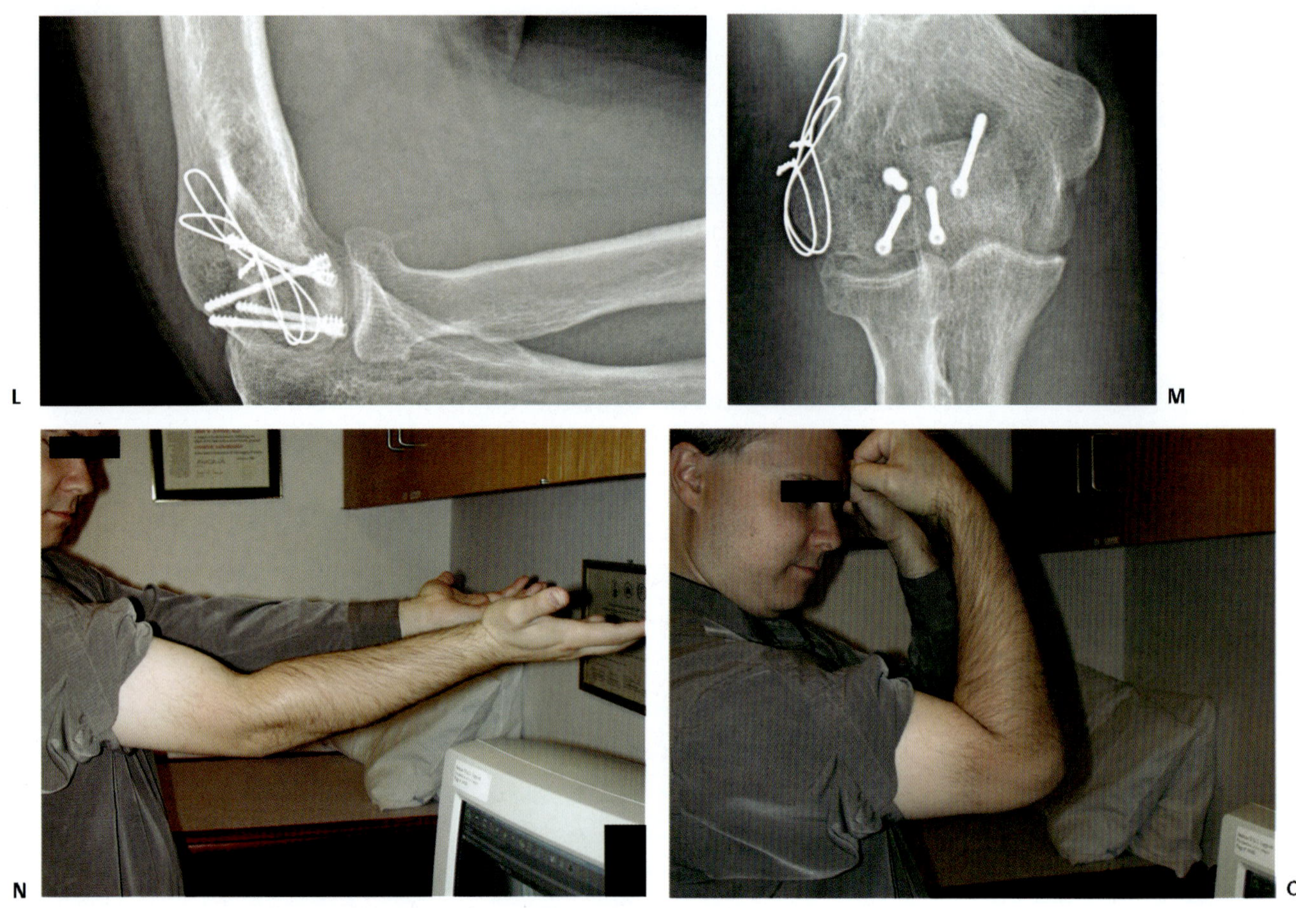

Figure 11–17 (*Continued*) **(L,M)** X-rays at 1-year follow-up. **(N,O)** An acceptable functional result.

flexion and extension. The surgeon should be alert to those patients who appear to be unable to gain motion due to ulnar neuritis pain, as this may be due to irritation of the ulnar nerve. What is sometimes problematic with this situation is the fact that the patient may not have any symptoms referable to the ulnar nerve except pain about the elbow.[97]

Complications

Nonunion

Nonunion following internal fixation of complex distal humeral fractures is well recognized and is the result, in most cases, of unstable internal fixation **(Fig. 11–21)**.[98–101] Pain, loss of motion and instability are commonplace, which can render the entire limb dysfunctional. It has become evident that the optimal result from the operative treatment of the nonunions will involve not only repeat internal fixation with or without autogenous bone graft, but also anterior and posterior capsulectomy, as well as ulnar nerve release.[102–104]

The outcome of operative repair of these nonunions has been remarkably good in several published series. This includes not only a high union rate (51 of 52 patients) in a series by Helfet et al, but also the recovery of a functional arc of motion.[105,106]

For the more complex nonunions associated with bone loss, articular degeneration, or an infirm patient, a total elbow arthroplasty should be considered.[107]

Ulnar Nerve Dysfunction

Ulnar nerve dysfunction is common following operative treatment and relatively underappreciated.[108] This may be due to excessive intraoperative traction, impingement on the nerve from the internal fixation, or fibrosis around the nerve, limiting its normal excursion during elbow flexion and extension. Most authors recommend mobilizing the nerve proximally to the level of the medial intermuscular septum and distally well into the two heads of the flexor carpi ulnaris. This will affect a subcutaneous transposition of the nerve.

A-C
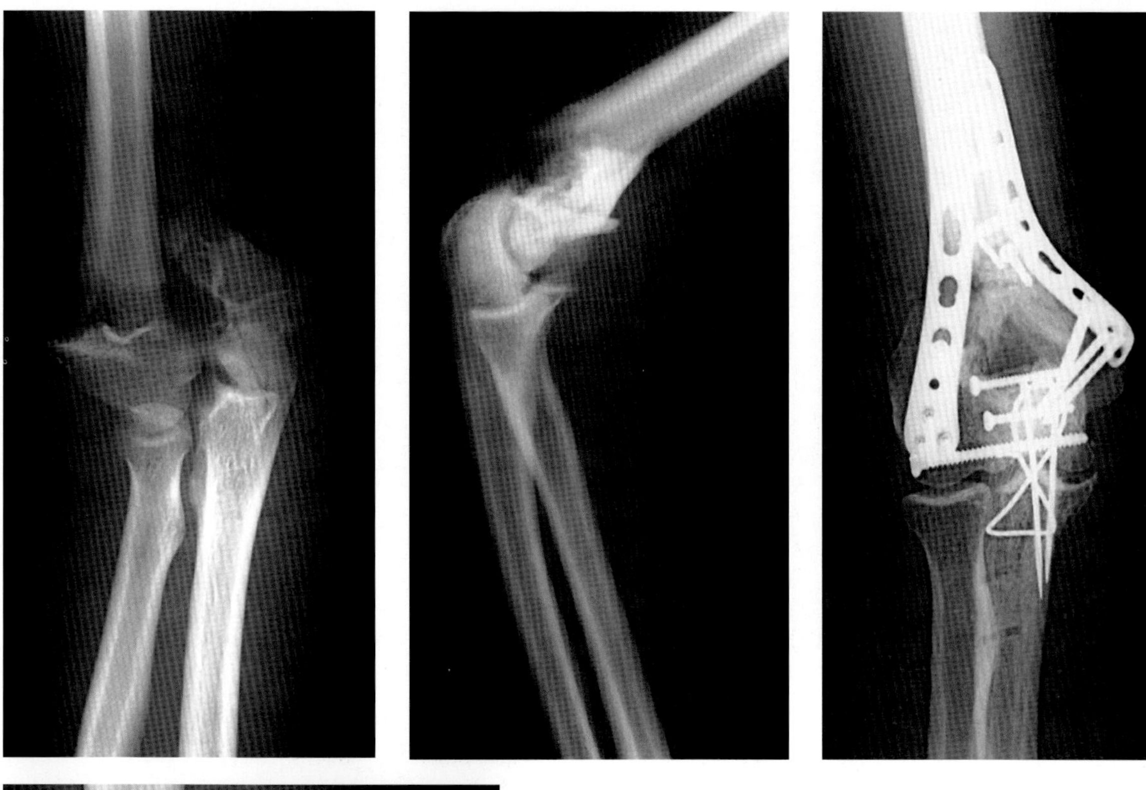

D
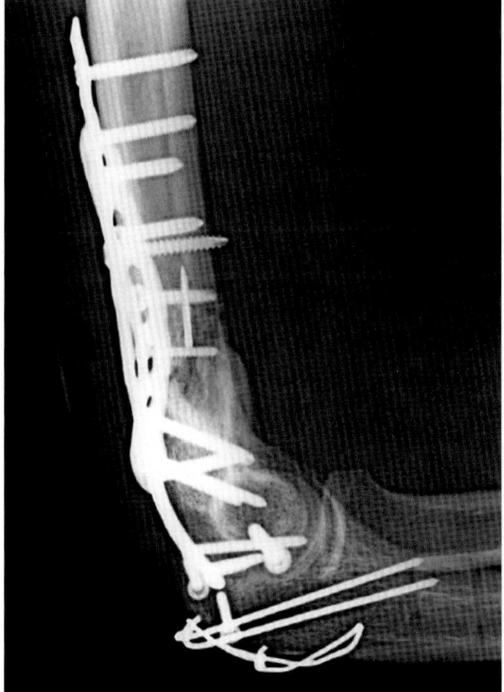

Figure 11–18 An open articular fracture in an active 40-year-old woman is secured using distal humeral plates with angular stable locking screws. **(A,B)** The preoperative radiographs. **(C,D)** Secure fixation is achieved with distal humeral locking plates.

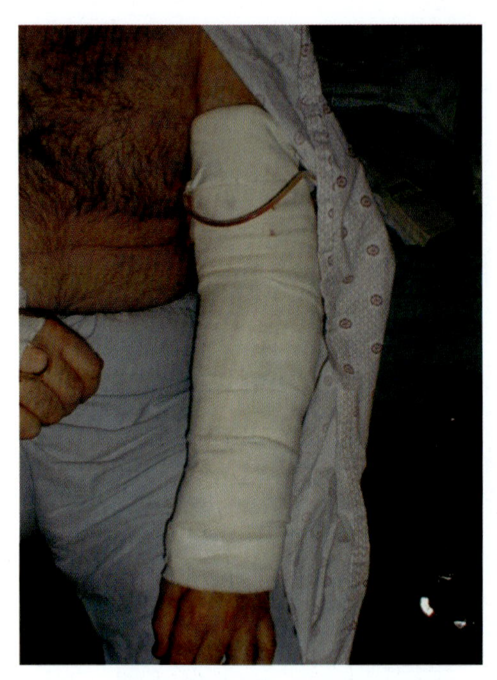

Figure 11–19 During the initial postoperative evening, the elbow is splinted in full extension.

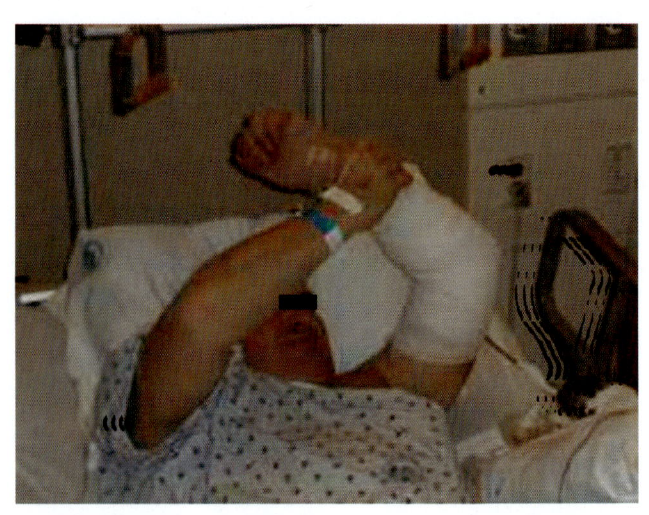

Figure 11–20 Active motion is initiated within 48 hours postsurgery using quantity-assisted exercises.

When attempting to surgically repair a nonunion or stiff elbow, the ulnar nerve will often require a meticulous dissection under high power loupe magnification to mobilize the nerve from surrounding fibrosis. It is especially important to mobilize the nerve prophylactically when performing an elbow release, when the preoperative range of motion is 40 degrees or less.

Elbow Contracture

Loss of motion is commonplace following surgical treatment of complex fractures of the distal humerus.[109] The decision to undertake surgical release should be based on failure to gain functional motion after an organized rehabilitation program, a stable soft tissue envelope, and a

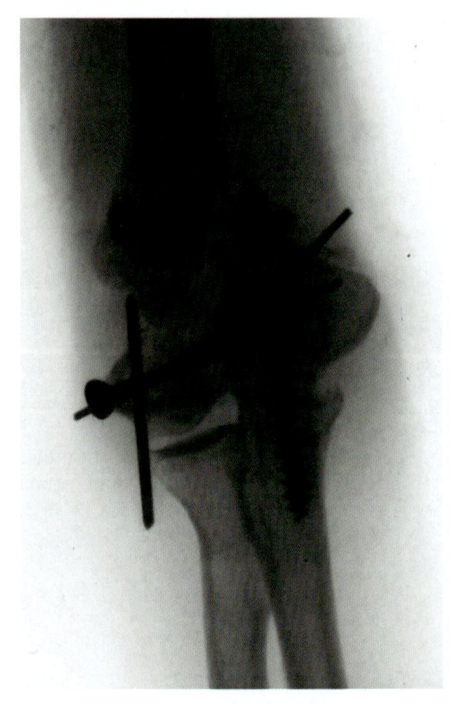

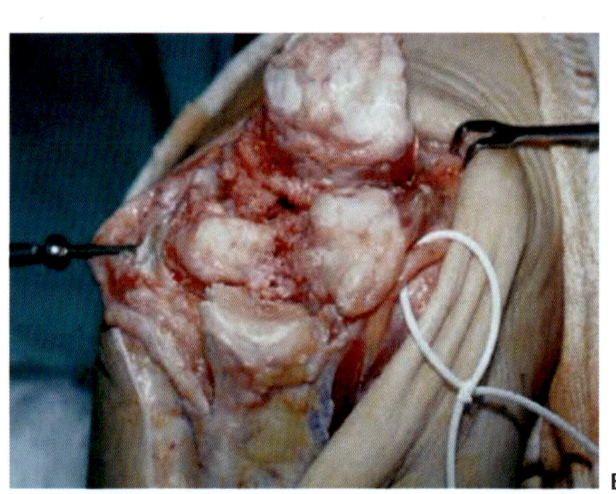

Figure 11–21 An intraarticular and supracondylar nonunion following an open distal humerus fracture and subsequent failed internal fixation. **(A)** A radiograph of the nonunion. **(B)** Intraoperative picture demonstrates the distorted articular fragments covered with granulation tissue.

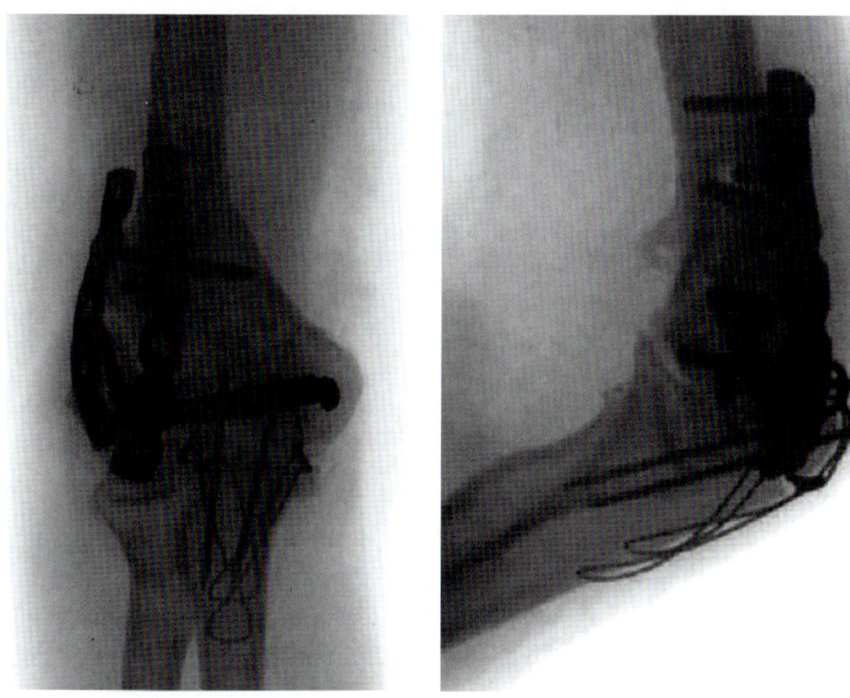

Figure 11–21 (*Continued*) **(C,D)** Stable internal fixation along with autogenous cancellous graft led to union with a functional outcome.

cooperative patient.[110,111] Generally, this should not be considered before a minimum of 4 months postsurgery. As greater experience has been generated the results of capsular release have been favorable with a low rate of complications.

Heterotopic ossification following fractures of the distal humerus is uncommon when operative excision is to be considered; prophylactic radiation treatment of one dose of 70 GY (7000 rad) is useful combined with an organized program of postoperative continuous passive motion.[112–114]

References

1. Aitken GK, Rorabeck CH. Distal humeral fractures in the adult. Clin Orthop Relat Res 1986;207:191–197
2. Anglen J. Distal humerus fractures. J Am Acad Orthop Surg 2005;13:291–297
3. Borrelli J Jr. Fractures of the Distal Humerus. 2nd ed. Rosemont, IL: American Academy of Orthopaedic Surgeons; 2000:33–38
4. Bryan RS. Fractures about the elbow in adults. Instr Course Lect 1981;30:200–223
5. Bryan RS, Bicket WH. "T" condylar fractures of distal humerus. J Trauma 1971;11:830–835
6. Brown RF, Morgan RG. Intercondylar T-shaped fractures of the humerus: results in ten cases treated by early mobilization. J Bone Joint Surg Br 1971;53:425–428
7. Ring D, Jupiter JB. Operative release of complete ankylosis of the elbow due to heterotopic bone in patients without severe injury of the central nervous system. J Bone Joint Surg Am 2003;85:849–857
8. Bryan RS, Morrey BF. Fractures of the distal humerus. In Morrey BF, ed. The Elbow and Its Disorders. Philadelphia, PA: WB Saunders; 1985:302–339
9. Caja VL, Moroni A, Vendemia V, et al. Surgical treatment of bicondylar fractures of the distal humerus. Injury 1994;25:433–438
10. Cassebaum WH. Open reduction of T & Y fractures of the lower end of the humerus. J Trauma 1969;9:915–925
11. Eralp L, Kocaoglu M, Sar C, Atalar AC. Surgical treatment of distal intraarticular humeral fractures in adults. Int Orthop 2001;25:46–50
12. Gabel GT, Hanson G, Bennett JB, et al. Intraarticular fractures of the distal humerus in the adult. Clin Orthop Relat Res 1987;216:99–108
13. Gofton WT, Macdermid JC, Patterson SD, et al. Functional outcome of AO type C distal humeral fractures. J Hand Surg [Am] 2003;28:294–308
14. Helfet DL, Schmeling GJ. Bicondylar intraarticular fractures of the distal humerus in adults. Clin Orthop Relat Res 1993;292:26–36
15. Henley MB, Bone LB, Parker B. Operative management of intra-articular fractures of the distal humerus. J Orthop Trauma 1987;1:24–35
16. Holdsworth BJ, Mossad MM. Fractures of the adult distal humerus: elbow function after internal fixation. J Bone Joint Surg Br 1990;72:362–365
17. Jupiter JB, Barnes KA, Goodman LJ, Saldana AE. Multiplane fracture of the distal humerus. J Orthop Trauma 1993;7:216–220

18. Kundel K, Braun W, Wieberneit J, Ruter A. Intraarticular distal humerus fractures: factors affecting functional outcome. Clin Orthop Relat Res 1996;332:200–208
19. Lansinger O, Mare K. Fracture of the capitulum humeri. Acta Orthop Scand 1981;52:39–44
20. McKee MD, Kim J, Kebaish K, et al. Functional outcome after open supracondylar fractures of the humerus: the effect of the surgical approach. J Bone Joint Surg Br 2000;82:646–651
21. Ray PS, Kakarlapudi K, Rajsekhar C, Bhamra MS. Total elbow arthroplasty as primary treatment for distal humeral fractures in elderly patients. Injury 2000;31:687–692
22. Reich RS. Treatment of intercondylar fractures of the elbow by means of traction. J Bone Joint Surg Am 1936;18:997–1004
23. Riseborough EJ, Radin EL. Intercondylar T fractures of the humerus in the adult. A comparison of operative and non-operative treatment in twenty-nine cases. J Bone Joint Surg Am 1969;51:130–141
24. Sodergard J, Sandelin J, Bostman O. Mechanical failures of internal fixation in T and Y fractures of the distal humerus. J Trauma 1992;33:687–690
25. Sodergard J, Sandelin J, Bostman O. Postoperative complications of distal humeral fractures: 27/96 adults followed up for 6 (2–10) years. Acta Orthop Scand 1992;63:85–89
26. Viola RW, Hastings H II. Treatment of ectopic ossification about the elbow. Clin Orthop Relat Res 2000;370:65–86
27. Wright TW, Wong AM, Jaffe R. Functional outcome comparison of semiconstrained and unconstrained total elbow arthroplasties. J Shoulder Elbow Surg 2000;9: 524–531
28. Ziran BH, Smith WR, Balk ML, Manning CM, Agudelo JF. A true triceps-splitting approach for treatment of distal humerus fractures: a preliminary report. J Trauma 2005;58:70–74
29. An KN, Morrey BF. Biomechanics of the elbow. In Morrey BF, ed. The Elbow and Its Disorders; vol 1. Philadelphia, PA: WB Saunders; 2005: 43–60
30. Hotchkiss RN. Fractures and dislocations of the elbow. In Rockwood CA Jr, Green DP, Bucholz RW, Heckman JD, eds. Rockwood and Green's Fractures in Adults. 4th ed. Philadelphia, PA: Lippincott-Raven; 1996: 929–1024
31. Jupiter JB. The surgical management of intraarticular fractures of the distal humerus. In Morrey BF, ed. The Elbow. 2nd ed. Philadelphia, PA: Lippincott Williams & Wilkins; 2002: 65–81
32. Jupiter JB, Goodman LF. The management of complex distal humerus nonunions in the elderly by elbow capsulectomy, triple plating, and ulnar nerve neurolysis. J Shoulder Elbow Surg 1992;1:37–46
33. Jupiter JB, Neff U, Holzach P, Allgöwer M. Intercondylar fractures of the humerus: an operative approach. J Bone Joint Surg Am 1985;67:226–239
34. Komurcu M, Yanmis I, Atesalp AS, Gur E. Treatment results for open comminuted distal humerus intra-articular fractures with Ilizarov circular external fixator. Mil Med 2003;168:694–697
35. London JT. Kinematics of the elbow. J Bone Joint Surg Am 1981;63:529–535
36. Martin J, Marsh JL, Nepola JV, Dirschl DR, Hurwitz S, DeCoster TA. Radiographic fracture assessments: which ones can we reliably make? J Orthop Trauma 2000;14: 379–385
37. Mehdian H, McKee MD. Fractures of capitellum and trochlea. Orthop Clin North Am 2000;31:115–127
38. O'Driscoll SW. The triceps-reflecting anconeus pedicle (TRAP) approach for distal humeral fractures and nonunions. Orthop Clin North Am 2000;31:91–101
39. O'Driscoll SW, Sanchez-Sotelo J, Torchia ME. Management of the smashed distal humerus. Orthop Clin North Am 2002;33:19–33
40. McKee M, Jupiter J, Toh CL, et al. Reconstruction after malunion and nonunion of intra-articular fractures of the distal humerus: methods and results in 13 adults. J Bone Joint Surg Br 1994;76:614–621
41. McKee M, Jupiter JB. Fractures of the distal humerus. In Browner BD, Jupiter JB, Levine AM, Trafton PG, eds. Skeletal Trauma: Basic Science, Management, and Reconstruction. Vol. 2. 3rd ed. Philadelphia, PA: WB Saunders; 2003; 1436–1480
42. Zagorski JB, Jennings JJ, Burkhalter WE, Uribe JW. Comminuted intraarticular fractures of the distal humeral condyles: surgical vs. nonsurgical treatment. Clin Orthop Relat Res 1986;202:197–204
43. Eastwood WJ. The T-shaped fracture of the lower end of the humerus. J Bone Joint Surg Am 1937;19:364–368
44. Evans EM. Supracondylar-Y fractures of the humerus. J Bone Joint Surg Br 1953;35:371–375
45. Morrey BF. Surgical treatment of extraarticular elbow contracture. Clin Orthop Relat Res 2000;370:57–64
46. Schatzker J. AO philosophy and principles. In: Ruedi TP, Murphy WM, eds. AO Principles of Fracture Management. Davos, Switzerland: AO Publishing, 2000:1–6
47. Morrey BF. Limited and extensile triceps reflecting and exposures of the elbow. In Morrey BF, ed. The Elbow. 2nd ed. Philadelphia: Lippincott Williams & Wilkins; 2002: 3–25
48. O'Driscoll SW, Jupiter JB, Cohen MS, Ring D, McKee MD. Difficult elbow fractures: pearls and pitfalls. Instr Course Lect 2003;52:113–134
49. Obremskey WT, Bhandari M, Dirschl DR, Shemitsch E. Internal fixation versus arthroplasty of comminuted fractures of the distal humerus. J Orthop Trauma 2003;17: 463–465
50. Jupiter JB, Neff U, Regazzoni P, Allgöwer M. Unicondylar fractures of the distal humerus: an operative approach. J Orthop Trauma 1988;2:102–109
51. Dushuttle RP, Coyle MP, Zawadsky JP, Bloom H. Fractures of the capitellum. J Trauma 1985;25:317–321
52. Grant IR, Miller JH. Osteochondral fracture of the trochlea associated with fracture-dislocation of the elbow. Injury 1975;6:257–260
53. McAuliffe JA, Wolfson AH. Early excision of heterotopic ossification about the elbow followed by radiation therapy. J Bone Joint Surg Am 1997;79:749–755
54. Pereles TR, Koval KJ, Gallagher M, Rosen H. Open reduction and internal fixation of the distal humerus: Functional outcome in the elderly. J Trauma 1997;43:578–584

55. Poynton AR, Kelly IP, O'Rourke SK. Fractures of the capitellum—a comparison of two fixation methods. Injury 1998;29:341–343
56. Dowdy PA, Bain GI, King GJ, Patterson SD. The midline posterior elbow incision: an anatomical appraisal. J Bone Joint Surg Br 1995;77:696–699
57. Liberman N, Katz T, Howard CB, Nyska M. Fixation of the capitellar fractures with the Herbert screw. Arch Orthop Trauma Surg 1991;110:155–157
58. Gainor BJ, Moussa F, Schott T. Healing rate of transverse osteotomies of the olecranon used in reconstruction of distal humerus fractures. J South Orthop Assoc 1995;4: 263–268
59. Hutchinson DT, Horwitz DS, Ha G, Thomas CW, Bachus KN. Cyclic loading of olecranon fracture fixation constructs. J Bone Joint Surg Am 2003;85(5):831–837
60. Ring D, Gulotta L, Chin K, Jupiter JB. Olecranon osteotomy for exposure of fractures and nonunions of the distal humerus. J Orthop Trauma 2004;18(7):446–449
61. Hausman M, Panozzo A. Treatment of distal humerus fractures in the elderly. Clin Orthop Relat Res 2004;425: 55–63
62. Cassebaum WH. Operative treatment of T & Y fractures of the lower end of the humerus. Am J Surg 1952;83:265–270
63. Ring D, Jupiter JB, Gulotta L. Articular fractures of the distal part of the humerus. J Bone Joint Surg Am 2003;85: 232–238
64. Wainwright AM, Williams JR, Carr AJ. Interobserver and intraobserver variation in classification systems for fractures of the distal humerus. J Bone Joint Surg Br 2000;82: 636–642
65. Alonso-Llames M. Bilaterotricipital approach to the elbow: its application in the osteosynthesis of supracondylar fractures of the humerus in children. Acta Orthop Scand 1972;43:479–490
66. Stamatis E, Paxinos O. The treatment and functional outcome of type IV coronal shear fractures of the distal humerus: a retrospective review of five cases. J Orthop Trauma 2003;17:279–284
67. Campbell WC. Incision for exposure of the elbow joint. Am J Surg 1932;15:65–67
68. Mills WJ, Hanel DP, Smith DG. Lateral approach to the humeral shaft: an alternative approach for fracture treatment. J Orthop Trauma 1996;10:81–86
69. Oppenheim W, Davlin LB, Leipzig JM, Johnson EE. Concomitant fractures of the capitellum and trochlea. J Orthop Trauma 1989;3:260–262
70. Bryan RS, Morrey BF. Extensive posterior exposure of the elbow: a triceps-sparing approach. Clin Orthop Relat Res 1982;166:188–192
71. Morrey BF, Chao EY. Passive motion of the elbow joint. J Bone Joint Surg Am 1976;58:501–508
72. Gerwin M, Hotchkiss RN, Weiland AJ. Alternative operative exposures of the posterior aspect of the humeral diaphysis with reference to the radial nerve. J Bone Joint Surg Am 1996;78:1690–1695
73. Morrey BF, Adams RA. Semiconstrained elbow replacement for distal humeral nonunion. J Bone Joint Surg Br 1995;77:67–72
74. McCarty LP, Ring D, Jupiter JB. Management of distal humerus fractures. Am J Orthop 2005;34:430–438
75. Helfet DL, Hotchkiss RN. Internal fixation of the distal humerus: a biomechanical comparison of methods. J Orthop Trauma 1990;4:260–264
76. Jupiter JB. Complex fractures of the distal part of the humerus and associated complications. Instr Course Lect 1995;44:187–198
77. Schildhauer TA, Nork SE, Mills WJ, Henley MB. Extensor mechanism-sparing paratricipital posterior approach to the distal humerus. J Orthop Trauma 2003;17:374–378
78. Soon JL, Chan BK, Low CO. Surgical fixation of intra-articular fractures of the distal humerus in adults. Injury 2004;35:44–54
79. Palvanen M, Kannus P, Niemi S, Parkkari J. Secular trends in the osteoporotic fractures of the distal humerus in elderly women. Eur J Epidemiol 1998;14:159–164
80. Palvanen M, Niemi S, Parkkari J, Kannus P. Osteoporotic fractures of the distal humerus in elderly women. Ann Intern Med 2003;139:W-W61
81. Johansson H, Olerud S. Operative treatment of intercondylar fractures of the humerus. J Trauma 1971;1:836–843
82. John H, Rosso R, Neff U, et al. Operative treatment of distal humeral fractures in the elderly. J Bone Joint Surg Br 1994;76:793–796
83. Mehne DK, Matta J. Bicolumn fractures of the adult humerus. Paper presented at: 53rd annual meeting of the American Academy of Orthopaedic Surgeons, 1986; New Orleans, LA
84. Ring D, Gulotta L, Jupiter JB. Unstable nonunions of the distal part of the humerus. J Bone Joint Surg Am 2003;85: 1040–1046
85. Mitsunaga MM, Bryan RS, Linscheid RL. Condylar nonunions of the elbow. J Trauma 1982;22:787–791
86. Sanchez-Sotelo J, Torchia ME, O'Driscoll SW. Principle-based internal fixation of distal humerus fractures. Tech Hand Up Extrem Surg 2001;5:179–187
87. Milch H. Fractures and fracture dislocations of the humeral condyles. J Trauma 1964;4:592–607
88. Dean GS, Holliger EHT, Urbaniak JR. Elbow allograft for reconstruction of the elbow with massive bone loss. Long-term results. Clin Orthop Relat Res 1997;341: 12–22
89. Cobb TK, Morrey BF. Total elbow arthroplasty as primary treatment for distal humerus fractures in elderly patients. J Bone Joint Surg Am 1997;79:826–832
90. Frankle MA, Herscovici D Jr, DiPasquale TG, et al. A comparison of open reduction and internal fixation and primary total elbow arthroplasty in the treatment of intraarticular distal humerus fractures in women older than age 65. J Orthop Trauma 2003;17:473–480
91. Gambirasio R, Riand N, Stern R, Hoffmeyer P. Total elbow replacement for complex fractures of the distal humerus: an option for the elderly patient. J Bone Joint Surg Br 2001;83:974–978
92. Garcia JA, Mykula R, Stanley D. Complex fractures of the distal humerus in the elderly: the role of total elbow replacement as primary treatment. J Bone Joint Surg Br 2002;84:812–816
93. Patterson SD, Bain GI, Mehta JA. Surgical approaches to the elbow. Clin Orthop Relat Res 2000;370:19–33

94. Perry CR, Gibson CT, Kowalski MF. Transcondylar fractures of the distal humerus. J Orthop Trauma 1989;3:98–106
95. Petraco DM, Koval KJ, Kummer FJ, Zuckerman JD. Fixation stability of olecranon osteotomies. Clin Orthop Relat Res 1996;333:181–185
96. Ring D, Jupiter JB. Complex fractures of the distal humerus and their complications. J Shoulder Elbow Surg 1999;8:85–97
97. Contreras MG, Warner MA, Charboneau WJ, Cahill DR. Anatomy of the ulnar nerve at the elbow: potential relationship of acute ulnar neuropathy to gender differences. Clin Anat 1998;11:372–378
98. Morrey BF, Askew LJ, Chao EY. A biomechanical study of normal functional elbow motion. J Bone Joint Surg Am 1981;63:872–877
99. Scharplatz D, Allgöwer M. Fracture-dislocations of the elbow. Injury 1975;7:143–159
100. Van Gorder GW. Surgical approach in supracondylar "T" fractures of the humerus requiring open reduction. J Bone Joint Surg Am 1940;22:278–292
101. Viola RW, Hanel DP. Early "simple" release of posttraumatic elbow contracture associated with heterotopic ossification. J Hand Surg [Am] 1999;24:370–380
102. Khoo D, Carmichael SW, Spinner RJ. Ulnar nerve anatomy and compression. Orthop Clin North Am 1996; 27:317–338
103. McKee MD, Wilson TL, Winston L, et al. Functional outcome following surgical treatment of intra-articular distal humeral fractures through a posterior approach. J Bone Joint Surg Am 2000;82:1701–1707
104. Ring D, Jupiter JB, Toh S. Salvage of contaminated fractured of the distal humerus with thin wire external fixation. Clin Orthop Relat Res 1999;359:203–208
105. Helfet DL, Kloen P, Anand N, Rosen HS. Open reduction and internal fixation of delayed unions and nonunions of fractures of the distal part of the humerus. J Bone Joint Surg Am 2003;85:33–40
106. Helfet DL, Kloen P, Anand N, Rosen HS. ORIF of delayed unions and nonunions of distal humeral fractures. Surgical technique. J Bone Joint Surg Am 2004;86:18–29
107. Müller ME, Nazarian S, Koch P, Schatzker J. The Comprehensive Classification of Fractures of Long Bones. Berlin: Springer-Verlag; 1990
108. Schemitsch EH, Tencer AF, Henley MB. Biomechanical evaluation of methods of internal fixation of the distal humerus. J Orthop Trauma 1994;8:468–475
109. Bruno RJ, Lee ML, Strauch RJ, Rosenwasser MP. Posttraumatic elbow stiffness: evaluation and management. J Am Acad Orthop Surg 2002;10:106–116
110. Müller ME, Allgöwer M, Willenegger H. Manual of Internal Fixation: Techniques Recommended by the AO-Group. Berlin, Germany: Springer-Verlag 1970
111. Wang KC, Shih HN, Hsu KY, Shih CH. Intercondylar fractures of the distal humerus: routine anterior subcutaneous transposition of the ulnar nerve in a posterior operative approach. J Trauma 1994;36:770–773
112. McKee MD, Jupiter JB, Bamberger HB. Coronal shear fractures of the distal end of the humerus. J Bone Joint Surg Am 1996;78:49–54
113. Ristic S, Strauch RJ, Rosenwasser MP. The assessment and treatment of nerve dysfunction after trauma around the elbow. Clin Orthop Relat Res 2000;370:138–152
114. Wilkinson JM, Stanley D. Posterior surgical approaches to the elbow: a comparative anatomic study. J Shoulder Elbow Surg 2001;10:380–382

12 Open Reduction and Internal Fixation for Fractures about the Elbow in the Elderly

Christian J. H. Veillette and Michael D. McKee

Fractures about the elbow in the elderly are often complicated by metaphyseal comminution, poor soft tissue quality, and diminished bone mineral density. A clear understanding of the surgical decision-making process in osteoporotic elbow fractures is important to prevent failures and optimize the independence of an elderly patient. The surgeon's ability to obtain stable fracture fixation and restore early function to the elbow has been enhanced by an improved understanding of elbow anatomy and newer techniques to optimize stability in elbow fracture fixation with improved implants. In this chapter, we will discuss the diagnosis, surgical treatment, and rehabilitation of fractures about the elbow in the elderly.

Fractures around the elbow in the elderly remain one of the most demanding challenges in surgical fracture treatment. Elbow fractures can lead to significant disability in the elderly due to the difficulties inherent in their treatment, poor tolerance for joint immobilization, and the fact that up to 30% of these patients develop complications.[1] Proper function of the elbow is central to positioning the hand in space for fine movements, powerful grasping, and serving as a fulcrum for the forearm.[2] Loss of basic elbow function can severely affect activities of daily living. For an elderly patient who may have comorbid illnesses and limited mobility, these injuries can lead to the loss of independence.

Fractures of the elbow comprise ~7% of adult fractures with less than half of all elbow fractures arising in the distal humerus. Recent evidence suggests that the age-adjusted incidence of elbow fractures in women older than 60 years has more than doubled from 1970 to 1995.[3] Although data on bone mineral density values for the elbow in large cohorts of patients are not available, from a clinical point of view, in elderly patients these fractures are often considered "osteoporotic fractures." The age-related osseous demineralization within the meta- and epiphyseal area of the distal humerus has been shown with preferential loss within the capitellar region.[4]

Anatomy of the Elbow

The elbow is a complex hinge joint that relies on a combination of bony articulations and soft tissue constraints to optimize stability and mobility.[5] The ulnohumeral articulation is the essential factor for osseous stability and mobility in the flexion-extension plane. The olecranon blocks the anterior translation of the ulna with respect to the distal humerus while an intact coronoid process resists posterior subluxation of the proximal ulna in extension beyond 30 degrees or greater.[6] The importance of the radial head as a secondary stabilizer to valgus stress and posterior translation is well recognized; however, the radial head also indirectly contributes to varus and posterolateral stability by creating tension in the lateral ligament complex.[7] The distal humerus consists of diverging medial and lateral columns joined at their most distal aspect by the "tie arch," consisting of the articular segment – the trochlea and the capitellum. The capitellum is the most distal portion of the lateral column; the nonarticular medial epicondyle is the most distal portion of the medial column. The trochlea is intermediate between the capitellum and the distal end of the medial column. The articular segment projects slightly anterior to the axis of the shaft at an angle of 40 degrees with the capitellum slightly further forward than the trochlea. The medial epicondyle is on the projected axis of the shaft, whereas the lateral epicondyle is projected slightly forward from the axis. Furthermore, soft tissue constraints play a major role in elbow stability. The anterior band of the ulnar collateral ligament acts as the major stabilizer to valgus stress.[8] The major stabilizer to varus or rotatory stress is the lateral collateral ligament complex, including the lateral ulnar collateral ligament.[9,10]

Epidemiology and Mechanisms of Injury

The majority of elbow fractures in the elderly are the result of a fall from a standing height after a tripping or slipping incident.[3] Fractures of the olecranon occur from direct or indirect trauma. A fall or blunt trauma on the posterior tip of the elbow may cause fracture directly. Indirect avulsion of the olecranon by forces generated within the triceps muscle may occur with eccentric contraction during a fall on a partially flexed elbow. In cases of severe force to the elbow, a fracture dislocation can occur with posterior displacement of the olecranon fragment and displacement of the distal ulnar fragment together with the head of the radius anterior to the humerus. Fractures of the distal humerus result from an axial load through the elbow with the joint flexed beyond 90 degrees. Cadaveric studies have shown that when the load is applied with the elbow at 90 degrees, an olecranon fracture is produced. Radial head fractures result from an axial load with maximum force transmission in full elbow extension with forearm pronation.[11]

Goals of Fracture Management in the Elderly

In the elderly, restoration of the complex anatomy of the elbow is often complicated by poor bone quality and associated metaphyseal and epiphyseal comminution. As a result, adequate fracture fragment fixation and stable joint reconstruction are often difficult to achieve, but are central to effective care. The primary goal of definitive fracture management in elderly patients is early restoration of function and independence. The tolerance for posttraumatic elbow immobilization is very poor in elderly patients with a duration of immobilization longer than 15 days leading in a high percentage of cases to significant stiffness and loss of function.[1] Therefore, the selected treatment should be prompt, definitive, and kept as simple as possible to minimize surgical time, blood loss, and physiologic stress. However, the presence of comorbid illnesses requires thorough evaluation before surgery. Although anatomic restoration is important for intraarticular fractures, in certain cases, a minor degree of incongruity may be preferred to prolonged immobilization. Metaphyseal and diaphyseal fractures are often best managed by attempts to primarily achieve stability rather than anatomic reduction.[12] Failure of screw purchase in bone, not implant breakage, is the primary mechanism of failure of internal fixation in osteoporotic bone. Decreased bone mineral density correlates with the holding power of the screws and may result in poor screw purchase.[13,14] For these reasons, fractures around the elbow in the elderly mandate a different algorithm for the surgical decision-making process and operative techniques compared with fractures in younger patients with superior bone quality and increased capacity for fracture repair.

Classification of Elbow Fracture

Fractures around the elbow in the elderly are best classified independently, but must be understood within the context of the overall injury. Associated ulna fractures can involve the coronoid process and/or the olecranon process. Regan and Morrey classified fractures of the coronoid process into three types, depending on the extent of involvement.[15] Type I fractures are a small fleck of bone sheared from the coronoid during subluxation or dislocation. Type II fractures involve up to 50% of the coronoid process. Type III fractures involve more than 50% of the coronoid. Recently, O'Driscoll has added an additional fracture pattern (type IV) to describe the sagittal plane fracture of the coronoid involving the attachment of the anterior bundle of the medial collateral ligament.[16] Colton's classification of olecranon fractures reflects displacement and the anatomy of the fracture, thus providing guidance as to the most biomechanically appropriate type of fixation. Fractures are described as nondisplaced and stable if they are displaced less than 2 mm, and exhibit no change in position with gentle flexion to 90 degrees or with extension against gravity. Displaced fractures can be further divided into avulsion fractures, transverse or oblique fractures, isolated comminuted fractures, or fractures with associated dislocations.[17]

Radial head fractures are classified based on the modified Mason's classification by Hotchkiss. Type I fractures represent nondisplaced or minimally displaced fractures (<2 mm) of the radial head or neck requiring no surgical intervention. Type II fractures are displaced fractures of the radial head or neck but can be fixed. Type III fractures are displaced radial head or neck fractures, but are not reconstructable.

The Orthopaedic Trauma Association (OTA)/AO classification system is most commonly used to describe distal humerus fractures and divides them into type A, nonarticular; type B, partial articular; and type C, complete articular. Based on the position and orientation of the fracture line and degree of comminution additional levels are appended.

Patient Assessment

History

Patients with a distal humeral, radial head, or proximal ulna fracture present with pain and swelling about the elbow. Those with displaced fractures usually have an obvious deformity, and attempted motion may elicit painful bony crepitus. The mechanism of injury as well as any associated neurovascular complications associated with the initial injury should be elicited from the patient. Thorough assessment for concurrent illnesses precipitating the injury (such as an arrhythmia) and a detailed account of comorbid conditions are important.

Clinical Examination

Physical examination should begin with assessment of the condition of the soft tissues around the elbow. Extensive swelling, ecchymosis, and any abrasions or lacerations should be noted and may influence the timing of surgery or location of incisions. An assessment of range of motion (ROM) or strength of the elbow should not be vigorously pursued. There may be a palpable sulcus at the site of an olecranon fracture, accompanied by painful and limited ROM. An important sign to be elicited with isolated olecranon fractures is the inability to extend the elbow actively against gravity. Although it may be difficult to get the patient's cooperation secondary to pain, this inability indicates discontinuity of the triceps mechanism. A careful neurovascular examination, especially of the ulnar nerve, is essential prior to any planned manipulation of the elbow.

Radiographic Assessment

Plain radiographs in the anteroposterior, true lateral, and oblique projections are usually sufficient to provide enough information for an accurate diagnosis. Severe comminution with displacement and overlap of the fracture fragments can obscure thorough determination of the fracture pattern. Thus, radiographs need to be good quality, out of splint, and obtained while maintaining gentle longitudinal traction with inclusion of the elbow joint on the film. Nontraction in the splint radiographs is not as well suited for accurate diagnosis, for classifying the fracture, and for formal preoperative planning. Rarely does computed tomography (CT) of the elbow provide additional information that alters decision making and preoperative planning.

Treatment

Distal Humerus Fractures

Historically, distal humerus fractures have been difficult to treat with unpredictable outcomes prior to the 1960s.[18] Nonoperative treatment, the "bag of bones" technique, was advocated by many authorities as the best treatment for fractures of the distal humerus, especially in elderly patients due primarily to the lack of adequate surgical techniques and implants. During the past few decades nonoperative treatment has been shown to result in poor outcomes with high rates of joint stiffness, malunion, or painful nonunion.[1,19,20] Advances in the theory, techniques, and instrumentation for operative management of intraarticular fractures has made open reduction and internal fixation (ORIF) the treatment of choice for displaced intraarticular distal humerus fractures in adults. Disagreements remain on how to treat these fractures in elderly patients as stable fracture fixation and early initiation of therapy can be difficult. Current controversy remains regarding the indications for performing a primary total elbow arthroplasty for the treatment of comminuted fractures of the distal humerus in the elderly (see Chapter 13). The rationale for ORIF is the limited longevity of arthroplasty compared with successful primary osteosynthesis. In addition, infection or implant failure is more difficult to manage in the context of arthroplasty.

The complete articular fractures (C-type) are the most commonly encountered in elderly patients. ORIF can be performed through several approaches such as the triceps-splitting approach, the posterior transolecranon approach, or the extensive triceps sparing approach.[21] In open distal humeral fractures, the wound is most commonly posterior or posterolateral with an associated defect in the triceps from the protrusion of the humeral shaft. In this scenario a triceps-splitting approach has been shown to have several advantages compared with olecranon osteotomy.[22] The plating construct that optimizes fracture fixation stiffness is two plates on separate distal humeral columns and in different planes.[23] This is commonly performed with a medially positioned reconstruction plate and a small fragment compression plate on the posterolateral surface or an anatomical lateral buttress "J" plate. Alternatively, precontoured anatomical plates can be placed directly medially and laterally with screws directed into the opposite column and the distal fragments further stabilized by the compressive effect of the plates.[24,25] The general principles are anatomic restoration of the articular surface, followed by restoration of joint shaft alignment, then stable fixation of the reduced distal fragment to the humeral shaft. Polymethylmethacrylate (PMMA) may be utilized to augment screw fixation proximally.[26,27]

Technique

The patient is placed in the lateral decubitus position with the arm at 90 degrees abduction and the elbow flexed at 90 degrees over a bolster. A midline posterior incision is made curving around the lateral tip of the olecranon. Full-thickness skin flaps are created laterally and medially with care taken to minimize soft tissue handling. The ulnar nerve is identified at the medial aspect of the triceps proximal to the injury and carefully exposed, including release of the cubital tunnel. A Penrose drain is placed around the nerve to assist in protection; however, traction is avoided. A midline split in the triceps muscle and tendon is created proximally and extended distally along the dorsal crest of the ulna. Meticulous sharp dissection is used to create full thickness flaps at the triceps insertion onto the ulna. Dissection is carried laterally and medially along the distal humerus to expose the lateral and medial column, respectively, taking care to protect the ulnar nerve medially and the radial nerve laterally. The fracture fragments are gently cleaned of clot and

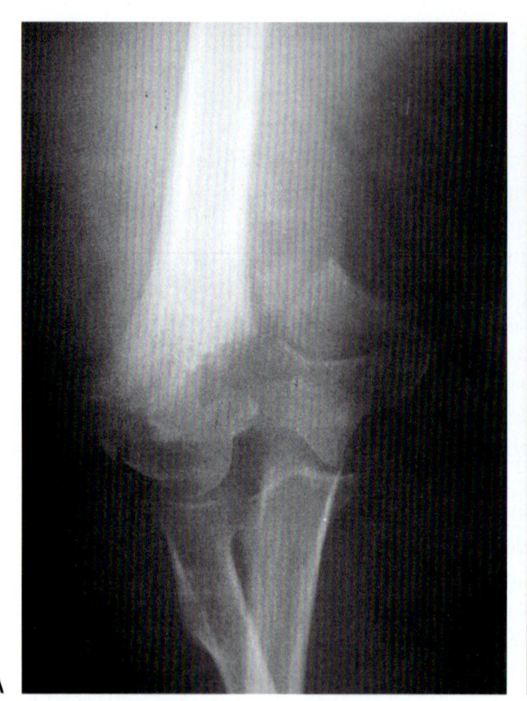
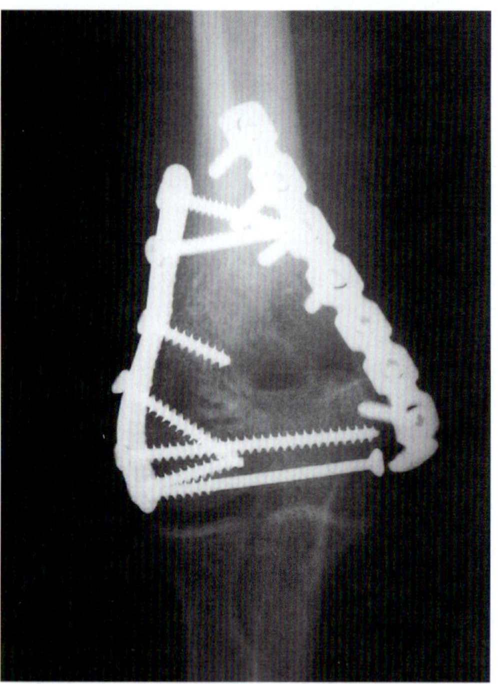

Figure 12–1 **(A)** Anteroposterior (AP) radiograph of a comminuted, intraarticular distal humerus fracture caused by a fall in an elderly patient. **(B)** AP radiograph following open reduction and internal fixation with a precontoured lateral J plate and a compression plate contoured to fit the medial column. Both plates "cradle" the distal fragments with good screw purchase distally.

debris and the distal humeral articular surface is reassembled and stabilized with Kirschner wires (K-wires). The articular fragment is stabilized with a transverse lag screw or fully threaded position screws when there is intercondylar comminution or bone loss to avoid narrowing the trochlea. The lateral plate, usually a 3.5-mm compression plate or specially designed anatomic lateral buttress "J" plate, is applied along the straight lateral column. The medial plate, usually a 3.5-mm reconstruction plate or compression plate, is contoured to lie directly over the medial epicondyle or more posteriorly along the medial column respectively **(Fig. 12–1)**.

Precontoured anatomical plates are available and may be helpful to provide a lower profile implant on the medial side. In addition, angular fixed locking plates have been introduced with the potential advantage of improved stability and pull-out strength within the osteoporotic bone of the distal fragment.[4,28] Regardless of implant choice, the distal placement of plates to "cradle" the distal fragments is imperative, thus relying on a combination of plate strength, placement of as many screws as possible in the distal fragment, and interdigitation of screws in the distal fragment to optimize stability.[24] A portable radiograph should be obtained following fixation. The triceps is reattached to the olecranon using three #2 Ethibond sutures (Ethicon, Inc., Somerville, NJ) passed through bone in a horizontal mattress fashion. The remainder of the triceps is reapproximated using interrupted figure-eight sutures. The ulnar nerve is transposed anteriorly to a subcutaneous position and prevented from migrating posteriorly with a suture between the fascia and subcutaneous tissue. The medial intermuscular septum is released and the nerve is checked to ensure there is no tethering or pressure in its transposed location. Subcutaneous tissue and skin are then closed in layers.

Proximal Ulnar Fractures

The subcutaneous location of the proximal ulna makes this area prone to fracture from a direct blow to the posterior surface of the elbow. This is a frequent mechanism suffered during falls in elderly patients and similar to distal humeral fractures can present a challenge because of associated comminution.

Nondisplaced fractures of the olecranon are treated nonoperatively. These fractures are defined by displacement less than 2 mm, no change in position with gentle flexion to 90 degrees or extension of the elbow against gravity. These fractures are immobilized in a long arm cast with the elbow in 90 degrees of flexion for 3 to 4 weeks followed by protected ROM exercises. Flexion past 90 degrees should be avoided until bone healing is complete radiographically at approximately 6 to 8 weeks.

In the elderly patient, ROM may be initiated earlier than 3 weeks if the patient can tolerate it, with the goal to prevent stiffness. A follow-up x-ray should be obtained within 5 to 7 days after cast application to ensure that displacement of the fracture has not occurred. Immobilization in full extension is not recommended because stiffness is more likely, and if the fracture requires full extension for reduction it should be treated operatively.

Displaced olecranon fractures require operative treatment to restore elbow extension, joint congruity, and elbow stability. In the elderly, the restoration of elbow extension is particularly important to allow independent standing from a seated position and use of canes or walkers. Transverse fractures without comminution are amenable to tension band wiring. The tension band wire construct converts the tensile distraction force of the triceps into a dynamic compressive force across the olecranon articular surface. Traditionally, K-wires have been used in the tension band construct. Intramedullary cancellous screw fixation should be avoided in elderly patients with underlying osteoporosis as the proximal fragment may fracture further if a single 6.5-mm cancellous screw is used to secure the longitudinal component of the fracture. In addition, poor purchase is often encountered in the wide osteoporotic medullary canal of elderly patients.

Technique

Two 1.6- or 2.0-mm K-wires are inserted into the olecranon tip to obtain proximal control; engagement distally in the anterior cortex of the ulna increases the stability of fixation.[29] Care should be taken to avoid overpenetration of the wires, as they may cause neurovascular damage, limitation in forearm rotation, or heterotopic ossification. The length of the wire should be noted at the point where it engages the second cortex. Once the wire penetrates the far cortex, it should be partially backed out and bent 180 degrees at the previously noted position and cut off. The fibers of the triceps tendon should be split sharply with a scalpel at the site of the K-wires to allow the cut and bent ends to be impacted against the cortex. A figure-eight loop of 1.5-mm or 18-gauge wire is positioned through a drill hole located distally approximately an equal distance from the fracture as the tip of the olecranon. The wire is then passed deep to the fibers of the triceps, adjacent to bone, beneath the K-wires. The wire is tightened by twisting in two places on opposite arms of the crossed portion of the figure eight for additional stability. The K-wires are seated firmly in the bone using an impactor and sutured beneath the fibers of the triceps to prevent wire migration.

In transverse fractures with comminution, the tension band technique will collapse the fragments together leading to a narrowed olecranon articulation that does not track properly. The optimal fixation for these fractures is offered with contoured, limited-contract dynamic compression (LCDC) plate fixation, with or without bone graft depending on the size of the comminuted region.[30] Similarly, a plate with lag screw fixation is preferable over the tension band construct for oblique fractures with and without comminution. Treatment with the tension band technique in this fracture pattern often results in displacement, as compression along the tension band causes shortening along the inclined plane of the obliquity.

The advantages of using the LCDC plate for fixation are several-fold.[31,32] The plate allows improved contouring and can be appropriately placed on the dorsal tension surface of the proximal ulna around the tip of the olecranon to help hold the proximal fragment when poor bone quality limits screw purchase. The redesigned screw holes allow greater angulation of screw placement and the option of compression from either side of the screw hole. In addition, its lower profile allows its use in subcutaneous situations where soft tissue coverage may be in question. The proximal fixation of the plate is often the greatest challenge in the elderly as the bone may be quite thin and thus cancellous screws rather than cortical screws should be used. The advent of newer precontoured plates allows for an increased number of fixation points in the proximal fragment and "cradles" the olecranon along its dorsal surface. In complex fractures of the proximal ulna a large coronoid fragment is often present. This fragment is very important to the final stability of the elbow and must be fixed with lag screws placed through or adjacent to the implanted plate to prevent early posterior subluxation of the elbow **(Figs. 12–2** and **12–3)**.[33]

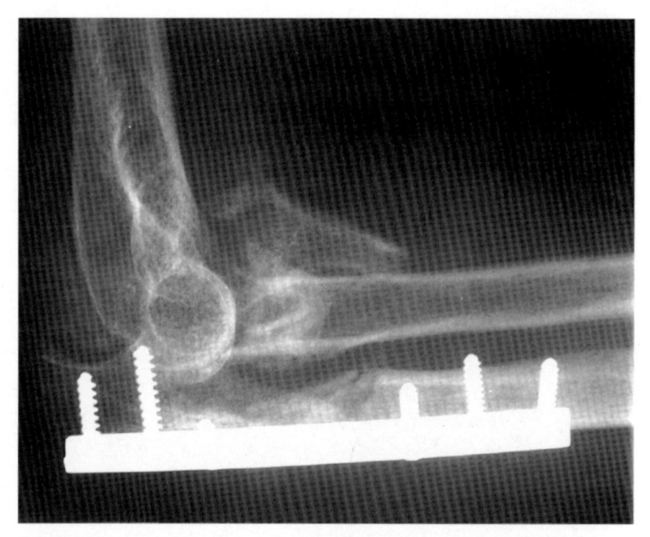

Figure 12–2 Technical errors in the management of a complex proximal ulna and radial head fracture resulted in early postoperative posterior elbow subluxation. The coronoid fragment was not repaired and the radial head has been excised and not reconstructed. When ligamentous disruption exists, the radial head and coronoid provide a critical buttress against posterior subluxation.

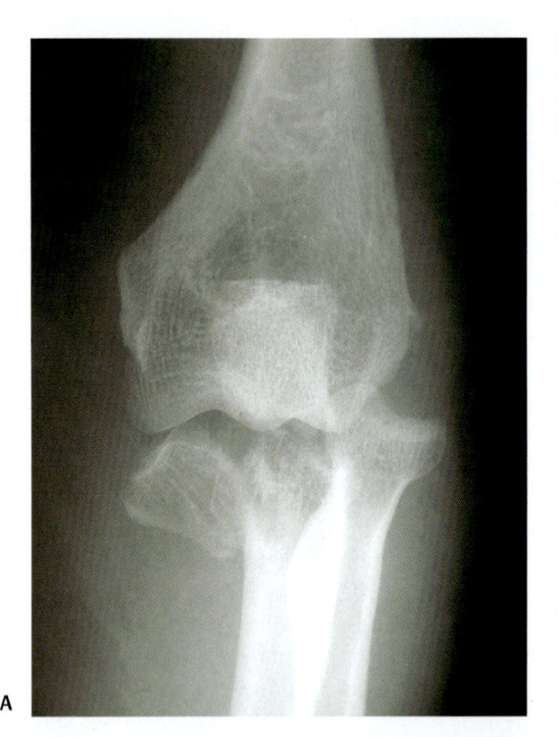

A

Figure 12–3 **(A)** Anteroposterior and **(B)** lateral radiograph of a complex elbow injury in an elderly patient with poor bone quality. There is a comminuted proximal ulna fracture with a large coronoid fragment, a small chip fracture of the radial head, and a posterior elbow subluxation. **(C)** Lateral radiograph following fixation with lag screw into coronoid, a contoured limited-contract dynamic compression (LCDC) plate, application, and a closed reduction of the radial head. **(D,E)** Final follow-up at one-year postinjury showed excellent clinical result, no pain, and full activities.

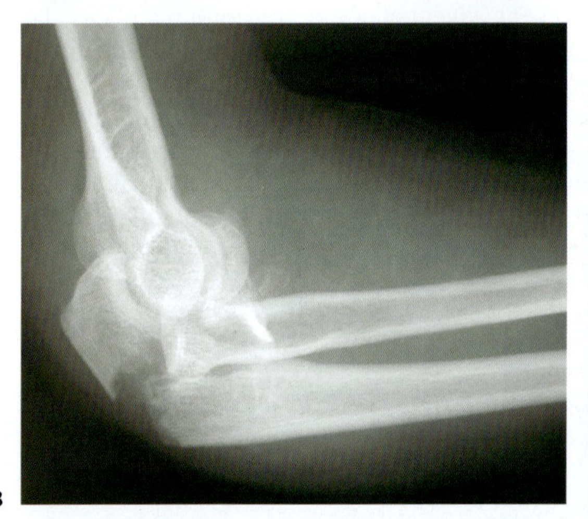

B

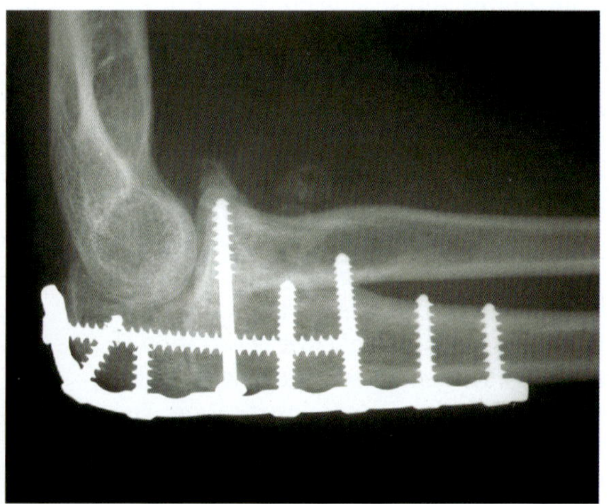

C

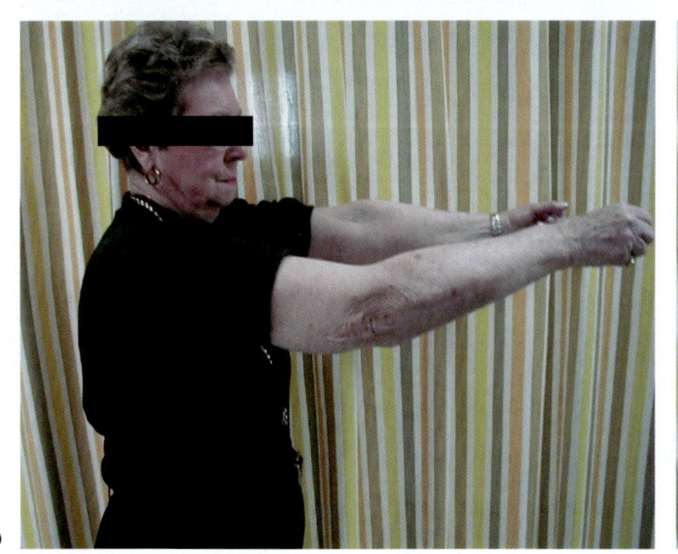

D

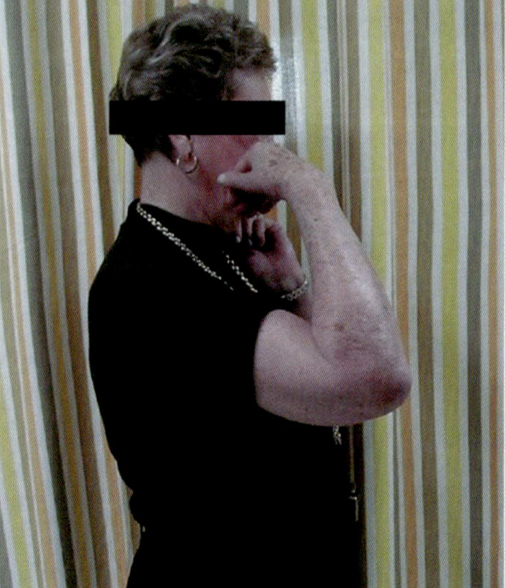

E

Technique

The patient is placed in a supine position on the operating room table with the injured arm on a bolster across the chest. A sterile tourniquet is placed on the upper arm after skin preparation and draping. A posterior midline incision centered on the olecranon is extended proximally 5 cm from the tip of the olecranon. The ulna is approached along its subcutaneous border and the anconeus can be elevated to approach the radial head if required. The coronoid can be visualized and reduced through the olecranon fracture by mobilizing the proximal olecranon fragment, as one would do with an olecranon osteotomy **(Fig. 12–4A)**. Impacted articular fragments are elevated and the coronoid is then reduced and provisionally fixed to the ulna with one or two K-wires **(Fig. 12–4B)**. The use of a heavy

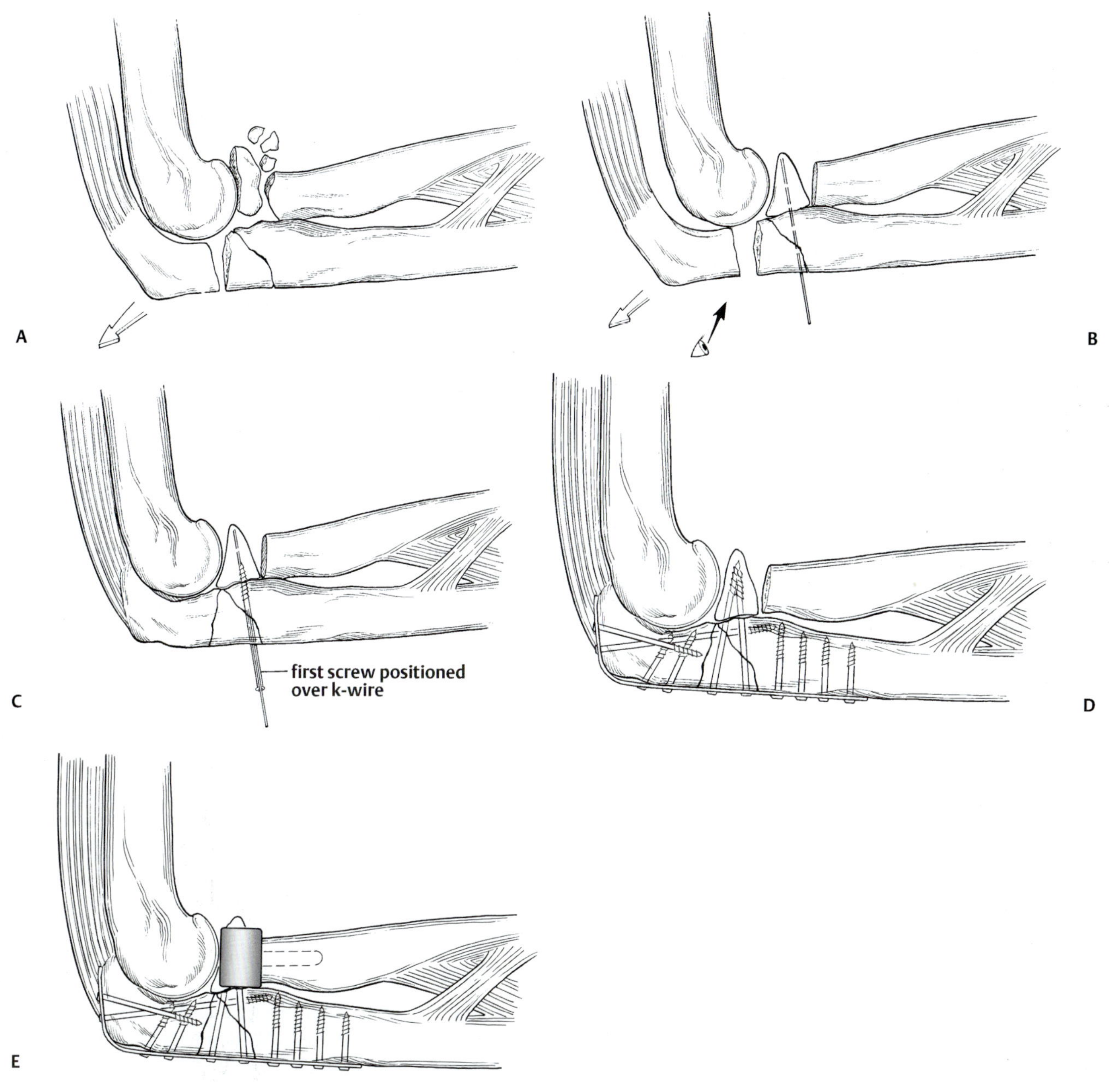

Figure 12–4 **(A)** Schematic of complex proximal ulnar fracture with coronoid and radial head fracture. **(B)** The radial head fragments are removed and the coronoid can be visualized and reduced through the olecranon fracture by mobilizing the proximal olecranon fragment as one would do with an olecranon osteotomy. The coronoid is reduced and provisionally fixed to the ulna with one or two Kirschner wires. **(C)** Definitive fixation of the coronoid should be performed with a small fragment screw prior to closure of the main ulnar fracture. **(D)** A narrow 3.5-mm LCDC plate is then contoured to fit the proximal ulna with the maximum bend, near 90 degrees, between the second and third screw holes of the plate. **(E)** A modular metallic implant should be used to replace the radial head.

suture passed around the coronoid fragment can assist with temporary reduction. Definitive fixation of the coronoid should be performed with a small fragment screw prior to closure of the main ulnar fracture **(Fig. 12–4C)**. A narrow 3.5-mm LCDC plate is then contoured to fit the proximal ulna with the maximum bend, near 90 degrees, between the second and third screw holes of the plate **(Fig. 12–4D)**. The plate must be of sufficient length to accommodate three or four screws distal to the fracture. Once fracture reduction is achieved, the contoured plate is applied to the dorsal aspect of the olecranon and the triceps fascia is incised to allow the implant to sit on the bone. The plate is secured proximally with one screw from the fourth or fifth hole obliquely upwards into the coronoid process in compression mode. A long cancellous screw is placed from the first or second hole across the fracture toward the proximal shaft at the base of the coronoid. Additional screws are placed proximally in the olecranon and the plate is secured distally to the shaft by three or four bicortical screws. The interlocking of screws maximizes purchase and stability.

In the osteoporotic olecranon, direct trauma to the posterior aspect of the elbow can result in an isolated severely comminuted fracture. Excision of the fracture fragments and reattachment of the triceps tendon may be indicated in a select group of elderly patients in whom the olecranon fracture fragments are too small or too comminuted for successful internal fixation. However, the coronoid and anterior soft tissues, collateral ligaments, and interosseus membrane must be intact otherwise instability will result. The triceps tendon is reattached adjacent to the articular surface with nonabsorbable sutures that are passed through drill holes in the remaining proximal ulna. Reattachment of the triceps in this manner creates a sling for the trochlea and a smooth congruent transition from the triceps tendon to the articular surface, but decreases the moment arm and may result in a weaker extensor mechanism but enhanced elbow stability. The amount of olecranon that can be excised safely has been debated. Based on in vitro[6] and clinical studies,[34,35] between 50 to 70% of the olecranon articular surface can be excised without compromising elbow stability provided the coronoid and distal trochlea are preserved.

Radial Head Fractures

In elderly patients, even low-energy impacts can result in a severely comminuted radial head fracture. The available bone stock may not be sufficient to allow internal fixation. However, the radial head is an important secondary stabilizer of the elbow and its role becomes critical in the presence of associated fractures and elbow instability. In type I fractures, forearm motion is limited only by pain and swelling and the patient is initially managed with a sling for 7 days followed by active forearm and elbow motion as soon as tolerated to prevent stiffness. Displacement can still occur and patient follow-up is required at regular intervals.

Type II fractures have limited motion due to intraarticular displacement and are best treated with ORIF. However, in elderly patients with severe osteoporosis the usual repertoire of mini-fragment screws and plates or countersunk Herbert screws may be unable to achieve sufficient purchase in the bone. Type III fractures have severe comminution of the radial head and/or neck and are not reconstructable with internal fixation. The treatment algorithm for type II and type III radial head fractures is therefore similar in elderly patients with poor bone mineral quality. ORIF of the radial head is best reserved for minimally comminuted fractures with three or fewer articular fragments when anatomic reduction, stable fixation, and early ROM can be achieved.[36,37]

The main options for management of comminuted radial head fracture in elderly patients are excision of the radial head or prosthetic replacement. In considering excision of the radial head, several criteria are required to prevent complications. The patient should have low functional demands, an isolated injury to the radial head, and no associated injuries to the distal radial ulnar joint and interosseus ligament. In addition, the medial and lateral collateral ligaments and coronoid process must be intact. The excision should be complete, and not limited to the displaced fragment, as higher contact forces through the remaining portion can lead to rapid development of degenerative arthritis. A careful repair of the lateral collateral ligament complex should be performed if it is damaged to prevent posterolateral rotatory instability.[10,38] A modular metallic implant should be used to replace the radial head if any of the above criteria for excision are not met. The use of a modular radial head implant provides multiple head diameters and heights and different stem sizes, which allow for a close approximation to normal anatomy. The different head heights can accommodate the extension of fractures into the proximal neck and also account for observed variability in head height.[39]

Technique

For management of comminuted radial head fractures with radial head prostheses, the patient is placed in either the supine or lateral position with a tourniquet on the upper arm and the operative arm placed over a padded bolster. A midline posterior or lateral elbow skin incision is used depending on the presence or absence of associated injuries, respectively. A full thickness fasciocutaneous flap is elevated and the fascial interval between the anconeus and extensor carpi ulnaris is exposed. This can typically be seen as a fine fascial line dividing the two muscle groups distal to the lateral epicondyle. The radial head is exposed by incising the lateral collateral ligament complex and annular ligament at the mid-axis of the radial head, thereby staying anterior to the lateral ulnar collateral ligament.[39] The radial collateral ligament and overlying extensor muscles are elevated anteriorly off the lateral epicondyle to expose the radial head. The surgical exposure of the radial head is simplified in more complex injuries by traumatic disruption of the lateral collateral ligament complex and common extensor mechanism from the lateral epicondyle. Access to the coronoid is facilitated by radial head excision, and thus coronoid fixation should be performed before radial head replacement in more complex injuries. Homan retractors are used to deliver the radial head laterally assisting canal preparation and subsequent implant insertion.

The fragments of the radial head are excised and the radial neck is prepared using a straight stem rasp. The neck is divided with an oscillating saw at the tuberosity. Bone-cutting forceps should not be used because they can splinter the bone. Care must be taken not to oversize the prosthesis and risk splitting the remaining radial neck. The radial neck planer is placed onto the trial stem and the neck is rasped to ensure good contact of the radial head with the radial neck. The radial head trial is slipped over the trial stem and the implant trials are evaluated for height, congruent tracking with the capitellum, and elbow stability. The trial components are removed and the definitive implants are inserted preassembled. The elbow is taken through its range of flexion–extension and pronation–supination. The radial collateral ligaments are repaired and reattached to the lateral epicondyle using nonabsorbable sutures through drill holes or with a suture anchor. The fascial interval between the anconeus and extensor carpi ulnaris should also be closed to augment lateral stability of the elbow. Hemostasis after tourniquet deflation should be performed before wound closure. After radial head replacement and lateral soft tissue closure as outlined above, the elbow should be placed through an arc of flexion–extension while carefully evaluating for elbow stability in pronation, neutral, and supination.

Complications

Distal Humerus Fractures

Postoperative ulnar neuritis due to nerve compression occurs in up to 15% of patients managed with ORIF for intraarticular fractures.[1,40] Korner et al found that 1 out of the 6 patients with initial neurological symptoms had persistent paresthesias in the distribution of the ulnar nerve, while the other 5 patients had complete resolution. These problems can be minimized by appropriately contouring the implants to conform to the bone surface, and to situate implants in such a way as to minimize their irritating effect on the nerve. It has been recommended that the ulnar nerve be transposed routinely when the nerve lies in contact with the hardware.[40] During the transposition of the ulnar nerve, the medial intermuscular septum and the fascia between and over the two heads of the flexor carpi ulnaris need to be adequately released to prevent sites of residual compression.

Hardware irritation is not uncommon once the swelling has subsided and the elbow has regained its ROM. The lower portion of the medial supracondylar ridge and medial epicondyle is a common site for prominent hardware in elderly patients who have minimal subcutaneous tissue in this area. Furthermore, loss of fixation in the distal fragment has been reported as a significant problem in elderly patients represented by distal screw loosening or implant failure.[1,24] This is most likely secondary to the age-dependent osseous demineralization within the metaphyseal and epiphyseal distal humerus region. Korner et al[1] reported implant failure and/or distal screw loosening in 12 of 45 patients with the majority of screw loosening appearing in the lateral column. This failure mechanism has been attributed to the repetitive varus torques that occur across the elbow with minimal-use activities, distracting the lateral column away from any fixation placed on its posterior surface.[24] Strict adherence to the guidelines discussed above for optimal fixation can minimize the occurrence of fixation failure.

Malunion or nonunion is often the result of inadequate fracture fixation or implant failure. It is more common in C-type fractures with incomplete consolidation in the meta-diaphyseal component of the fracture. Removal of the retained hardware and reosteosynthesis with medial and lateral column compression plating can be performed in instances where adequate bone stock is present. Cancellous bone graft or bone substitute should be used to maximize healing potential of the nonunion site. Anterior and/or posterior capsular releases should be performed if elbow joint motion is significantly compromised.[41] In elderly patients with hardware failure and inadequate bone stock for reosteosynthesis, total elbow arthroplasty is the procedure of choice to maximize timely return to function.[42]

Loss of motion is the most common problem after fractures about the elbow, especially in elderly patients. Elderly patients with isolated injuries to the distal humerus typically lose 20 degrees of extension and 20 degrees of flexion, with a pronation/supination deficit of 30 degrees.[1]

Proximal Ulnar Fractures

Painful hardware irritation requiring removal is one of the most common complications after internal fixation of olecranon fractures. Complaints related to prominent hardware have been reported in 3 to 80% of cases. A higher incidence of prominent painful hardware has been reported after tension-band wiring than compression plating with fewer cases of symptomatic hardware irritation after LCDC plating.[30,31,43]

Nonunion of olecranon fractures have been reported to occur in up to 5% with typical symptoms of pain, instability, or loss of motion.[30,44] Treatment options for olecranon nonunions in the elderly include excision, osteosynthesis with a LCDC plate, or elbow arthroplasty in the presence of severe posttraumatic arthritis. Excision of the proximal portion of the pseudarthrosis and repair of the triceps tendon is an acceptable method of management in elderly patients ensuring that the coronoid and anterior soft tissues are intact.

Radial Head Fractures

Wound healing problems are occasionally seen, most commonly in the elderly because of pressure over the posterior aspect of the elbow. Stiffness caused by capsular contracture of the elbow is most commonly seen in patients with associated fractures and delayed initiation of mobilization. Redislocation of the elbow can be seen in patients in whom concomitant coronoid or collateral ligament injuries are present and were not addressed at the time of the initial procedure. Late complications include implant loosening and elbow osteoarthritis. Although radiographic lucencies are often seen around the implant stems at follow-up, symptomatic implant loosening is rare with current implant designs.

Postoperative Rehabilitation

Early initiation of physical therapy is one of the most important issues in elbow surgery of elderly patients. Korner et al[1] in their retrospective series of distal humeral fractures in 45 patients, aged 60 and older, showed that a duration of immobilization longer than 15 days correlated with more significant impairment in ROM. An initial posterior plaster slab with the elbow flexed to 90 degrees can be applied in the operating room to assist in immediate postoperative pain management. The posterior slab is removed on day 1 or 2 if the soft tissue is reasonable; otherwise, it is discontinued at 7 to 10 days and a removable splint is provided. Gentle active-assisted and passive motion is then started with the patient instructed to support the wrist with the opposite hand and gently flex and extend the elbow, gradually increasing the ROM. The patient is instructed to take the arm out of the splint several times daily for these exercises and to let gravity work on extending the elbow. Active motion against resistance is avoided until callous formation is evident, usually at 8 to 10 weeks.

Results

Several studies have shown that the treatment of distal humerus fractures in elderly patients with ORIF can achieve functional results that are good to excellent in 75 to 80% of patients.[1,45–48] Pereles et al evaluated 18 patients, aged 63 to 85 years, in a retrospective review of plate and screw fixation for distal humerus fractures. They found that the general health status, as measured by the SF-36 Health Survey, was comparable to the published norms for U.S. male and female populations of similar age.[49] John et al found good to excellent functional results in 85% of patients in their retrospective analysis of internal fixation of distal humerus fractures in 49 patients over 75 years of age with a mean follow-up time of 18 months.[45] Recently, Korner et al have reviewed the outcome of 45 patients older than age 60 that underwent ORIF of distal humerus fractures with a minimum follow-up of 24 months.[1] In 60% of patients, elbow function was scored as good to excellent according to the Mayo Elbow Score. In 6 patients, results at follow-up were scored as poor and 12 of 19 patients with fair or poor results were found to have been immobilized for 14 days or longer. Together these studies suggest that an average arc of motion of 100 to 112 degrees for flexion/extension and 150 to 160 degrees for pronation/supination can be achieved. Although prospective studies using validated outcome measures are not available for ORIF of distal humerus fractures in elderly patients, it appears that strict adherence to the principles of meticulous joint restoration, stable primary fracture fixation, and early mobilization are of decisive importance for good functional results.

Gartsman et al performed a retrospective study of 107 patients with isolated olecranon fractures with 53 patients treated by excision and 54 treated by internal fixation.[35] Pain, function, ROM, elbow stability, extensor function, and incidence of degenerative joint changes were similar for each group at an average of 3.6 years. However, 13 local complications occurred in the patients who underwent open reduction internal fixation compared with two in the patients who had primary excision.

Fracture dislocations of the olecranon often are complex fractures of the proximal ulna or complex combined injuries of the radial head, coronoid, and collateral ligament complexes. Doornberg et al[33] reported a retrospective review of 26 patients with fracture-dislocations of the elbow composed of 10 anterior and 16 posterior fracture dislocations. Only 1 patient in the anterior fracture-dislocation group was over 60 years of age; in the posterior fracture-dislocation group, 8 of the 16 patients were 60 years or older. All of these elderly patients had an associated coronoid fracture and all but 1 patient had an associated radial head fracture (Mason type II or III). The average score on the American Shoulder and Elbow Surgeons elbow evaluation method[50] was 87 points (range 72.5 to 100) with three excellent, five good, and one fair result according to the system of Broberg and Morrey[51]. Thus, careful attention to stable restoration of the trochlear notch leads to a good functional outcome in these complex injuries in the majority of elderly patients.

Moro et al[52] evaluated the functional outcomes of arthroplasties with a metal radial head implant for the treatment of 25 displaced, nonreconstructable fractures of the radial head in 24 consecutive patients at a minimum of 2 years. Eight of these 24 patients were older than 60 years with 6 women and 2 men. The average Mayo Elbow Performance Index[53] was 86 with three excellent, four good, and one fair result. The ROM in these patients was similar to the entire cohort with elbow flexion of the injured extremity averaging 141 degrees; extension, −9 degrees; pronation, 77 degrees; and supination, 68 degrees. The use of metal radial head implants for the management of comminuted radial head fractures appears to provide reliable outcomes and patient satisfaction.

Summary

Fractures about the elbow in the elderly and their associated challenges will become increasingly common with our aging population. Increased comminution, diminished bone quality for fixation, and poor tolerance of immobilization in the elderly require strict adherence to principles of elbow surgery and fracture fixation. Advanced age is not a contraindication for ORIF because functional outcome is good or excellent in the majority of patients. A good result and avoidance of complications often dictate their ability to perform basic daily tasks and their independence.

Ongoing research is evaluating the role of new implants and techniques in the management of osteoporotic elbow fractures. Total elbow arthroplasty may play a larger role in the surgical management of comminuted distal humerus fractures and newer precontoured anatomical plate designs with angular locking screws may increase fixation options in patients with poor bone quality. The role of bone substitutes with intrinsic stability will play an increased role in the management of regions of comminution and bony defects. However, well-conducted prospective studies using a combination of patient-oriented and functional outcome instruments are still required to determine the efficacy of these operative interventions and surgical decision-making processes in the management of fractures about the elbow in elderly patients.

References

1. Korner J, Lill H, Muller LP, et al. Distal humerus fractures in elderly patients: results after open reduction and internal fixation. Osteoporos Int 2005;16(Suppl 2):S73–S79
2. Morrey BF, Askew LJ, Chao EY. A biomechanical study of normal functional elbow motion. J Bone Joint Surg Am 1981;63:872–877
3. Palvanen M, Kannus P, Parkkari J, et al. The injury mechanisms of osteoporotic upper extremity fractures among older adults: a controlled study of 287 consecutive patients and their 108 controls. Osteoporos Int 2000;11:822–831
4. Korner J, Lill H, Muller LP, Rommens PM, Schneider E, Linke B. The LCP-concept in the operative treatment of distal humerus fractures–biological, biomechanical and surgical aspects. Injury 2003;34(Suppl 2):B20–B30
5. Morrey BF, An KN. Articular and ligamentous contributions to the stability of the elbow joint. Am J Sports Med 1983;11:315–319
6. An KN, Morrey BF, Chao EY. The effect of partial removal of proximal ulna on elbow constraint. Clin Orthop Relat Res 1986;209:270–279
7. Morrey BF, Tanaka S, An KN. Valgus stability of the elbow. A definition of primary and secondary constraints. Clin Orthop Relat Res 1991;265:187–195
8. Hotchkiss RN, Weiland AJ. Valgus stability of the elbow. J Orthop Res 1987;5:372–377
9. Cohen MS, Hastings H II. Rotatory instability of the elbow. The anatomy and role of the lateral stabilizers. J Bone Joint Surg Am 1997;79:225–233
10. O'Driscoll SW, Bell DF, Morrey BF. Posterolateral rotatory instability of the elbow. J Bone Joint Surg Am 1991;73:440–446
11. Morrey BF, An KN, Stormont TJ. Force transmission through the radial head. J Bone Joint Surg Am 1988;70:250–256
12. Cornell CN. Internal fracture fixation in patients with osteoporosis. J Am Acad Orthop Surg 2003;11:109–119
13. Stromsoe K, Kok WL, Hoiseth A, Alho A. Holding power of the 4.5-mm AO/ASIF cortex screw in cortical bone in relation to bone mineral. Injury 1993;24:656–659
14. Alho A. Mineral and mechanics of bone fragility fractures. A review of fixation methods. Acta Orthop Scand 1993;64:227–232
15. Regan W, Morrey B. Fractures of the coronoid process of the ulna. J Bone Joint Surg Am 1989;71:1348–1354
16. Sanchez-Sotelo J, O'Driscoll SW, Morrey BF. Medial oblique compression fracture of the coronoid process of the ulna. J Shoulder Elbow Surg 2005;14:60–64

17. Colton CL. Fractures of the olecranon in adults: classification and management. Injury 1973;5:121–129
18. Riseborough EJ, Radin EL. Intercondylar T fractures of the humerus in the adult. A comparison of operative and non-operative treatment in twenty-nine cases. J Bone Joint Surg Am 1969;51:130–141
19. Miller WE. Comminuted fractures of the distal end of the humerus in the adult. J Bone Joint Surg Am 1964;46: 644–657
20. Zagorski JB, Jennings JJ, Burkhalter WE, Uribe JW. Comminuted intraarticular fractures of the distal humeral condyles. Surgical vs. nonsurgical treatment. Clin Orthop Relat Res 1986;202:197–204
21. Bryan RS, Morrey BF. Extensive posterior exposure of the elbow. A triceps-sparing approach. Clin Orthop 1982;166: 188–192
22. McKee MD, Kim J, Kebaish K, Stephen DJ, Kreder HJ, Schemitsch EH. Functional outcome after open supracondylar fractures of the humerus. The effect of the surgical approach. J Bone Joint Surg Br 2000;82:646–651
23. Schemitsch EH, Tencer AF, Henley MB. Biomechanical evaluation of methods of internal fixation of the distal humerus. J Orthop Trauma 1994;8:468–475
24. O'Driscoll SW. Optimizing stability in distal humeral fracture fixation. J Shoulder Elbow Surg 2005;14:186S–194S
25. O'Driscoll SW, Sanchez-Sotelo J, Torchia ME. Management of the smashed distal humerus. Orthop Clin North Am 2002;33:19–33 vii
26. Struhl S, Szporn MN, Cobelli NJ, Sadler AH. Cemented internal fixation for supracondylar femur fractures in osteoporotic patients. J Orthop Trauma 1990;4:151–157
27. Motzkin NE, Chao EY, An KN, Wikenheiser MA, Lewallen DG. Pull-out strength of screws from polymethylmethacrylate cement. J Bone Joint Surg Br 1994;76:320–323
28. Korner J, Diederichs G, Arzdorf M, et al. A biomechanical evaluation of methods of distal humerus fracture fixation using locking compression plates versus conventional reconstruction plates. J Orthop Trauma 2004;18:286–293
29. Prayson MJ, Williams JL, Marshall MP, Scilaris TA, Lingenfelter EJ. Biomechanical comparison of fixation methods in transverse olecranon fractures: a cadaveric study. J Orthop Trauma 1997;11:565–572
30. Hak DJ, Golladay GJ. Olecranon fractures: treatment options. J Am Acad Orthop Surg 2000;8:266–275
31. Simpson NS, Goodman LA, Jupiter JB. Contoured LCDC plating of the proximal ulna. Injury 1996;27:411–417
32. McKee MD, Seiler JG, Jupiter JB. The application of the limited contact dynamic compression plate in the upper extremity: an analysis of 114 consecutive cases. Injury 1995;26:661–666
33. Doornberg J, Ring D, Jupiter JB. Effective treatment of fracture-dislocations of the olecranon requires a stable trochlear notch. Clin Orthop Relat Res 2004;429:292–300
34. Inhofe PD, Howard TC. The treatment of olecranon fractures by excision or fragments and repair of the extensor mechanism: historical review and report of 12 fractures. Orthopedics 1993;16:1313–1317
35. Gartsman GM, Sculco TP, Otis JC. Operative treatment of olecranon fractures. Excision or open reduction with internal fixation. J Bone Joint Surg Am 1981;63:718–721
36. Ring D, Quintero J, Jupiter JB. Open reduction and internal fixation of fractures of the radial head. J Bone Joint Surg Am 2002;84-A:1811–1815
37. King GJ, Evans DC, Kellam JF. Open reduction and internal fixation of radial head fractures. J Orthop Trauma 1991;5: 21–28
38. Hall JA, McKee MD. Posterolateral rotatory instability of the elbow following radial head resection. J Bone Joint Surg Am 2005;87:1571–1579
39. King GJ. Management of comminuted radial head fractures with replacement arthroplasty. Hand Clin 2004;20: 429–441, vi
40. Jupiter JB, Neff U, Holzach P, Allgower M. Intercondylar fractures of the humerus. An operative approach. J Bone Joint Surg Am 1985;67:226–239
41. McKee M, Jupiter J, Toh CL, Wilson L, Colton C, Karras KK. Reconstruction after malunion and nonunion of intra-articular fractures of the distal humerus. Methods and results in 13 adults. J Bone Joint Surg Br 1994;76: 614–621
42. McKee MD, Jupiter JB. Semiconstrained elbow replacement for distal humeral nonunion. J Bone Joint Surg Br 1995;77:665–666
43. Wolfgang G, Burke F, Bush D, et al. Surgical treatment of displaced olecranon fractures by tension band wiring technique. Clin Orthop Relat Res 1987;224:192–204
44. Mezera K, Hotchkiss R. Fractures and dislocations of the elbow. In: Bucholz RW, Heckman JD, eds. Rockwood and Green's Fractures in Adults. 5th ed. Philadelphia, PA: Lippincott Williams & Wilkins; 2001:921–952
45. John H, Rosso R, Neff U, Bodoky A, Regazzoni P, Harder F. Distal humerus fractures in patients over 75 years of age. Long-term results of osteosynthesis. Helv Chir Acta 1993;60:219–224
46. Kocher M, Melcher GA, Leutenegger A, Ruedi T. Elbow fractures in elderly patients. Swiss Surg 1997;3:167–171
47. Huang TL, Chiu FY, Chuang TY, Chen TH. The results of open reduction and internal fixation in elderly patients with severe fractures of the distal humerus: a critical analysis of the results. J Trauma 2005;58:62–69
48. Jupiter J, Morrey BF. Fractures in the distal humerus in the adult. In: Morrey BF, ed. The Elbow and Its Disorders. 2nd ed. Philadelphia, PA: WB Saunders; 1993: 328–366.
49. Pereles TR, Koval KJ, Gallagher M, Rosen H. Open reduction and internal fixation of the distal humerus: functional outcome in the elderly. J Trauma 1997;43:578–584
50. King GJW, Richards RR, Zuckermann JD, et al. A standardised method for assessment of elbow function. J Shoulder Elbow Surg 1999;8:351–4
51. Broberg MA, Morrey BF. Results of delayed excision of the radial head after fracture. J Bone Joint Surg 1986;68: 669–674
52. Moro JK, Werier J, MacDermid JC, Patterson SD, King GJ. Arthroplasty with a metal radial head for unreconstructible fractures of the radial head. J Bone Joint Surg Am 2001;83-A:1201–1211
53. Morrey BF, An KN, Chao EYS. Functional evaluation of the elbow. In: Morrey BF, ed. The Elbow and Its Disorders. 2nd ed. Philadelphia: W. B. Saunders; 1993:86–97

13 Total Elbow Arthroplasty for Distal Humeral Fractures

Joseph A. Abboud and Matthew L. Ramsey

As the populations of North America and Europe continue to age, the number of patients having comminuted displaced intraarticular distal humerus fractures is expected to increase. Palvanen et al[1] reported an age adjusted increase in incidence of such fractures resulting from moderate trauma from 12 in 100,000 in 1970 to 28 in 100,000 in 1995. The study concluded that if this trend continued, a threefold increase in the number of distal humerus fractures would occur by 2030.[1] Although fractures of the distal humerus account for only a small percentage of adult fractures (1 to 2%), traditional methods of fixation have been associated with a significant number of complications and poor outcomes.[2,3] In addition, the greater the age, the worse the result of open reduction and internal fixation.[4] Therefore, a difficult orthopedic problem may become increasingly common over the next 20 years.

Classification

The most commonly used classification system for distal humerus fractures is the Association for the Study for Internal Fixation (ASIF).[5] The principle is to divide the fracture type into three subsets based on the anatomic level of the fracture and relative involvement of the articular surface **(Fig. 13–1)**. These fracture types are as follows: type A, completely extraarticular fracture; type B, intraarticular fracture involving only one condyle; and type C, intraarticular fracture with bicondylar disruption and loss of metaphyseal continuity with the humeral shaft. Each type can be further subdivided based on various fracture patterns and comminution.[5] As with any classification system in orthopedics, this system has been used in an attempt to compare fracture patterns, the difficulties of their treatment, and the outcomes between various studies.

Until the 1960s, most orthopedic surgeons believed that the preferred treatment for distal humerus fractures was nonoperative.[2] This involved lengthy periods of immobilization and resulted in unacceptable outcomes. Nonoperative treatment often resulted in either a malunion with associated joint stiffness, chronic pain, and poor function, or nonunion of the fracture with a subsequent painful pseudarthrosis.[3,6–8] Early attempts at open reduction and internal fixation also provided poor results. However, in the 1970s the AO group introduced instrumentation and surgical techniques that allowed accurate anatomic reduction and stable internal fixation of distal humerus fractures.[9] The AO principles of anatomic reduction, rigid internal fixation, minimal soft tissue disruption, and early active range of motion (ROM) were shown to be critical in elbow fracture reconstruction.[9] These principles eventually allowed early mobilization of the joint and provided for improved outcomes.

Operative fixation in the elbow is a technically challenging endeavor. It requires knowledge of multiple surgical exposures, an understanding of the complex regional anatomy, and the ability to achieve fixation that allows early ROM. If adequate stability is not achieved, nonunion, malunion, posttraumatic arthritis, and stiffness of the elbow may result. The current data on internal fixation of distal humerus fractures indicate that complications such as failure of fixation, persistent pain and/or stiffness, heterotopic ossification, ulnar nerve entrapment, nonunion, malunion, and posttraumatic arthritis are common despite adhering to AO principles.[6,10–12]

The difficulties of anatomic reduction and internal fixation are compounded in elderly patients because of the increased comminution and osteopenia. Caja et al[4] reported on a group of 22 patients with bicondylar fractures of the distal humerus treated with osteosynthesis and found that the ROM and functional outcome were most dependent on the age of the patient. They concluded that even if early mobilization was achieved the results were worse in older patients.

It is not surprising that in the presence of osteopenia, internal fixation that is sufficiently stable to allow early mobilization is often the exception. Insufficient internal fixation for these fractures results in extensive immobilization and subsequent stiffness. Therefore, it is fair to conclude that the treatment of comminuted fractures of the distal humerus in elderly patients is associated with a high rate of complications and generally yields a poorer result than equivalent fractures in younger patients.[2,3,7,8,13,14]

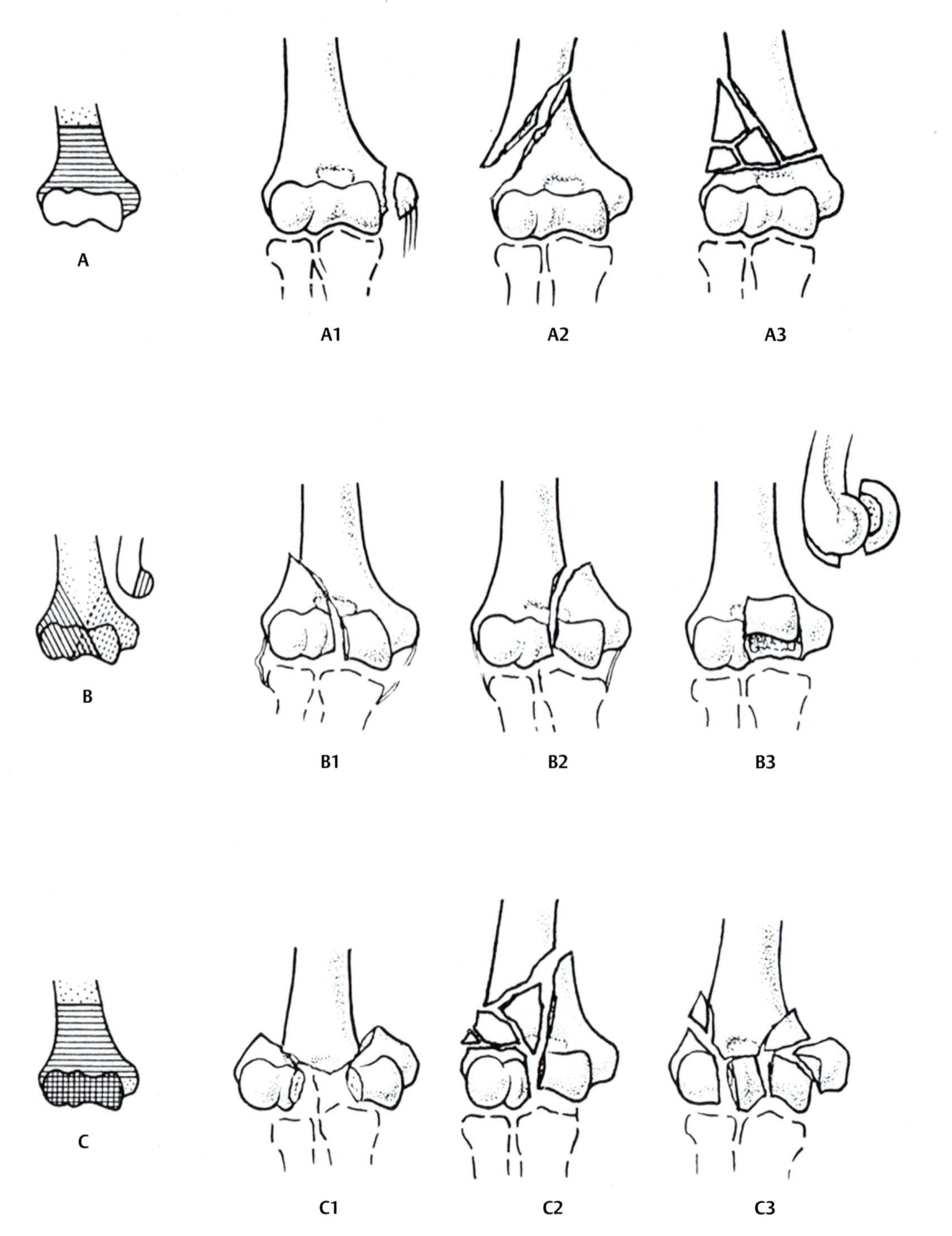

Figure 13–1 The AO classification of distal humerus fractures. (From Muller ME, Nazarian S, Koch P, et al. Comprehensive Classification of Fractures of Long Bones. New York: Springer-Verlag; 1990. Reprinted by permission.)

Outcomes of Open Reduction and Internal Fixation

Jupiter and Morrey[8] reviewed 846 procedures from 13 different reports on open reduction and internal fixation (ORIF) for fractures of the distal humerus and found that 20% of patients had an unsatisfactory outcome. They concluded that in the elderly patients, osteopenic bone and increased comminution compounded the difficulties of achieving an anatomical reduction and stable fixation.

John et al[7] reported the results of surgical stabilization of 49 patients with supracondylar fractures of the humerus whose mean age was 80 years (75 to 90); 41 (84%) were intraarticular fractures, and 39 patients were evaluated at a mean follow-up of 18 months. A very good result was reported for 31% of patients, a good result for 49%, and a fair or poor result for 20%. Constant pain was reported in 5% of patients. Complications included fracture of the plate or screws in 4 patients, symptoms related to the ulnar nerve in 6, and nonunion at the site of the osteotomy of the olecranon in 2 patients. Ten patients assessed their result as fair or poor.[7]

Pereles et al[15] performed a retrospective review of fractures of the distal humerus in 18 patients over the age of 60 years. They reported that at a minimum follow-up of 1 year, 12 patients had a good clinical outcome while 5 patients (28%) complained of moderate pain during activity for which medication was required.

Helfet and Schmeling[6] reviewed the results of nine published studies and reported less-than-good results in 25% of the patients. The complications included heterotopic ossification in 3 to 30% of the patients, infection in 3 to 7%, ulnar nerve palsy in 7 to 15%, failure of fixation in 5 to 15%, and nonunion in 1 to 11%.[6]

These reports showing a high rate of complications, residual pain, and limited function in a large percentage of patients has raised the question about the effectiveness of osteosynthesis in elderly patients and emphasized the need for better methods of treatment. It is in comparison to these outcome studies that total elbow arthroplasty (TEA) for fracture should be evaluated.

Treatment

The use of total hip arthroplasty in elderly patients who have a fracture of the femoral neck is well accepted. Total elbow replacement was thus suggested as an option for similarly comminuted elbow fractures in elderly patients.[16] Elbow replacement has proven effective in traumatic conditions of the elbow including posttraumatic arthritis[11] and in the salvage of distal humeral nonunions.[10,12] As an extension of these successes, Cobb and Morrey reported their results of TEA for fractures of the distal humerus in a select patient population.[16] Since then, total elbow arthroplasty has been used in cases of distal humerus fracture in the elderly.

TEA has undergone numerous changes in the past 20 years. The marked improvement in the results are due to improvements in the design of the implants, the operative technique, and the selection of patients.[12–14,16–25] The indications for TEA have likewise changed, and good results have been reported for carefully selected patients who have posttraumatic conditions of the elbow.

Fracture classification is clearly an important factor when considering the appropriate treatment. A good rule of thumb is to expect more fracture comminution than that appreciated on preoperative radiographs. However, extensive intraarticular comminution is not the only determining factor. Extensive osteopenia and underlying inflammatory arthropathies are significant factors when considering TEA. Appropriate selection of ORIF or TEA at the time of primary treatment cannot be overstated. The decision to attempt fixation with the strategy of later converting to a TEA if the fixation fails often yields inferior results as compared with primary TEA. In a retrospective study of patients older than 65 years of age with complex elbow fractures, those who were treated with primary TEA had better results than those converted to TEA after the primary open reduction and internal fixation failed.[13,18]

Surgical Treatment

As with any orthopedic problem, the assessment of every distal humerus fracture begins with a thorough history and physical examination. Specific details in the history should include age, handedness, mechanism of injury, prior level of function of the affected extremity, history of any inflammatory arthropathies, work demands, and associated medical comorbidities.

Physical examination should include documentation of a careful baseline neurologic examination. The cervical spine, ipsilateral shoulder and wrist should be examined for associated injuries. A thorough evaluation of the skin and soft tissue around the elbow is critically important. A good soft tissue envelope is essential to being able to replace the elbow and prevent infection, stiffness, or early failure. In addition, an open fracture (particularly Gustilo types II and III) is a relative contraindication to an acute arthroplasty. However, an open fracture may benefit from arthroplasty once the soft tissue envelope has been appropriately managed.

Radiographic evaluation involves orthogonal anteroposterior (AP) and lateral x-rays **(Fig. 13–2)**. These are usually all you need for evaluating the fracture pattern and deciding on a surgical treatment plan. A computed tomography (CT) scan is occasionally ordered if a more detailed description of the intraarticular comminution is felt to be necessary. Magnetic resonance imaging (MRI) is generally not needed in assessing these fractures.

The physician needs to provide both patient and family with appropriate counseling about this injury and the prognosis. The presence of realistic patient expectations should be confirmed by the physician before any treatment recommendations are made. In our experience, this makes postoperative management much simpler for the

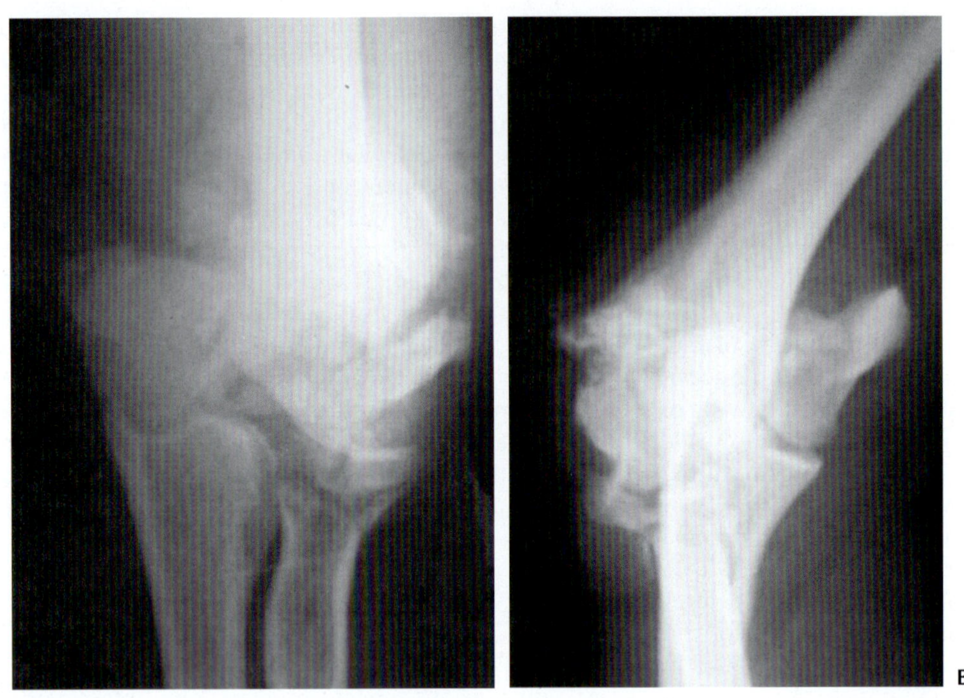

Figure 13–2 **(A)** Anteroposterior and **(B)** lateral radiographs of a comminuted intraarticular distal humerus fracture in a 72-year-old woman.

patient and for the surgeon. In addition, in those patients in whom TEA is being considered, a clear understanding of the limitations imposed following surgery is necessary. Inform the patient that these prostheses do not tolerate the large mechanical stresses often associated with lifting and repetitive use of the arm and that lifelong activity restrictions will be required.

The determination to perform a TEA is made prior to surgery and is usually not based on intraoperative findings. However, there are some seemingly fixable fractures that prove unfixable and the surgeon should be prepared to convert to a TEA if required. Contraindications to TEA include active infection, a contaminated open fracture, or a neurologic injury that impairs elbow flexion.

Technique

Implant Selection

A linked "semiconstrained" implant system is preferred for the management of acute fractures. Resection of the fracture fragments of the distal humerus compromises the collateral ligament attachments, making unlinked designs ineffective for this indication. Several features of implant design are important to consider. The presence of an anterior flange on the humeral component helps counter posteriorly directed forces and provides rotational control of the implant. Additionally, the anterior flange establishes the depth of insertion of the implant as it rests against the anterior humeral cortex **(Fig. 13–3)**.

The physical linkage between the humeral and ulnar components stabilizes the implant. The articulation is a semiconstrained linkage. This "sloppy hinge" design allows

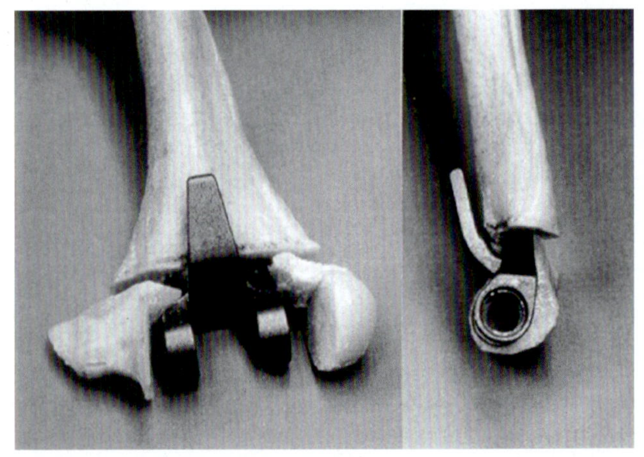

Figure 13–3 The depth of the humeral component is established as the anterior flange engages the anterior cortex at the level of the roof of the olecranon fossa. The depth of insertion is independent of the presence or absence of distal humeral bone stock. (From Morrey BF. The Elbow and Its Disorders. 3rd ed. Philadelphia, PA: WB Saunders; 2000: 657, Fig. 53-3 A/C. Reprinted by permission.)

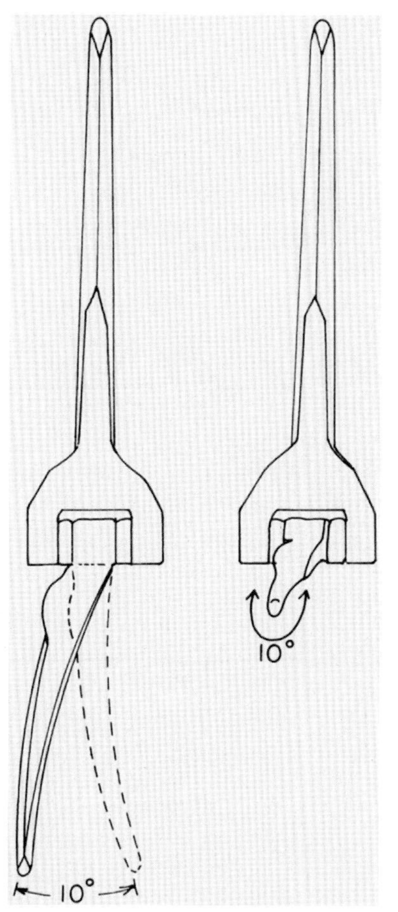

Figure 13–4 Linked "semiconstrained" implant designs allow several degrees of varus-valgus and rotational laxity. (From Morrey BF. The Elbow and its Disorders. 3rd ed. Philadelphia, PA: WB Saunders; 2000: 617, Fig 49-1. Reprinted by permission.)

various degrees of varus-valgus and rotational laxity such that a portion of the forces across the elbow are dissipated by the soft tissues of the elbow **(Fig. 13–4)**.

All of the studies of TEA for acute fracture have utilized linked semiconstrained implants. Several studies have highlighted the success of linked implants in the management of distal humerus fractures.[12,18,20,25,29–32]

Overview of Triceps Management

A posterior surgical approach is recommended; however, management of the triceps tendon differs.[26–28] In an approach described by Bryan and Morrey,[26] the ulnar nerve is isolated and subcutaneously transposed. Subsequently, the triceps is subperiosteally reflected laterally off of the olecranon in continuity with the anconeus muscle producing a continuous myofascial sleeve **(Fig. 13–5)**. The triceps is reattached to the olecranon at the end of the case through drill holes with heavy nonabsorbable sutures **(Fig. 13–6)**. The advantage of this approach is that continuity of the extensor mechanism to the anconeus is maintained. The disadvantage is possible failure of the triceps mechanism to heal, resulting in loss of active extension.[17]

An alternate exposure to the joint leaves the triceps attached to the olecranon by developing the medial and lateral borders of the triceps to expose the fracture site. Release of the flexor pronator and common extensor muscle groups from the fracture fragments permits exposure to the distal humerus and proximal ulna. Morrey and Adams[12] have described this approach for TEA in patients who have a nonunion of the distal aspect of the humerus. The advantage is that the triceps mechanism remains undisturbed and therefore concerns about postoperative triceps tendon failure are minimized. The disadvantage of this approach is the relative difficulty in visualizing the ulnar component to assess its appropriate orientation.

Authors' Preferred Approach

The patient is placed supine on the operating table with a bump under the scapula of the operated arm. The arm is prepped and draped in standard fashion. A sterile tourniquet is preferred over a nonsterile tourniquet because it increases the zone of sterility. The arm is brought across the chest over a bolster, and a straight posterior skin incision is made off the lateral aspect of the tip of the olecranon **(Fig. 13–7)**. Medial and lateral subcutaneous flaps are elevated exposing the margins of the triceps. The ulnar nerve is identified and dissected from proximally to the first motor branch to the flexor carpi ulnaris. The nerve is routinely transposed into an anterior subcutaneous position. The medial intramuscular septum defines the anterior from the posterior compartment of the brachium. The medial border of the triceps is developed from high in the arm to the medial triceps insertion on the olecranon. Similarly, the lateral border of the triceps is developed along the lateral supracondylar column to the lateral triceps attachment on the olecranon. The common flexors are sharply released from the medial fracture fragments, which are then removed. The common extensors are released from the lateral fragments and these are excised as well.[21]

The humerus is delivered through the void created by excision of the fracture fragments along the lateral margin of the triceps **(Fig. 13–8)**. The humeral canal is readily prepared with intramedullary rasps. Depending on the implant system to be used, the remaining distal humerus may need to be modified to some degree. Release of the capsule from the olecranon along with the medial portion

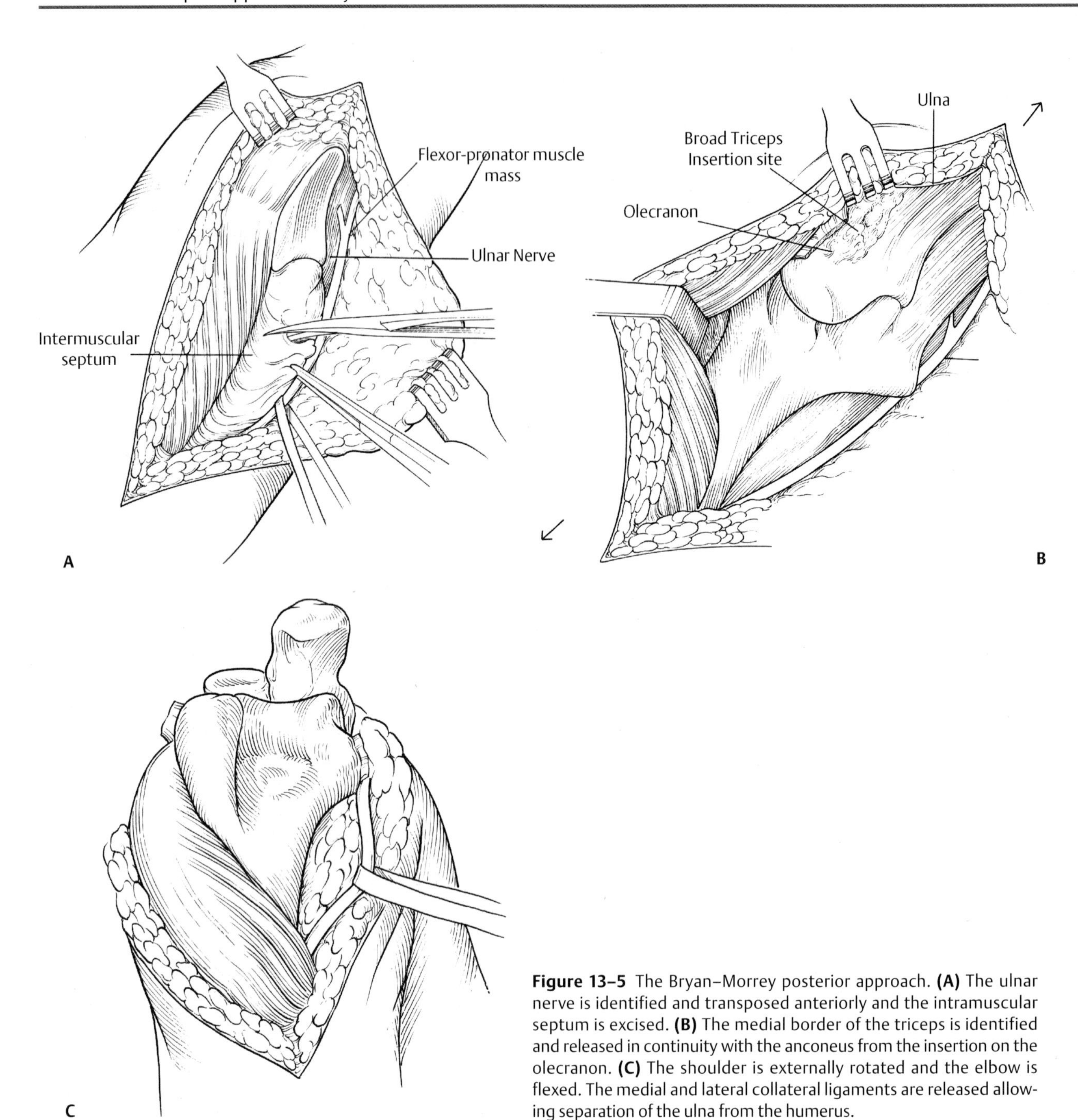

Figure 13–5 The Bryan–Morrey posterior approach. **(A)** The ulnar nerve is identified and transposed anteriorly and the intramuscular septum is excised. **(B)** The medial border of the triceps is identified and released in continuity with the anconeus from the insertion on the olecranon. **(C)** The shoulder is externally rotated and the elbow is flexed. The medial and lateral collateral ligaments are released allowing separation of the ulna from the humerus.

of the attachment of the triceps allows the ulna to be exposed through supination of the forearm **(Fig. 13–9)**.

The tip of the olecranon is excised allowing a parallel approach to the medullary canal of the ulna. The medullary canal is entered at the base of the coronoid with a high speed burr angled 45 degrees to the ulna in line with the medullary canal **(Fig. 13–10)**. The medullary canal is sequentially enlarged in preparation for trial reduction. Proper axial orientation of the ulna is obtained by placing the rasp handle perpendicular to the flat portion of the proximal part of the ulna **(Fig. 13–11)**.[21] Trial reduction of the ulna and humerus is performed to be sure full ROM is possible and the component remains aligned throughout the flexion–extension arc.

A cement restrictor is placed in the humerus and ulna. The medullary canals are prepared with pulse lavage and packed. Cement is deployed with a narrow nozzle delivered via an injector system. The nozzle is cut to the length of the longest planned implant. The ulnar component is inserted to a depth such that the articulation rests

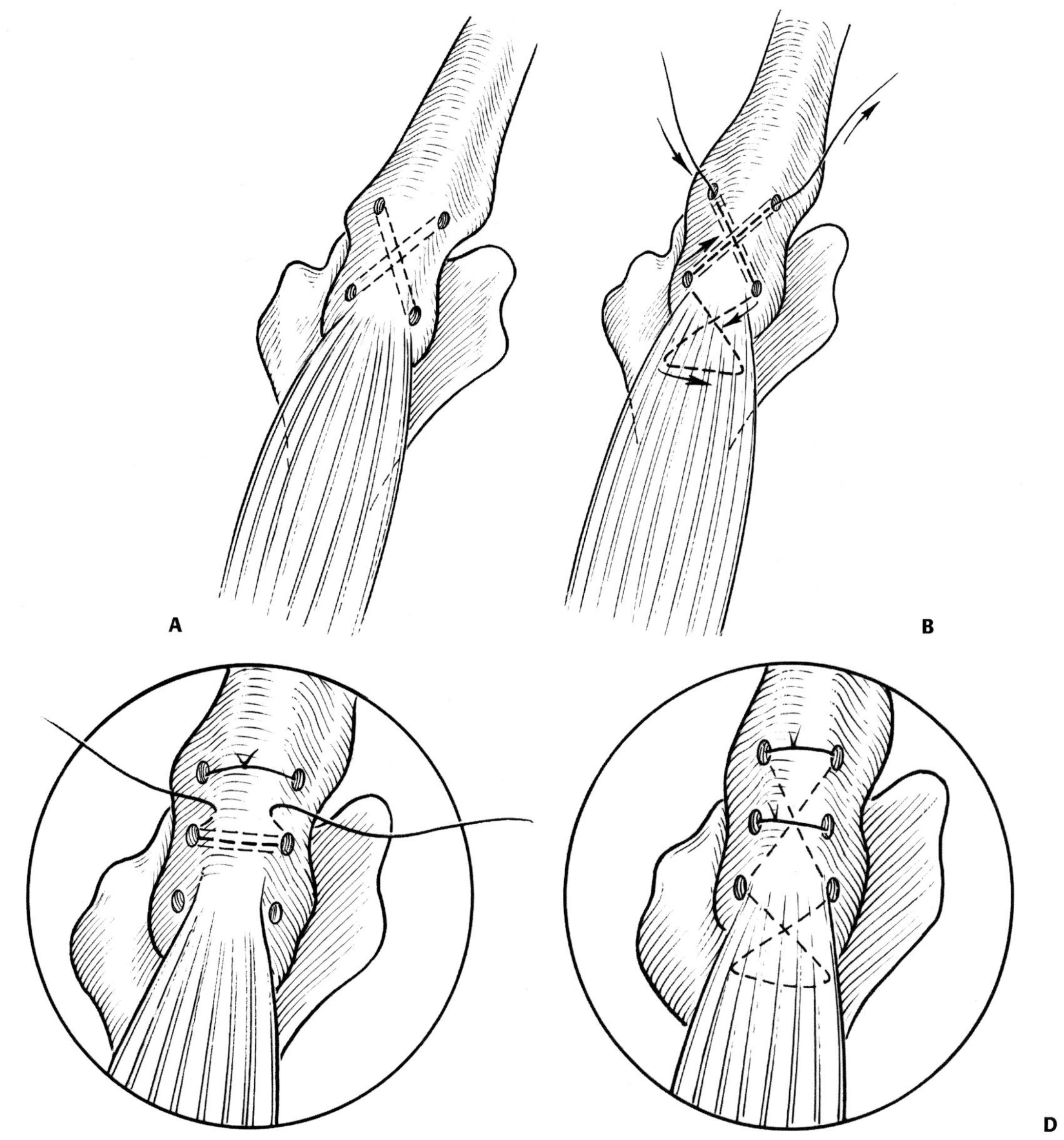

Figure 13–6 (A–D) The triceps is reconstructed through cruciate drill holes in the ulna and a supplemental transverse drill hole in the ulna. The sutures should be tied with the elbow in 90 degrees of flexion.

approximately midway between the tips of the olecranon and the coronoid **(Fig. 13–12)**. The bone graft is placed anterior to the anterior humeral cortex and is captured by the flange as the humeral component is driven into place **(Fig. 13–13)**. Because the medial and lateral columns of the distal humerus are missing, it is not critical to link the components before placing them at their final depth. Once the cement has hardened, the implants are articulated.

The flexor and extensor musculotendinous origins are repaired to the medial and lateral aspects of the triceps, respectively. Subcutaneous tissues are closed over a drain and skin is closed with staples. A bulky cotton dressing is applied and the arm is immobilized in extension with an anterior plaster splint. The arm is elevated for 1 to 2 days. When the drainage is minimal, the dressings are removed and rehabilitation is initiated.

Postoperative Rehabilitation

Postoperative rehabilitation concentrates on managing swelling while encouraging use of the extremity. Patients are fitted with an elastic sleeve to minimize edema of the operative extremity and asked to maintain the extremity elevated as much as possible to facilitate drainage of the arm.

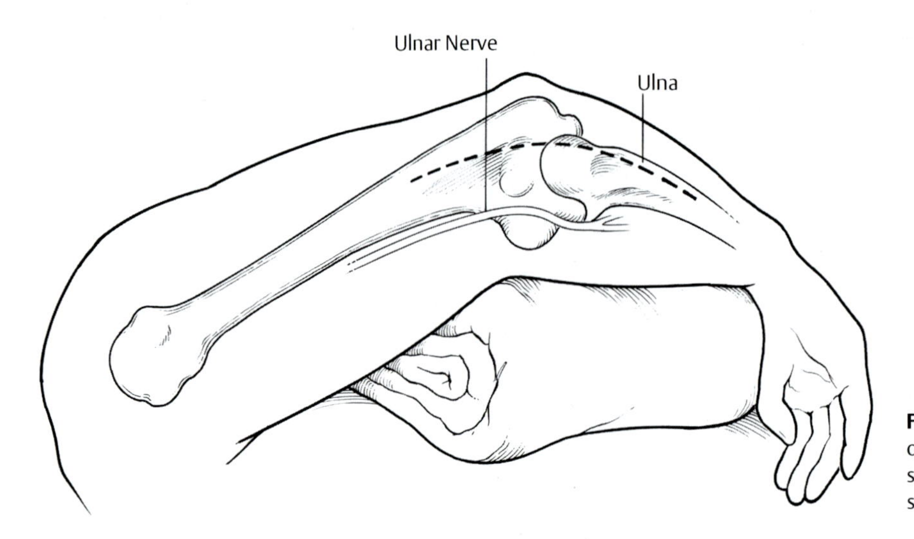

Figure 13–7 The patient is placed supine on the operating table with a bump under the involved scapula. The arm is brought across the chest and supported on a bolster.

The ROM program prescribed postoperatively depends on the management of the triceps during surgery. If the triceps is left attached to the olecranon, as is our preference, active-assisted ROM is initiated without the need to protect the triceps. If a triceps-reflecting approach is used, active assisted flexion, pronation, and supination are allowed immediately. However, active extension is avoided in the first 6 weeks while the triceps heals. Gravity-assisted and passive extension are allowed in this period.

Excellent functional ranges of motion are usually obtained in TEA for acute fractures with the program described above. Formal physical therapy sessions generally are not necessary.

Results

Cobb and Morrey[16] were the first to report their results of TEA as the primary index operation for acute fractures of the distal humerus in elderly patients. A retrospective review over 10 years included 129 acute distal humerus fractures (125 adults) that presented for care. However, only 21 patients with acute distal humerus

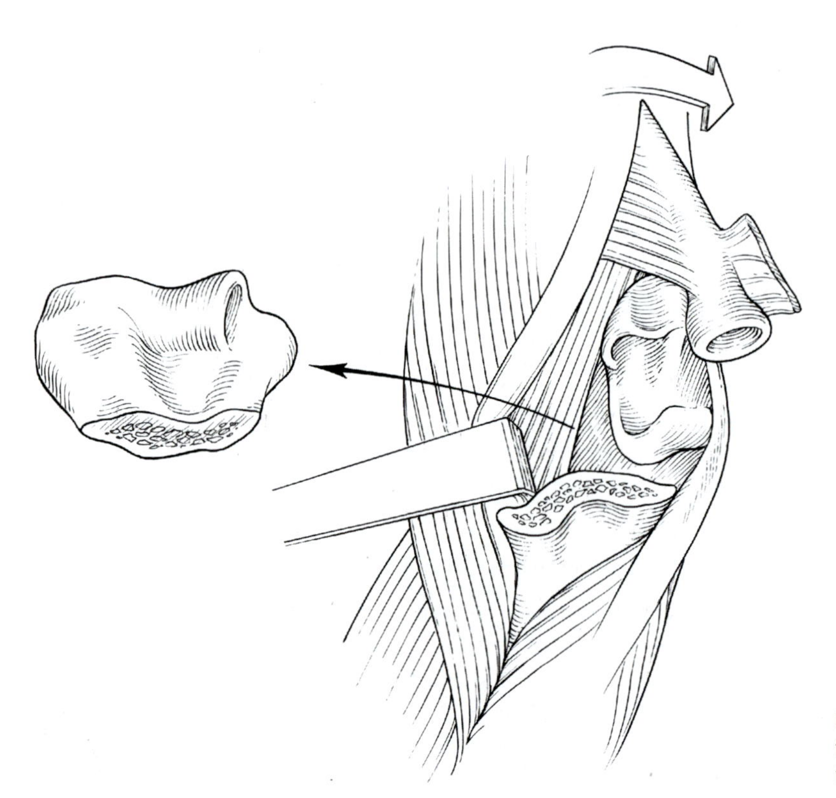

Figure 13–8 The humerus is delivered through the defect created along the lateral triceps once the fracture fragments have been excised.

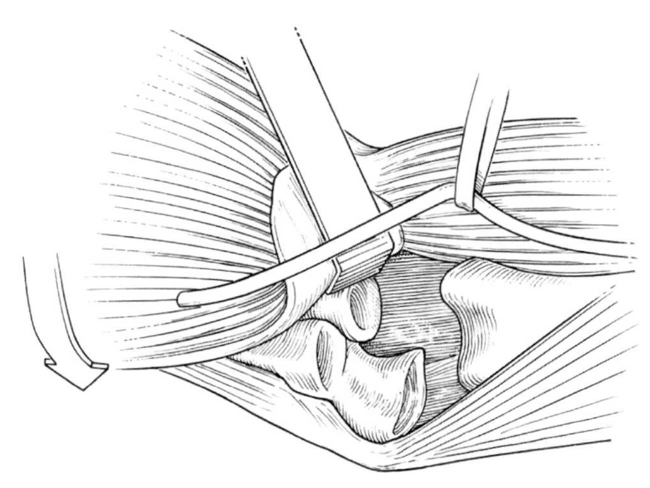

Figure 13–9 The ulna is delivered through the defect created along the medial triceps once the fracture fragments have been excised. The forearm is supinated, which turns the triceps tendon inside out allowing exposure of the greater sigmoid notch.

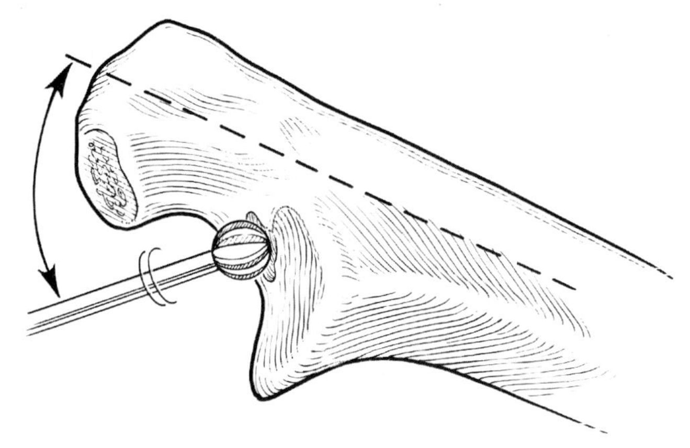

Figure 13–10 The intramedullary canal of the ulna is entered using a high-speed burr angled at 45 degrees to the long axis of the ulna. The burr is directed in line with the subcutaneous border of the ulna.

fractures at the Mayo Clinic were treated with arthroplasty over these 10 years. The indications for arthroplasty were an extensively comminuted acute fracture and underlying articular destruction from rheumatoid arthritis (RA) in 9 patients or 10 elbows. The remaining 11 patients did not have RA, but were far older than age 65 years. Five out of the 11 had an AO classification type C3 distal humerus fracture. The mean flexion arc postoperatively was 25 to 130 degrees. There was no evidence of loosening on the radiographs. Postoperative complications included fracture of the ulnar component in 1 patient, ulnar neuropraxia in 3 patients, and reflex sympathetic dystrophy in one. They suggested that TEA could be successfully used for severely comminuted fractures of the distal humerus in older patients.

A smaller study by Ray et al reported 7 patients who had TEA as primary treatment for fracture of the distal humerus. They had a mean age of 81.7 years and all had good results at a follow-up between 2 and 4 years. Three of those 7 patients had associated RA.[32]

In 2001, Gambirasio et al[18] evaluated the functional outcome of 10 older patients (mean age 85) treated with primary TEA for comminuted, intraarticular distal humerus fractures. Follow-up was a minimum of 1 year. All patients were women who had suffered a simple fall, but had significant comminution and osteopenia. Eight patients had excellent results; 2 patients had good results using the Mayo Elbow Performance Score. The mean arc of flexion–extension was 23.5 to 125.5 degrees.[33]

In 2002, Garcia et al[34] reported on 16 patients (none with inflammatory arthropathies) treated with primary TEA after a mean follow-up of 3 years. Their ages ranged

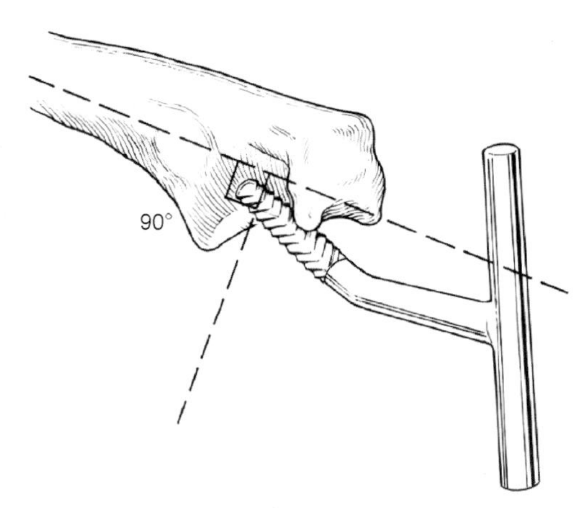

Figure 13–11 The ulna is prepared to allow proper orientation relative to the axis of rotation of the elbow. The rasp handle should be perpendicular to the posterior flat portion of the proximal ulna.

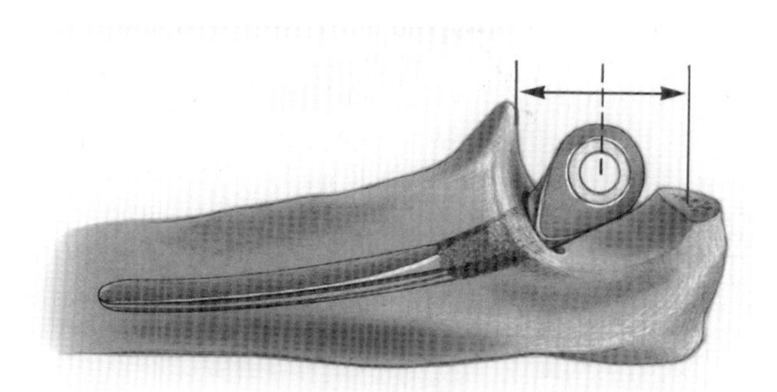

Figure 13–12 The ulna is inserted to a depth that recreates the center of rotation in the center of the greater sigmoid notch. (From the Mayo Foundation for Medical Education and Research, Rochester, MN.)

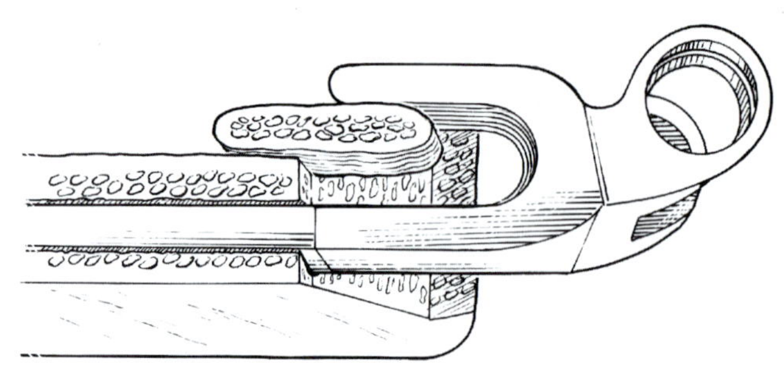

Figure 13–13 The humerus is inserted with a bone graft behind the anterior flange. The anterior flange engages the anterior cortex of the humerus at the level of the roof of the olecranon fossa.

from 61 to 95 years. Eleven patients had AO fracture classification type C3. Fifteen patients were satisfied with their outcome, and the mean Mayo Elbow Performance Score was 93. The mean flexion arc was 24 to 125 degrees. Garcia's study involved the largest reported group of nonrheumatoid patients undergoing TEA for fractures of the distal humerus. This patient population most closely resembled osteoarthritic or posttraumatic patients who had undergone TEA.

Frankle and associates[13] compared ORIF to TEA for comminuted intraarticular fractures of the distal humerus in women older than 65 years of age. In the group treated with TEA, 11 elbows were rated excellent, and 1 elbow was rated as good using the Mayo Elbow Performance Score. The mean arc of flexion–extension was 15 to 125 degrees. Six patients had no pain, and 1 had only mild pain complaints. In their study, despite the superimposed comorbidities, patients treated with TEA scored higher (as determined by the Mayo Elbow Performance Score) than the 75% of patients successfully treated with osteosynthesis. They concluded that initial TEA provided more-predictable outcomes over the short term. They cautioned, however, that the disadvantages of this procedure must be considered, including excessive loss of bone stock, the stringent weight restrictions TEA patients need to follow, and the devastating problem of mechanical failure or infections. Despite the disadvantages, results of this study led the authors to conclude that they would preferentially treat comminuted and displaced intraarticular fractures of the distal humerus in older women with associated comorbidities with a primary TEA.

Complications

The patient with an acute fracture treated with primary TEA usually carries the same significant comorbidities associated with any elderly fracture population (i.e., cardiovascular disease, diabetes, cancer). A common comorbidity in this group of patients is RA. With progressive destruction of the elbow, the supracondylar columns of the distal humerus and proximal ulna become very thin. These patients are at increased risk for pathologic fracture of the distal humerus even with minor trauma to the elbow. Postoperative complications include the risk of heterotopic ossification, reflex sympathetic dystrophy, neuropraxia, superficial and deep wound infection, stiffness, and aseptic loosening.[16,20,23,24,32] Complications in posttraumatic total elbow replacement group are more commonly seen than in the RA group undergoing elbow arthroplasty.[11] This should not be surprising as patients who have posttraumatic elbow replacement are more active than patients who have TEA for inflammatory arthropathy; therefore, they have a higher risk of component loosening and bushing wear.

In addition, anyone with multiple prior surgeries on their elbow is at greater risk for developing chronic pain syndromes, loss of bone stock, nerve injury, wound infection, and significant stiffness after TEA. Ulnar and median neuropathies can also present either after the initial trauma or after the primary treatment; if this happens it can make patient satisfaction nearly impossible.

Summary

The outcomes of distal humerus fractures in patients treated by ORIF and TEA demonstrate that with the proper indication either operative treatment can restore reasonable function and provide adequate pain relief. However, patients undergoing ORIF have the advantage of maintaining bone stock, and when bony healing is complete, long-lasting function without the need for any further major reconstructive surgery. In an older patient with adequate bone stock and without associated comorbidities, such as osteoporosis or RA, ORIF performed by experienced surgeons is still the preferred method of treatment.

In those patients that are unlikely to do as well with an ORIF, total elbow replacement as the primary treatment of acute distal humerus fractures offers an immediate alternative. This is in contrast to revising a previously failed ORIF to a TEA, which does not fair as well. Immediate arthroplasty of a distal humerus fracture appears to be supported in those individuals that are physiologically older than age 65 years, have significant underlying joint arthrosis, such as RA, and have severely comminuted fractures such as AO classified type C3 distal humerus fractures.

The indications for replacement arthroplasty as the primary treatment of extensively comminuted intraarticular fractures of the distal aspect of the humerus in elderly patients are strengthened by the unreliable results and the high rate of complications of open reduction and internal fixation, especially in patients who have RA or extensive comminution. Our recommendations should not be misinterpreted to suggest that we support the use of TEA rather than open reduction and internal fixation in patients who have an acute fracture of the distal aspect of the humerus. However, TEA is an option when adequate fixation of a fracture in an elderly patient is difficult because of comminution and poor-quality bone.

References

1. Palvanen M, Kannus P, Niemi S, Parkkari J. Secular trends in the osteoporotic fractures of the distal humerus in elderly women. Eur J Epidemiol 1998;14:159–164
2. Riseborough EJ, Radin EL. Intercondylar T fractures of the humerus in the adult. A comparison of operative and non-operative treatment in twenty-nine cases. J Bone Joint Surg Am 1969;51:130–141
3. Zagorski JB, Jennings JJ, Burkhalter WE, Uribe JW. Comminuted intraarticular fractures of the distal humeral condyles. Surgical vs. nonsurgical treatment. Clin Orthop Relat Res 1986;202:197–204
4. Caja VL, Moroni A, Vendemia V, Sabato C, Zinghi G. Surgical treatment of bicondylar fractures of the distal humerus. Injury 1994;25:433–438
5. Muller M, Nazarian S, Koch P, et al. The Comprehensive Classification of Fractures of Long Bones. Berlin, Germany: Springer; 1990
6. Helfet DL, Schmeling GJ. Bicondylar intraarticular fractures of the distal humerus in adults. Clin Orthop Relat Res 1993;292:26–36
7. John H, Rosso R, Neff U, Bodoky A, Regazzoni P, Harder F. Operative treatment of distal humeral fractures in the elderly. J Bone Joint Surg Br 1994;76:793–796
8. Jupiter J, Morrey BF, Eds. Fractures in the Distal Humerus in the Adult. The Elbow and Its Disorders. Philadelphia, PA: WB Saunders; 1993
9. Muller ME, Allgower M, Schneider R, et al. Manual of Internal Fixation Techniques Recommended by the AO-ASIF Group. New York, NY: Springer; 1995
10. Figgie MP, Inglis AE, Mow CS, Figgie HE III. Salvage of nonunion of supracondylar fracture of the humerus by total elbow arthroplasty. J Bone Joint Surg Am 1989;71:1058–1065
11. Morrey BF, Adams RA, Bryan RS. Total replacement for post-traumatic arthritis of the elbow. J Bone Joint Surg Br 1991;73:607–612
12. Morrey BF, Adams RA. Semiconstrained elbow replacement for distal humeral nonunion. J Bone Joint Surg Br 1995;77:67–72
13. Frankle MA, Herscovici D Jr, DiPasquale TG, Vasey MB, Sanders RW. A comparison of open reduction and internal fixation and primary total elbow arthroplasty in the treatment of intraarticular distal humerus fractures in women older than age 65. J Orthop Trauma 2003;17:473–480
14. McCarty LP, Ring D, Jupiter JB. Management of distal humerus fractures. Am J Orthop 2005;34:430–438
15. Pereles TR, Koval KJ, Gallagher M, Rosen H. Open reduction and internal fixation of the distal humerus: functional outcome in the elderly. J Trauma 1997;43:578–584
16. Cobb TK, Morrey BF. Total elbow arthroplasty as primary treatment for distal humeral fractures in elderly patients. J Bone Joint Surg Am 1997;79:826–832
17. Frankle M, Fisher D, Mighell M, Eds. Replacement Arthroplasty for Acute Fractures. Shoulder and Elbow Arthroplasty. Philadelphia, PA: Lippincott, Williams & Wilkins; 2005
18. Gambirasio R, Riand N, Stern R, Hoffmeyer P. Total elbow replacement for complex fractures of the distal humerus. An option for the elderly patient. J Bone Joint Surg Br 2001;83:974–978
19. Gill DR, Morrey BF. The Coonrad-Morrey total elbow arthroplasty in patients who have rheumatoid arthritis. A ten to fifteen-year follow-up study. J Bone Joint Surg Am 1998;80:1327–1335
20. Hastings H II, Theng CS. Total elbow replacement for distal humerus fractures and traumatic deformity: results and complications of semiconstrained implants and design rationale for the Discovery Elbow System. Am J Orthop 2003;32:20–28
21. Kamineni S, Morrey BF. Distal humeral fractures treated with noncustom total elbow replacement. Surgical technique. J Bone Joint Surg Am 2005;87:41–50
22. Kozak TK, Adams RA, Morrey BF. Total elbow arthroplasty in primary osteoarthritis of the elbow. J Arthroplasty 1998;13:837–842
23. Morrey BF. Fractures of the distal humerus: role of elbow replacement. Orthop Clin North Am 2000;31:145–154
24. Muller LP, Kamineni S, Rommens PM, Morrey BF. Primary total elbow replacement for fractures of the distal humerus. Oper Orthop Traumatol 2005;17:119–142
25. Wright TW, Hastings H. Total elbow arthroplasty failure due to overuse, C-ring failure, and/or bushing wear. J Shoulder Elbow Surg 2005;14:65–72
26. Bryan RS, Morrey BF. Extensive posterior exposure of the elbow. A triceps-sparing approach. Clin Orthop Relat Res 1982;166:188–192
27. Shahane SA, Stanley D. A posterior approach to the elbow joint. J Bone Joint Surg Br 1999;81:1020–1022
28. Wolfe SW, Ranawat CS. The osteo-anconeus flap. An approach for total elbow arthroplasty. J Bone Joint Surg Am 1990;72:684–688
29. Armstrong AD, Yamaguchi K. Total elbow anthroplasty and distal humerus elbow fractures. Hand Clin 2004;20:475–483

30. Athwal GS, Chin PY, Adams RA, Morrey BF. Conrad-Morrey total elbow arthroplasty for tumours of the distal humerus and elbow. J Bone Joint Surg Br 2005;87:1369–1374
31. Morrey BF, Bryan RS. Complications of total elbow arthroplasty. Clin Orthop Relat Res 1982;170:204–212
32. Ray PS, Kakarlapudi K, Rajsekhar C, Bhamra MS. Total elbow arthroplasty as primary treatment for distal humeral fractures in elderly patients. Injury 2000;31: 687–692
33. Schneeberger AG, Adams R, Morrey BF. Semiconstrained total elbow replacement for the treatment of post-traumatic osteoarthrosis. J Bone Joint Surg Am 1997;79: 1211–1222
34. Garcia JA, Mykula R, Stanley D. Complex fractures of the distal humerus in the elderly. The role of total elbow replacement as primary treatment. J Bone Joint Surg Br 2002;84:812–816

14 Acute Fracture-Dislocations about the Elbow

Christian J. H. Veillette and Michael D. McKee

Elbow dislocation is the second most common type of dislocation encountered in the adult upper extremity and constitutes 10 to 25% of all injuries to the elbow.[1] When an isolated elbow dislocation occurs without an associated fracture (simple dislocation), closed reduction of the elbow with short-term immobilization and early range of motion (ROM; within 2 weeks) can provide a stable joint with good functional outcome.[2–4] However, an elbow dislocation with concomitant intraarticular fracture of the radial head, olecranon, or coronoid process is termed a *complex dislocation;* its treatment requires strict adherence to a systematic stepwise treatment approach to obtain reliable patient satisfaction and functional results.[5,6] Acute elbow fracture-dislocations are a challenge to treat because they are prone to acute recurrent instability, chronic instability, stiffness, posttraumatic arthrosis, and pain.[7,8] Operative procedures for reconstruction of elbow fracture-dislocations are technically demanding because of the complex anatomy, the interplay between soft tissue and osseous injuries, and the proximity of crucial neurovascular structures. In this chapter, we will discuss the diagnosis, standard surgical approach, and rehabilitation of acute fracture-dislocations about the elbow.

The elbow is an inherently stable joint. However, the stability of the elbow becomes compromised and more difficult to control as the soft tissue injury becomes more extensive or with associated fractures.[9] As we have gained more experience treating elbow fracture-dislocations, it has become evident that careful attention must be paid to both the bony and soft tissue disruption associated with the injury.

In 1987, Broberg and Morrey[10] reported radiographic arthrosis in 22 of 24 patients with a fracture-dislocation of the elbow treated without repair or replacement of the radial head at an average of 10 years postoperatively. In 1989, Josefsson et al[11] reported the long-term (3 to 34 years) outcome in 23 patients who had sustained an elbow dislocation with a displaced radial head fracture. They reported a high prevalence of osteoarthrosis in 12 of 19 patients who had been treated with radial head excision following elbow fracture-dislocation. In addition, they noted redislocation in 4 patients, all of whom had an untreated fracture of the coronoid process. In 1989, Regan and Morrey[12] reported on the Mayo Clinic experience in 35 patients who had a fracture of the coronoid process of the ulna. In their series, treatment of type II fractures resulted in worse outcomes with an associated radial head fracture or elbow instability, and 4 of the 5 patients with a type III fracture had a poor result secondary to stiffness, pain, and recurrent instability. In 2002, Ring et al[13] reviewed 11 patients with posterior dislocation and associated radial head and coronoid fractures, the so-called terrible triad of the elbow. Nine patients had the radial head treated by internal fixation (5 patients) or excision (4 patients), with reattachment of the lateral collateral ligament complex (LCLC) in only 3 patients. All coronoid fractures were less than 50% and were not fixed. Five elbows redislocated in the splint postoperatively including all four with radial head excision. The result of treatment was rated as unsatisfactory for 7 of the 11 patients. Together these studies highlight (1) the difficulties in the management of these complex injuries, (2) the reduction of the coronoid fragment is critical to restore elbow stability, and (3) resection of the radial head is contraindicated when the elbow is unstable.

It is well recognized that prolonged immobilization following an episode of acute elbow instability is associated with poor outcome.[4] The dilemma in management of complex elbow fracture-dislocations is that, without appropriate surgical reconstruction, instability rapidly ensues with attempted motion, but prolonged cast immobilization leads to unacceptable stiffness. In addition, immobilization in a cast does not ensure concentric reduction of the elbow.[13] In previous studies, standard reconstruction protocols based on restoring both osseous and soft tissue structures were not used to optimize elbow stability, leading to high rates of prolonged cast immobilization and resultant stiffness and arthrosis.[11,13,14]

An improved understanding of the mechanism of elbow instability, the primary and secondary constraints providing stability, the patterns of soft tissue disruption, and improved techniques for surgical repair have led to the development of a surgical strategy for these injuries.

Anatomy

The elbow is a complex hinge joint that relies on a combination of bony articulations and soft tissue constraints to optimize stability and mobility.[15] The ulnohumeral articulation is the essential factor for osseous stability and mobility in the flexion-extension plane. It has been shown that the osseous articulation provides 30% resistance to valgus stress and 75% resistance to varus stress with the elbow at 90 degrees of flexion.[15] The olecranon blocks the anterior translation of the ulna with respect to the distal humerus while an intact coronoid process provides an anterior buttress resisting posterior subluxation of the proximal ulna in extension beyond 30 degrees or greater.[16] It has been shown that ~50% of the coronoid is required to maintain stability against a direct posterior force in an otherwise intact elbow.[17] The medial facet of the coronoid is especially crucial to stability in varus stress.[18] The importance of the radial head as a secondary stabilizer to valgus stress and posterior translation is well recognized; however, the radial head also indirectly contributes to varus stability by creating tension in the lateral ligament complex.[19]

Schneeberger et al[20] have recently evaluated the concurrent role that the radial head and the coronoid process have as posterolateral rotatory stabilizers of the elbow and the stabilizing effect of radial head replacement and coronoid reconstruction. The posterolateral rotatory displacement of the ulna was measured after application of a valgus and supinating torque in seven cadaveric elbows. Resection of the radial head with an intact LCLC showed a significant increase in rotatory instability compared with intact elbows. The clinical correlation of this finding was recently reported by Hall and McKee,[21] who described posterolateral rotatory instability (PLRI) in 7 patients following radial head resection. Additional removal of 30% of the height of the coronoid fully destabilized the elbows, always resulting in ulnohumeral dislocation despite intact ligaments. The implantation of a rigid radial head without reconstruction of the coronoid restored stability to the elbow. However, the elbows with a defect of 50 or 70% of the coronoid, loss of the radial head, and intact ligaments could not be stabilized by radial head replacement alone, but additional coronoid reconstruction restored stability. This study highlights the importance of the radial head for elbow stability and further illustrates the necessity for coronoid reconstruction in more complex injuries.

Treatment

The treatment of elbow fracture-dislocations has traditionally focused on management of the bony injuries. However, it has become apparent that equal attention should be paid to the dynamic and static soft tissue stabilizers. Soft tissue constraints about the elbow are responsible for as much as 40 and 50% of the resistance to valgus stress and varus stress in the extended position, respectively.[22] McKee et al[23] have defined the patterns of soft tissue disruption in 61 patients (62 elbows) requiring operative repair for a dislocation (10 cases) or fracture-dislocation (52 cases) of the elbow. In the 52 fracture-dislocations, the associated fractures were coronoid (n = 39), radial head (n = 36), proximal ulna (n = 14), and distal humerus (n = 6). Disruption of the LCLC was seen in all 62 elbows in one of six patterns: proximal avulsion (52%), bony avulsion of lateral condyle (8%) **(Fig. 14–1)**, midsubstance rupture (29%), ulnar detachment (5%), ulnar bony avulsion (5%), or combined (2%). Rupture of the common extensor origin was seen in 66% of the patients. Medial side injuries were confirmed in 80% of cases by direct visualization, intraoperative stress testing, or radiographs. The exact role that the dynamic stabilizers, such as the common extensors, play in providing stability to the elbow has not been clearly defined; however, active ROM of the elbow is inherently more stable than passive ROM.[24] The anterior band of the ulnar collateral ligament acts as the major stabilizer to valgus stress. The major stabilizer to varus or rotatory stress is the LCLC, including the lateral ulnar collateral ligament.[25,26]

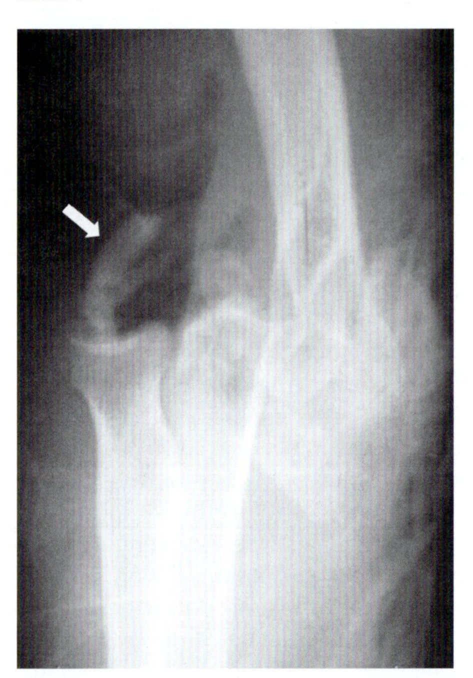

Figure 14–1 Acute disruption of the lateral collateral ligament complex (LCLC) occurs in one of six patterns. Although proximal soft tissue avulsion is the most common, bony avulsion (*white arrow*) can also occur as illustrated in this anteroposterior radiograph of a posterolateral elbow fracture-dislocation. Repair of the LCLC, posterolateral capsule, and common extensor origin is a critical step in the operative technique to obtain and maintain a stable congruent joint.

Etiology and Mechanism of Injury

Posterior dislocations of the elbow are commonly caused by a fall on the outstretched hand or wrist with either a hyperextension or posterolateral rotatory mechanism. In the hyperextension mechanism, an anterior force is generated that levers the ulna out of the trochlea as force is transmitted from the fall to the extended elbow. As the joint progressively hyperextends, the anterior capsule and collateral ligaments are placed under increasing tension and eventually fail. O'Driscoll et al have described a combination of valgus stress and forearm supination with axial compression through the lateral column of the elbow as a mechanism for elbow dislocation. This posterolateral dislocation causes a sequential soft tissue and possibly bony disruption from lateral to medial and has been classified into three stages. In stage 1, the LCLC is disrupted resulting in PLRI; stage 2 involves further soft tissue disruption of the anterior and posterior capsule resulting in incomplete posterolateral dislocation; and stage 3 involves further soft tissue disruption and instability subdivided into three degrees (3A, anterior band medial collateral ligament [MCL] intact; 3B, anterior band of MCL disrupted; 3C, entire distal humerus stripped of all soft tissue).[26,27] The more uncommon anterior dislocation may be caused by impact on the posterior forearm in a slightly flexed position.

Classification

Most acute elbow dislocations are posterior and involve both the radius and ulna. The distinction between posterior, posterolateral, and posteromedial is sometimes difficult to determine and seldom influences treatment. The other positions of dislocation – anterior, medial, lateral, and divergent – are rare and require individualized care.[22] No single universally accepted classification scheme exists for elbow fracture-dislocations. However, the type of injury can be determined based on the injury acuity, direction of dislocation, and extent of ligamentous disruption and associated fractures.

Associated Radial Head Fractures

Radial head fractures are classified based on the modified Mason's classification: type I fractures represent nondisplaced or minimally displaced fractures (less than 2 mm) of the radial head or neck; type II fractures are displaced fractures of the radial head or neck but fixable; and type III fractures are displaced radial head or neck fractures, but unreconstructable. Type IV injuries are defined as a fracture of the radial head with dislocation of the ulnohumeral joint.[28,29] Failure to restore the contact of the radial head with the capitellum may compromise not only immediate elbow stability, but also the ability of the LCL and MCL complexes to heal with proper physiologic tension.[9,29] Excision of the radial head without replacement can lead to progressive valgus instability, deformity, PLRI, and arthrosis in the setting of concomitant MCL injury. Therefore, the current recommendation is for reconstruction or replacement of the radial head in this setting.[28,30,31]

Associated Proximal Ulna Fractures

Associated proximal ulna fractures can involve the coronoid process and/or the olecranon process. The integrity of the coronoid process of the ulna plays a substantial, if not essential, role in elbow stability.[17] Regan and Morrey[12] classified fractures of the coronoid process into three types, depending on the extent of involvement. Type I fractures are a small fleck of bone sheared from the coronoid during subluxation or dislocation; type II fractures involve up to 50% of the coronoid process; and type III fractures involve more than 50% of the coronoid. Recently, Sanchez-Sotelo and colleagues[18] have added an additional fracture pattern (type IV) to describe the sagittal plane fracture of the coronoid involving the attachment of the anterior bundle of the MCL. This medial oblique compression fracture occurs with an axial load and probable varus force. The depressed anteromedial fragment causes a pathognomonic double subchondral density on the lateral radiograph, which has been termed the double crescent sign. It has been suggested that 50% of the coronoid can be fractured before instability develops in the intact elbow situation; however, in the setting of an elbow dislocation, even type I coronoid fractures are important for stability. It has become apparent that even these small fragments provide important stability through their attachment to the anterior capsule.[32]

The subcutaneous position of the ulna makes it vulnerable to direct trauma that can result in complex fractures of the proximal ulna. In cases of severe force to the elbow, a fracture dislocation can occur with posterior displacement of the olecranon fragment and displacement of the distal ulnar fragment together with the head of the radius anterior to the humerus. An associated coronoid fracture is not infrequent and typically is triangular and involves 50 to 100% of the coronoid process. It is important to restore a stable trochlear notch for effective treatment of transolecranon fracture-dislocations of the elbow.[33]

In complex proximal ulna fractures with comminution, the tension band technique will collapse the fragments together leading to a narrowed olecranon articulation that does not track properly. The optimal fixation for these fractures is offered with contoured, limited-contract dynamic compression (LCDC) plate fixation, with or without bone graft depending on the size of the comminuted region.[34] The advantages of using the LCDC plate for fixation are several-fold.[35,36] The plate allows improved contouring and can be appropriately placed on the dorsal tension surface of the proximal ulna around the tip of the olecranon to help hold the proximal fragment when poor bone quality limits screw purchase. The redesigned screw holes allow greater angulation of screw placement and the option of compression from either side of the screw hole. In addition, its lower profile allows its use in subcutaneous situations where soft tissue coverage may be in question. The proximal fixation of the plate is often the greatest challenge and cancellous screws rather than cortical screws should be used. The advent of newer precontoured plates allows for an increased number of fixation points in the proximal fragment and "cradles" the olecranon along its dorsal surface.

The Terrible Triad

The "terrible triad" injury of the elbow classically refers to a combined injury involving an elbow dislocation in association with a radial head and coronoid fracture because of the difficulties inherent in treatment and the consistently poor reported outcomes. There are few published reports specifically addressing the management and outcome of this injury complex.[7,8] Most available information has been gleaned from small subsets of patients in larger series of elbow injuries that developed acute recurrent instability, stiffness, and posttraumatic arthrosis. Recent literature has focused on a standard surgical protocol to minimize complications associated with this injury complex. With this improved understanding of the terrible triad, it has been proposed that the definition of this injury complex be revised to elbow dislocation with radial head and coronoid fracture, LCLC injury ± MCL injury, ± common extensor and flexor pronator origin injury, ± osteochondral injury to the capitellum/trochlea. Effective treatment of this injury complex requires correctly addressing both the bony and soft tissue injuries to attain and maintain a stable congruent joint that allows early ROM.

Monteggia Lesion

Fractures of the proximal third of the ulna with dislocation of the radial head are termed *Monteggia fracture-dislocations*.[37] These injuries have been classified by Bado into four types according to the direction of the displacement of the radial head: type I, anterior; type II, posterior; type III, lateral; and type IV, associated radial shaft fracture. It is the character of the ulnar fracture, however, rather than the direction of radial head dislocation, that is useful in determining the optimal treatment of Monteggia fractures in adults.[38] The posterior (Bado type II) fracture is the most common in adults and three distinct components of this injury have been identified: a comminuted fracture of the ulna near the coronoid (frequently involving a triangular or quadrangular fragment); a posterior dislocation of the proximal radius; and a triangular chip fracture of the radial head.[38] This injury complex closely resembles a variation of posterior dislocation of the elbow, except that failure occurs through the proximal ulna with proximal radioulnar dissociation. Stable anatomical fixation of the ulnar fracture (including associated fractures of the coronoid process) with compression plate and screw fixation **(Fig. 14–2)** leads to a satisfactory result in most adults who have a Monteggia fracture.[35,39,40] Problems with the elbow related to fractures of the coronoid process and the radial head, which are common with Bado type II Monteggia fractures, remain the most challenging elements in the treatment of these injuries.[38,40]

Patient Assessment

History

Patients with an elbow fracture-dislocation present after an acute injury with pain, soft tissue swelling, and deformity about the elbow. The injured elbow has a limited ROM and attempted motion may elicit painful bony crepitus. The mechanism of injury as well as any associated neurovascular complications associated with the initial injury should be elicited from the patient. Thorough assessment for concurrent illnesses precipitating the injury and a detailed account of comorbid conditions are important, especially in elderly patients.

Physical Examination

Physical examination should begin with assessment of the condition of the soft tissues around the elbow. Extensive swelling, ecchymosis, and any abrasions or lacerations should be noted and may influence the timing of surgery or location of incisions. An assessment of ROM or strength of the elbow should not be vigorously pursued. The relationship between the two epicondyles, the radial head, and the olecranon can provide information about the likely type of dislocation. There may be a palpable sulcus at the site of an olecranon fracture or dislocated radial head, accompanied by a painful and limited ROM. The wrist and shoulder should be examined to rule out a concomitant upper extremity injury, which occurs in 10 to 15% of cases. The distal radioulnar joint and the interosseous membrane of the forearm should be examined for tenderness and instability to rule out an interosseous

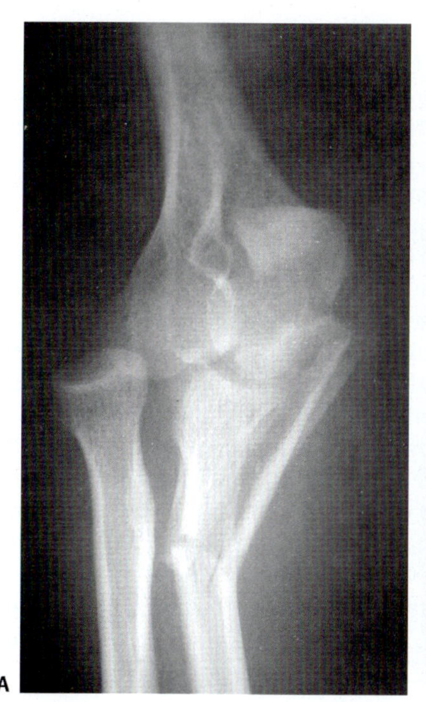

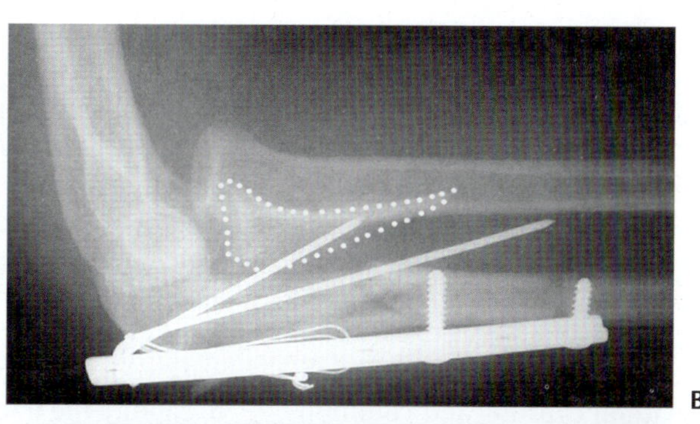

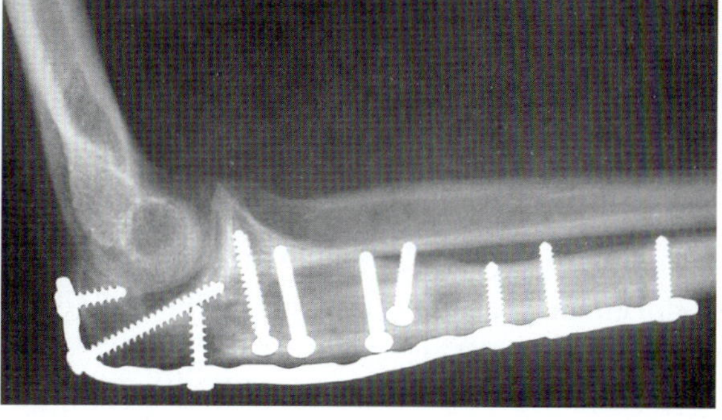

Figure 14–2 (A) Monteggia variant injury demonstrating complex proximal ulna fracture with large coronoid fragment and dislocated radial head. **(B)** Inadequate reduction and fixation of the proximal ulna and associated coronoid fragment (*white dotted line*) with tension-band wiring resulted in residual anterior subluxation of the radial head and an incongruous ulno-trochlearjoint. **(C)** At revision surgery, the coronoid was visualized through the main proximal ulna fracture line and fixed with lag screws, followed by limited-contact dynamic compression (LCDC) plate fixation contoured around the tip of the olecranon to stabilize the comminuted proximal ulna fracture and restore joint congruity.

membrane disruption and possible Essex–Lopresti injury. A careful neurovascular examination is essential especially prior to any planned manipulation or intervention of the elbow.

Radiographic Assessment

Plain radiographs in the anteroposterior, true lateral, and oblique projections are usually sufficient to provide enough information to determine the direction of the dislocation and to identify associated periarticular fractures. Severe comminution with displacement and overlap of the fracture fragments can obscure thorough determination of the fracture patterns. Thus, radiographs need to be good quality, out of splint, and obtained while maintaining gentle longitudinal traction with inclusion of the elbow joint on the film. Rarely does computed tomography (CT) provide additional information that alters decision-making and preoperative planning. Postreduction radiographs should be carefully evaluated to document concentric reduction of the elbow joint in two planes. Widening of the joint space may indicate entrapped osteochondral fragments or residual PLRI.

Treatment

Indications for Surgery

The specific indications for operative intervention are a displaced intraarticular fracture, an inability to obtain or maintain a concentric reduction in a closed fashion, and residual instability of the elbow in a functional (30 to 130 degrees) arc of motion following closed reduction.[5,6]

Surgical Treatment

A standard surgical protocol has been developed to provide more reliable outcomes and minimize complications associated with elbow fracture-dislocations. The general approach is to repair the damaged structures sequentially from deep to superficial, as visualized from the lateral approach (coronoid to anterior capsule to radial head to lateral ligament complex to common extensor origin). The goal is concentric stability with no observed posterior or posterolateral subluxation through a flexion-extension arc of 20 to 130 degrees with the forearm in neutral rotation. Instability is typically most evident in extension and supination and if persistent the MCL should be repaired and/or a hinged external fixator shoulder be applied. Isolated valgus instability is not an indication for repair of the MCL or application of a hinged fixator; this rarely seems to result in clinically evident valgus instability postoperatively.

There are five principles of the operative technique in the management of an elbow-fracture dislocation: (1) restore coronoid and proximal ulna stability; (2) restore radial head stability; (3) restore lateral stability through repair of the LCLC, posterolateral capsule, and common extensor origin; (4) repair the MCL and flexor pronator origin in patients with residual posterior instability; and (5) apply a hinged external fixator if sufficient joint stability is not achieved to allow early mobilization.

Techniques

The surgical approach starts with either a posterior (universal) incision with subcutaneous dissection laterally (and medially if required) or an extended lateral approach with a separate medial approach if required. Full thickness fasciocutaneous flaps are elevated to expose the interval between anconeus and extensor carpi ulnaris. The LCLC and common extensor origin are often avulsed from the posterolateral aspect of the humerus,[23] and every effort should be made to preserve intact soft tissue structures and work through any soft tissue disruption created by the trauma **(Fig. 14–3)**.

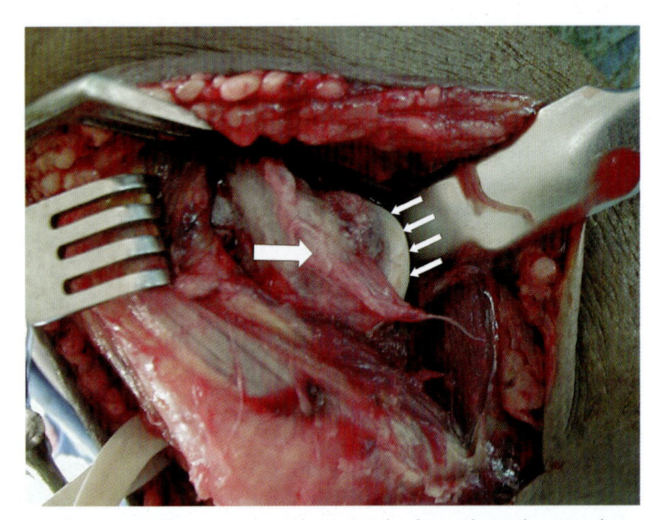

Figure 14–3 Intraoperative photograph after a lateral surgical approach to an elbow with a terrible triad injury. There is characteristic stripping of the lateral collateral ligament complex from the distal part of the humerus (lateral epicondyle, *large arrow*; capitellum, *small arrows*) with only a shred of lateral collateral ligament remaining attached. There has been minimal surgical dissection (skin, subcutaneous tissue, fascia); the extensive soft tissue disruption has been done by the injury itself.

The coronoid is the first structure addressed. Visualization is improved by resection of a radial head with an irreparable fracture, as described below. In addition, the coronoid can be visualized and reduced through a proximal ulna fracture, if present, by mobilizing the proximal olecranon fragment as one would do with an olecranon osteotomy. The injury to the coronoid is typically a transverse fracture and large fragments (type II or III coronoid fracture) can be reduced and fixed with one or two cannulated lag screws from the posterior surface of the ulna to capture the fracture fragment. In comminuted fractures, an attempt should be made to fix the largest fragment possible to fix, which is typically the articular portion. Type I coronoid fractures are too small to be fixed with screws and are repaired by placing lasso-type sutures around the fragment and the attached anterior capsule and tying these sutures to the base of the coronoid through drill holes made with an eyed Kirschner wire. If comminution of type II and type III fractures precludes stable internal fixation with screws, then repair with suture around the fragments and/or capsule should be performed.

Next, the radial head fracture is evaluated. The primary goal should be to fix the fracture when there are one or two fracture fragments of the head. A combination of mini-fragment plates and screws or countersunk Herbert screws is useful for fixation. If fracture comminution (three or more fragments), impaction, cartilage damage, or an associated radial neck fracture precludes a stable anatomic reduction, the radial head is excised pending radial head replacement with a modular metal implant.[41] Minor fragments (<25% of the head) that are too small or damaged to fix can be débrided and the residual intact radial head left in situ. Excision of the radial head without replacement is contraindicated in the setting of elbow dislocation.

In the presence of a proximal ulna fracture, a narrow 3.5-mm LCDC plate is then contoured to fit the proximal ulna with the maximum bend, near 90 degrees, between the second and third screw holes of the plate. The plate must be of sufficient length to accommodate three or four screws distal to the fracture. Once fracture reduction is achieved, the contoured plate is applied to the dorsal aspect of the olecranon and the triceps fascia is incised to allow the implant to sit on the bone. The plate is secured proximally with one screw from the fourth or fifth hole obliquely upwards into the coronoid process in compression mode. A long cancellous screw is placed from the first or second hole across the fracture toward the proximal shaft at the base of the coronoid. Additional screws are placed proximally in the olecranon and the plate is secured distally to the shaft by three or four bicortical screws. The interlocking of screws in the proximal fragment maximizes purchase and stability.

After addressing the bony injuries, the assessment and treatment of the soft tissue disruptions is required. Avulsion of the lateral ligament complex from the humerus is repaired with nonabsorbable sutures placed through bone tunnels in the distal part of the humerus (isometric point) or with suture anchors. Midsubstance tears can be repaired with a nonabsorbable suture and tendon grafts; ligament augmentation is not routinely required. The common extensor origin may be an important secondary constraint and should be repaired in a similar manner if involved.

Stability of the elbow is then assessed under fluoroscopic guidance through a flexion-extension arc of 20 to 130 degrees with the forearm in neutral rotation. The effect of forearm position on elbow stability should also be assessed as the elbow may be most stable with the forearm in pronation if the medial structures are intact. However, forearm pronation may worsen the instability if the medial soft tissues are involved and neutral forearm rotation may correct the problem. If stability of the elbow has not been achieved, then the MCL and flexor pronator origin are exposed and repaired in similar fashion. If the elbow still remains unstable, then a hinged external fixator is applied to help maintain concentric reduction of the elbow while allowing early ROM.[14,42]

Complications

Chronic Instability

Chronic instability usually results from inadequate initial treatment of the entire bony and soft tissue injuries associated with the elbow fracture-dislocation (**Fig. 14–4**). The radial head fracture may not be reduced or fixed adequately to provide support against posterior redisplacement, the coronoid fragment may not be restored, and the lateral ligament repair may be omitted or poorly performed. The most common cause of instability following elbow fracture-dislocation is PLRI. Repair of the lateral ligamentous complex, restoration of radial head and coronoid stability, and application of a hinged external fixator provide effective treatment in these situations. McKee et al[14] reported good results in 16 patients with posttraumatic elbow instability treated with a hinged external fixator for an average of 6 weeks. The mean arc of flexion/extension was 105 degrees and the mean Mayo Elbow Performance Score[43] was 84 at an average follow-up of 23 months (range 14 to 40 months). Cobb and Morrey[44] have also reported success in 6 of 7 patients with unstable fracture-dislocations of the elbow treated with a joint distraction device at a minimum of 2 years. The mean arc of flexion before surgery was 33 degrees and the arc increased to 88 degrees after surgery.

Stiffness of the Elbow

Stiffness is a common complication following simple and complex elbow dislocations. In general, it can be managed conservatively with aggressive active assisted physiotherapy and either static or dynamic extension/flexion splinting. Even with optimal care, a mean arc of flexion–extension of 112 degrees with a mean flexion contracture of 19 degrees can be expected. Pugh et al[6]

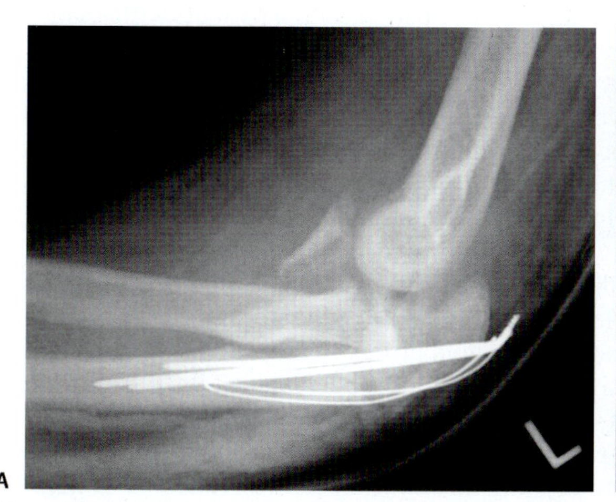

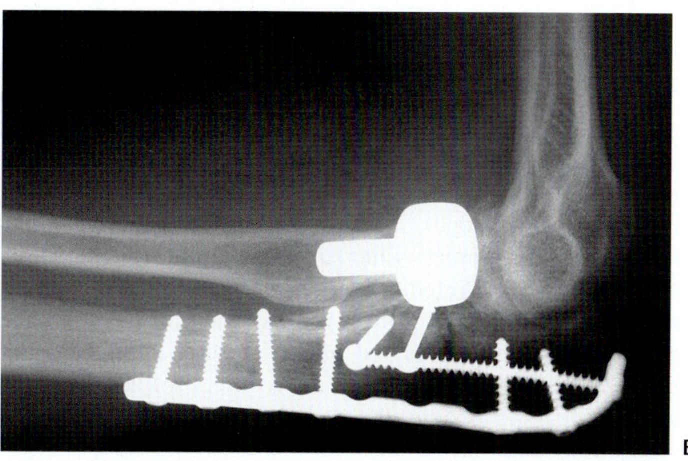

Figure 14–4 Technical errors in the management of a complex proximal ulna fracture-dislocation with associated radial head fracture. **(A)** The coronoid fracture fragment was not fixed, the radial head fragments were excised and not replaced, and the comminuted proximal ulna fracture was inappropriately treated with tension-band wiring. It can be anticipated that the lateral collateral ligament complex was not repaired and is incompetent. The elbow rapidly subluxated posteriorly. **(B)** Reconstruction of the trochlear notch, replacement of the radial head with a modular metal implant, fixation of the proximal ulna with a contoured limited-contact dynamic compression plate, and lateral ligament repair restored elbow stability and allowed early motion, enhancing the functional result.

were able to achieve a functional arc of motion, according to the criteria of Morrey et al (a flexion–extension arc of 30 degrees to 130 degrees and 100 degrees of forearm rotation)[45] in 80% of patients. If a final functional arc of motion is not obtained, excision of any heterotopic ossification and anterior and/or posterior capsular resection followed by immediate aggressive ROM has a high success rate in restoring function. Pugh et al[6] reported a mean gain in flexion–extension of 35 degrees (range: 25 to 60 degrees) and a mean gain in forearm rotation of 25 degrees (range: 0 to 50 degrees) after elbow release.

Heterotopic Ossification

Heterotopic ossification or periarticular calcification can be seen in up to 55% of elbow dislocations.[46] Although calcifications in the medial and lateral ligaments are common, radiographically evident synostosis of the forearm that requires reoperation occurs in only 5% of complex elbow fracture-dislocations.[6] The use of indomethacin, 25 mg orally three times daily for 2 to 3 weeks postoperatively, may help lower the risk of heterotopic ossification. However, Pugh et al[6] were unable to detect a difference in the rate of synostosis or heterotopic ossification between the group that received indomethacin and the group that did not with the numbers available in their study. Previous studies have suggested waiting for the heterotopic ossification to "mature," as indicated by bone scans or radiographs before resection and elbow release. However, this often resulted in delays of 18 to 24 months and severe, irreversible stiffness, contracture, and disability resulted. Recent studies have suggested that resection can be done much earlier, from 6 to 9 months postinjury, when soft tissue equilibrium has been reached.[46,47]

Postoperative Rehabilitation

A well-padded posterior plaster splint with the elbow flexed to 90 degrees and the forearm pronated (to protect the lateral repair) is applied in the operating room to assist in immediate postoperative pain management. If both the medial and lateral soft tissues have been repaired, the forearm should be splinted in neutral rotation. Conventionally, the posterior slab is discontinued at 7 to 10 days after the surgery and supervised motion is begun. Earlier mobilization, typically on the first or second postoperative day, appears to be tolerated well without additional complications and may result in improved ROM. Active and active-assisted ROM exercises are then started with the patient instructed to support the wrist with the opposite hand and gently flex and extend the elbow, gradually increasing the ROM. Flexion and extension exercises are allowed with the forearm in pronation and active forearm rotation exercises are done with the elbow at 90 degrees. The terminal 30 degrees of extension are avoided until 4 weeks after the surgery. Hinged splints or casts are not routinely required and heterotopic ossification prophylaxis with Indocid (Merck, Sharpe, & Dohme, Inc., Whitehouse Station, NJ) or radiation may be considered in at-risk individuals.

Results

Ring et al[13] reported on 11 patients with the terrible triad injury after a minimum of 2 years. The radial head fracture had been repaired in 5 patients, and the radial head had been resected in 4 patients. None of the coronoid fractures had been repaired, and the lateral collateral ligament had been repaired in only 3 patients. Seven elbows (64%) redislocated in a splint after manipulative reduction. Five elbows (45%), including all four treated with resection of the radial head, redislocated after operative treatment. At the time of final follow-up, 3 patients were considered to have a failure of the initial treatment. One of them had recurrent instability, which was treated with a total elbow arthroplasty after multiple unsuccessful operations; one had severe arthrosis and instability resembling neuropathic arthropathy; and one had an elbow flexion contracture and proximal radioulnar synostosis requiring reconstructive surgery. The remaining 8 patients, who were evaluated at an average of 7 years after injury, had mean ulnohumeral motion of 92 degrees and 126 degrees of forearm rotation. The average Broberg and Morrey[48] functional score was 76 points (range: 34 to 98 points), with two results rated as excellent, two rated as good, three rated as fair, and one rated as poor. Overall, the result of treatment was rated as unsatisfactory for 7 of the 11 patients. All 4 patients with a satisfactory result had retained the radial head, and 2 patients had undergone repair of the lateral collateral ligament. Seven of the 10 patients who had retained the native elbow had radiographic signs of advanced ulnohumeral arthrosis.

In comparison, Pugh et al[6] retrospectively reviewed the results of a standard surgical protocol, at two university affiliated teaching hospitals, in 36 patients with an elbow dislocation and associated fractures of both the radial head and coronoid process (terrible triad of the elbow).[6] At a mean of 34 months postoperatively, the mean flexion–extension arc of the elbow was 112 degrees (±11 degrees) and forearm rotation averaged 136 degrees (±16 degrees). The mean flexion contracture was 19 degrees (±9 degrees). The mean Mayo Elbow Performance Score was 88 points with 15 excellent results, 13 good results, 7 fair results, and 1 poor result. Concentric reduction of both the ulnotrochlear and the radiocapitellar articulations was achieved in 34 of the 36 patients. Eight patients had complications requiring reoperation that included two proximal radioulnar synostoses, one recurrent posterolateral instability, four hardware removals with concomitant elbow releases, and one wound infection.

Fracture dislocations of the olecranon often are complex fractures of the proximal ulna or complex combined injuries of the radial head, coronoid, and collateral ligament complexes. Doornberg et al[33] reported a retrospective review of 26 patients with fracture-dislocations of the elbow comprising of 10 anterior and 16 posterior fracture dislocations. Five of 10 patients with anterior injuries and all of the patients with posterior injuries had an associated fracture of the coronoid process of the ulna. One of 10 patients with anterior and 13 of 16 patients with posterior injuries had fracture of the radial head. Interestingly, only one patient had a true dislocation of the ulnohumeral joint; the articular surfaces remained apposed in the other 25 patients. All 26 patients were treated operatively and followed up for at least 3 years (average, 6 years). The results were good or excellent in 21 of 26 patients according to the system of Broberg and Morrey.[48] The five unsatisfactory results were related to inadequate fixation of the coronoid with subsequent arthrosis (3 patients), proximal radioulnar synostosis (3 patients), and a subsequent fracture of the distal humerus (1 patient). Thus, careful attention to stable restoration of the trochlear notch leads to a good functional outcome in these complex injuries in the majority of patients.

Summary

The treatment of fracture-dislocations of the elbow is difficult and challenging. These injuries are prone to recurrent instability, stiffness, and late arthrosis. There are two main goals for the orthopedic surgeon treating these injuries: restoration of a stable concentric reduction of the elbow joint and initiation of early motion to help prevent stiffness and maximize functional outcome. Our better understanding of the entire bony and soft tissue disruptions associated with these injuries should improve our ability to obtain and maintain a stable congruent joint. A systematic stepwise surgical protocol should be applied to acute fracture-dislocations about the elbow based on five principles of the operative technique: (1) restore coronoid and proximal ulna stability; (2) restore radial head stability; (3) restore lateral stability through repair of the LCLC, posterolateral capsule, and common extensor origin; (4) repair the MCL and flexor pronator origin in patients with residual posterior instability; and (5) apply a hinged external fixator if sufficient joint stability is not achieved to allow early mobilization.

References

1. Cohen MS, Hastings H II. Acute elbow dislocation: evaluation and management. J Am Acad Orthop Surg 1998;6: 15–23
2. Josefsson PO, Gentz CF, Johnell O, Wendeberg B. Surgical versus non-surgical treatment of ligamentous injuries following dislocation of the elbow joint: a prospective randomized study. J Bone Joint Surg Am 1987;69:605–608
3. Josefsson PO, Johnell O, Gentz CF. Long-term sequelae of simple dislocation of the elbow. J Bone Joint Surg Am 1984;66:927–930
4. Mehlhoff TL, Noble PC, Bennett JB, Tullos HS. Simple dislocation of the elbow in the adult: results after closed treatment. J Bone Joint Surg Am 1988;70:244–249
5. McKee MD, Pugh DM, Wild LM, Schemitsch EH, King GJ. Standard surgical protocol to treat elbow dislocations with radial head and coronoid fractures: surgical technique. J Bone Joint Surg Am 2005;87(Suppl 1):22–32
6. Pugh DM, Wild LM, Schemitsch EH, King GJ, McKee MD. Standard surgical protocol to treat elbow dislocations with radial head and coronoid fractures. J Bone Joint Surg Am 2004;86-A:1122–1130
7. O'Driscoll SW, Jupiter JB, King GJ, Hotchkiss RN, Morrey BF. The unstable elbow. Instr Course Lect 2001;50:89–102
8. Zagorski JB. Complex fractures about the elbow. Instr Course Lect 1990;39:265–270
9. Ring D, Jupiter JB. Fracture-dislocation of the elbow. Hand Clin 2002;18:55–63
10. Broberg MA, Morrey BF. Results of treatment of fracture-dislocations of the elbow. Clin Orthop Relat Res 1987; 216:109–119
11. Josefsson PO, Gentz CF, Johnell O, Wendeberg B. Dislocations of the elbow and intraarticular fractures. Clin Orthop Relat Res 1989;246:126–130
12. Regan W, Morrey B. Fractures of the coronoid process of the ulna. J Bone Joint Surg Am 1989;71:1348–1354
13. Ring D, Jupiter JB, Zilberfarb J. Posterior dislocation of the elbow with fractures of the radial head and coronoid. J Bone Joint Surg Am 2002;84-A:547–551
14. McKee MD, Bowden SH, King GJ, et al. Management of recurrent, complex instability of the elbow with a hinged external fixator. J Bone Joint Surg Br 1998;80:1031–1036
15. Morrey BF, An KN. Articular and ligamentous contributions to the stability of the elbow joint. Am J Sports Med 1983;11:315–319
16. An KN, Morrey BF, Chao EY. The effect of partial removal of proximal ulna on elbow constraint. Clin Orthop Relat Res 1986;209:270–279

17. Closkey RF, Goode JR, Kirschenbaum D, Cody RP. The role of the coronoid process in elbow stability. A biomechanical analysis of axial loading. J Bone Joint Surg Am 2000;82-A:1749–1753
18. Sanchez-Sotelo J, O'Driscoll SW, Morrey BF. Medial oblique compression fracture of the coronoid process of the ulna. J Shoulder Elbow Surg 2005;14:60–64
19. Morrey BF, Tanaka S, An KN. Valgus stability of the elbow. A definition of primary and secondary constraints. Clin Orthop Relat Res 1991;265:187–195
20. Schneeberger AG, Sadowski MM, Jacob HA. Coronoid process and radial head as posterolateral rotatory stabilizers of the elbow. J Bone Joint Surg Am 2004;86-A:975–982
21. Hall JA, McKee MD. Posterolateral rotatory instability of the elbow following radial head resection. J Bone Joint Surg Am 2005;87:1571–1579
22. Mezera K, Hotchkiss R. Fractures and dislocations of the elbow. In: Bucholz RW, Heckman JD, eds. Rockwood and Green's Fractures in Adults. 5th ed. Philadelphia, PA: Lippincott Williams & Wilkins; 2001:921–952
23. McKee MD, Schemitsch EH, Sala MJ, O'Driscoll SW. The pathoanatomy of lateral ligamentous disruption in complex elbow instability. J Shoulder Elbow Surg 2003;12: 391–396
24. Armstrong AD, Dunning CE, Faber KJ, Duck TR, Johnson JA, King GJ. Rehabilitation of the medial collateral ligament-deficient elbow: an in vitro biomechanical study. J Hand Surg [Am] 2000;25:1051–1057
25. Cohen MS, Hastings H II. Rotatory instability of the elbow. The anatomy and role of the lateral stabilizers. J Bone Joint Surg Am 1997;79:225–233
26. O'Driscoll SW, Bell DF, Morrey BF. Posterolateral rotatory instability of the elbow. J Bone Joint Surg Am 1991;73: 440–446
27. O'Driscoll SW, Morrey BF, Korinek S, An KN. Elbow subluxation and dislocation: a spectrum of instability. Clin Orthop Relat Res 1992;280:186–197
28. Frankle MA, Koval KJ, Sanders RW, Zuckerman JD. Radial head fractures associated with elbow dislocations treated by immediate stabilization and early motion. J Shoulder Elbow Surg 1999;8:355–360
29. Ring D, Jupiter JB. Fracture-dislocation of the elbow. J Bone Joint Surg Am 1998;80:566–580
30. Popovic N, Gillet P, Rodriguez A, Lemaire R. Fracture of the radial head with associated elbow dislocation: results of treatment using a floating radial head prosthesis. J Orthop Trauma 2000;14:171–177
31. Sanchez-Sotelo J, Romanillos O, Garay EG. Results of acute excision of the radial head in elbow radial head fracture-dislocations. J Orthop Trauma 2000;14:354–358
32. Armstrong AD. The terrible triad injury of the elbow. Curr Opin Orthop 2005;16:267–270
33. Doornberg J, Ring D, Jupiter JB. Effective treatment of fracture-dislocations of the olecranon requires a stable trochlear notch. Clin Orthop Relat Res 2004;429: 292–300
34. Hak DJ, Golladay GJ. Olecranon fractures: treatment options. J Am Acad Orthop Surg 2000;8:266–275
35. Simpson NS, Goodman LA, Jupiter JB. Contoured LCDC plating of the proximal ulna. Injury 1996;27:411–417
36. McKee MD, Seiler JG, Jupiter JB. The application of the limited contact dynamic compression plate in the upper extremity: an analysis of 114 consecutive cases. Injury 1995;26:661–666
37. Bado JL. The Monteggia lesion. Clin Orthop Relat Res 1967;50:71–86
38. Ring D, Jupiter JB, Simpson NS. Monteggia fractures in adults. J Bone Joint Surg Am 1998;80:1733–1744
39. Ring D, Hannouche D, Jupiter JB. Surgical treatment of persistent dislocation or subluxation of the ulnohumeral joint after fracture-dislocation of the elbow. J Hand Surg [Am] 2004;29:470–480
40. Ring D, Tavakolian J, Kloen P, Helfet D, Jupiter JB. Loss of alignment after surgical treatment of posterior Monteggia fractures: salvage with dorsal contoured plating. J Hand Surg [Am] 2004;29:694–702
41. Moro JK, Werier J, MacDermid JC, Patterson SD, King GJ. Arthroplasty with a metal radial head for unreconstructible fractures of the radial head. J Bone Joint Surg Am 2001;83-A:1201–1211
42. Ring D, Jupiter JB. Compass hinge fixator for acute and chronic instability of the elbow. Oper Orthop Traumatol 2005;17:143–157
43. Morrey BF, An KN, Chao EYS. Functional evaluation of the elbow. In: Morrey BF, ed. The Elbow and Its Disorders, 2nd ed. Philadelphia: W.B. Saunders, 1993:86–97
44. Cobb TK, Morrey BF. Use of distraction arthroplasty in unstable fracture dislocations of the elbow. Clin Orthop Relat Res 1995;312:201–210
45. Morrey BF, Askew LJ, Chao EY. A biomechanical study of normal functional elbow motion. J Bone Joint Surg Am 1981;63:872–877
46. Hildebrand KA, Patterson SD, King GJ. Acute elbow dislocations: simple and complex. Orthop Clin North Am 1999;30:63–79
47. Ring D, Jupiter JB. Operative release of ankylosis of the elbow due to heterotopic ossification: surgical technique. J Bone Joint Surg Am 2004;86-A(Suppl 1):2–10
48. Broberg MA, Morrey BF. Results of delayed excision of the radial head after fracture. J Bone Joint Surg 1986;68A:669–674

15 Reconstruction of Posttraumatic Stiffness and Instability

David C. Ring and Diego L. Fernandez

Instability and stiffness are common complications of complex elbow trauma. Chronic lateral collateral ligament (LCL) insufficiency is unusual and is characterized by a mobile, functional elbow that is prone to intermittent symptomatic subluxation or dislocation.[1] In contrast, persistent subluxation and dislocation after trauma are more common and are usually associated with articular fractures and stiffness.[2] Other contributors to elbow stiffness include contractures of skin, capsule, and muscle; heterotopic ossification; nerve compression; malpositioned implants; articular damage; and fracture nonunion or malunion.[3] Isolated LCL instability is effectively treated by reconstructing the ligament with a tendon graft. The treatment of stiffness, subluxation, and dislocation are less predictable and determined largely by the relative preservation of the trochlear notch and the articular surfaces.

Patient Assessment

Morrey and colleagues found that 15 daily activities could be accomplished with an arc of ulnohumeral motion between 30 and 130 degrees of flexion and an arc of forearm rotation from 50 degrees of pronation to 50 degrees of pronation.[4] These numbers should not, however, be used to decide when to operate on elbow stiffness. Patients can adapt to and function very well with much less motion,[5] perhaps more so when the stiffness is in the nondominant elbow. Therefore, the indication for operative contracture release is a combination of diminished elbow motion and disability directly related to stiffness in a patient who understands and agrees to the operative risks.

It is helpful to be aware of the details of prior trauma, burn, or central nervous system injury, as well as any prior surgeries. In patients with prior central nervous system injury, one must determine the ability of the patient to participate in a postoperative rehabilitation protocol.[6] A painful contracture suggests arthritis or ulnar neuropathy. Numbness and dexterity problems suggest ulnar neuropathy.

Patients with malunion, nonunion, subluxation, or dislocation are at risk of articular surface injury and progressive arthrosis. They usually have severe stiffness. Patients with chronic LCL insufficiency present with good elbow function, but either recurrent dislocation or symptomatic subluxation.

Physical Examination

The quality of the skin is important, particularly in postburn contractures.[7] The status of the skin with respect to prior injury and operative treatment will influence the operative tactics. When planning operative treatment of a posttraumatic contracture, the authors prefer to wait until the skin and scar are mobile and soft, and no longer edematous or adherent (usually about 3 or 4 months). A complete motor and sensory examination of the ulnar nerve along with Tinel's sign and an elbow flexion test should be performed.

Tests for posterolateral rotatory instability are best performed in a very relaxed or anesthetized patient. These tests are intended to provoke a clunk or a skin divot consistent with subluxation of the elbow joint. Pain alone is too nonspecific to be considered a positive test.

A posterolateral rotatory stress can be applied to the elbow by applying axial compression, valgus, and supination. This can be done with the patient supine and the arm externally rotated – a position that helps to both relax the patient and to prevent humeral rotation when the stress is applied.[1,8] As stress is applied, the elbow is brought from extension into flexion. A clunk indicates relocation of a subluxated elbow. Alternatively, a posterolateral rotatory stress is produced when a patient is asked to support their body weight on the maximally externally rotated and supinated arms in a sitting position.[9] In our opinion and experience, unless patients have learned how to provoke subluxation with certain positions and stresses, these tests are not definitive in an awake patient. Posterolateral rotatory instability is very uncommon and elbow pain and dysfunction are very common. Therefore, only a clearly positive and reproducible test should be considered positive.

Radiographic Assessment

Standard anteroposterior and lateral radiographs of the elbow are usually sufficient to identify and characterize arthritis, heterotopic ossification, and nonunions, but computed tomography (CT) is occasionally of use. In more complex cases, the CT scan can help with preoperative planning.[6] The authors find three-dimensional reconstructions particularly easy to interpret. CT scans may be especially useful for characterizing malunion of the articular surface of the distal humerus.[10]

Laboratory Studies

Neurophysiological testing should be considered when there is any possibility of preoperative ulnar neuropathy. In the presence of nonunion, infection should be considered and investigated with laboratory and imaging studies when appropriate, and possibly a diagnostic aspiration.

Treatment

Simple capsular contracture (no heterotopic bone, no malunion or nonunion, no implants blocking motion, no ulnar neuropathy, etc.) usually responds to time, reassurance, encouragement of exercises, and static progressive or dynamic elbow splinting.[11] Therefore, one should never rush into operative treatment of capsular contracture as long as progress is being made: Patience and frequent visits for reassurance and encouragement are worthwhile. Obvious hindrances to motion, including heterotopic bone, malunion, nonunion, prominent implants, ulnar neuropathy, subluxation, or dislocation merit prompt operative treatment. Heterotopic ossification can be resected within 4 months of injury (when radiographically mature and the skin is mobile and has little or no edema) regardless of activity on bone scans.[6,7,12,13] Stiffness associated with advanced arthrosis or unsalvageable nonunion or nonunion should be treated by interpositional or prosthetic elbow arthroplasty.[3,14]

Elbow capsulectomy can be performed simultaneously with débridement of a deep infection. It also forms an integral part of the treatment of malunion,[10] nonunion,[15] and instability.[2] Unstable skin can be treated with either prior or concomitant procedures to improve soft tissue coverage.[7]

Patients with capsular contracture that desire extension can be treated with lateral capsulectomy.[16,17] Patients with concomitant ulnar neuropathy or limitation of elbow flexion are best treated with medial capsulectomy so that the ulnar nerve can be addressed.[18,19] Patients with heterotopic bone, prominent implants, or complex contracture that cannot be adequately released from medial or lateral alone may benefit from a combined medial and lateral release.[7,19] Preoperative radiation therapy, a single 7-gray (700-rad) dose, is administered to patients with heterotopic bone to be excised.

Direct anterior release[20] is rarely the best choice because the anterior capsule can be more safely excised from medial or lateral. A posterior release with splitting of the triceps and fenestration of the olecranon fossa for access to the anterior elbow is used primarily for débridement of primary elbow arthrosis[21] rather than posttraumatic stiffness or arthrosis. In this chapter, we will describe an elbow capsulectomy through lateral and medial intervals.

The best candidate for an arthroscopic elbow contracture release is a patient with capsular contracture with or without osteophytes, but no ulnar nerve problem, heterotopic bone, implants, etc. Because such patients are uncommon and because arthroscopic elbow contracture release is more difficult and more dangerous than open contracture release, arthroscopic contracture release should only be done by surgeons with sufficient training and experience.[22–26]

Chronic posterolateral rotatory instability is treated with ligament reconstruction using a tendon graft.[8] Subluxation and dislocation are treated with open realignment, reconstruction of articular insufficiency due to fractures, and ligament repair. Ligament reconstruction is not usually necessary. The reconstruction is often protected with hinged external fixation.[2,27] In the presence of advanced articular injury, interposition arthroplasty may be considered.

Surgical Treatment

Elbow Stiffness

Open elbow contracture release can be performed under general anesthesia or brachial plexus block. The patient is supine and the arm is supported on a hand table. A sterile tourniquet is applied to the upper arm.

The skin incision can be straight and directly over the muscle interval to be utilized or posterior[28,29] with a skin flap elevated to expose the muscle interval **(Fig. 15–1A)**. If both medial and lateral intervals are to be used, a single posterior or both medial and lateral incisions can be used. In the unusual case of a direct anterior release, a direct anterior skin incision is used and should cross the flexion crease obliquely.

Hinged external fixation has not been particularly helpful and has not been necessary after elbow contracture release.[30] In the stiff elbow, slight instability is well tolerated (such as that which occurs when an ossified medial collateral ligament is fractured) and does not merit hinged external fixation.

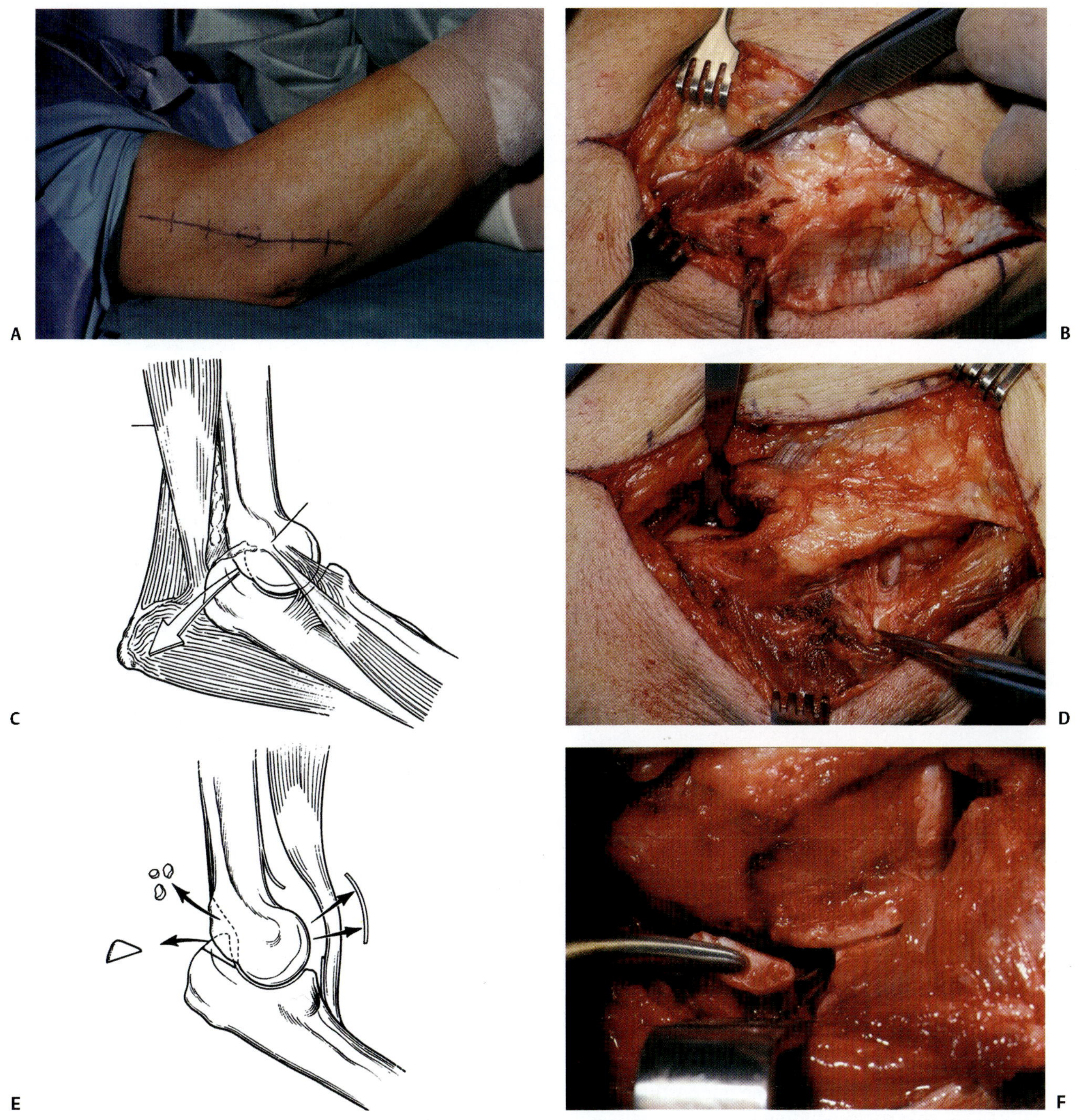

Figure 15–1 Open elbow contracture release through a lateral muscular interval. **(A)** A lateral or posterior skin incision can be used. **(B)** Identification of the supracondylar ridge orients the surgeon and helps with the initiation of the release. The origin of the extensor carpi radialis longus is incised and elevated off of the anterior surface of the distal humerus. **(C)** The triceps and anconeus are elevated off of the posterior surface of the distal humerus. **(D)** The posterior capsule is exposed and excised. **(E)** The olecranon fossa is cleared. **(F)** The tip of the olecranon is excised if it is felt that this will enhance elbow extension.

Lateral Elbow Capsulectomy

Release of elbow stiffness from the lateral side preserves the common wrist and digit extensors overlying the LCL. The skin is mobilized off of the fascia to help identify the appropriate deep muscle interval **(Fig. 15–1B)**. Deep dissection begins by identifying the supracondylar ridge, dividing the overlying fascia, and exposing the ridge. The triceps is elevated off of the posterior humerus and elbow capsule **(Fig. 15–1C)**. The posterior dissection continues distally in the interval between the anconeus and extensor carpi ulnaris. The anconeus is elevated off of the

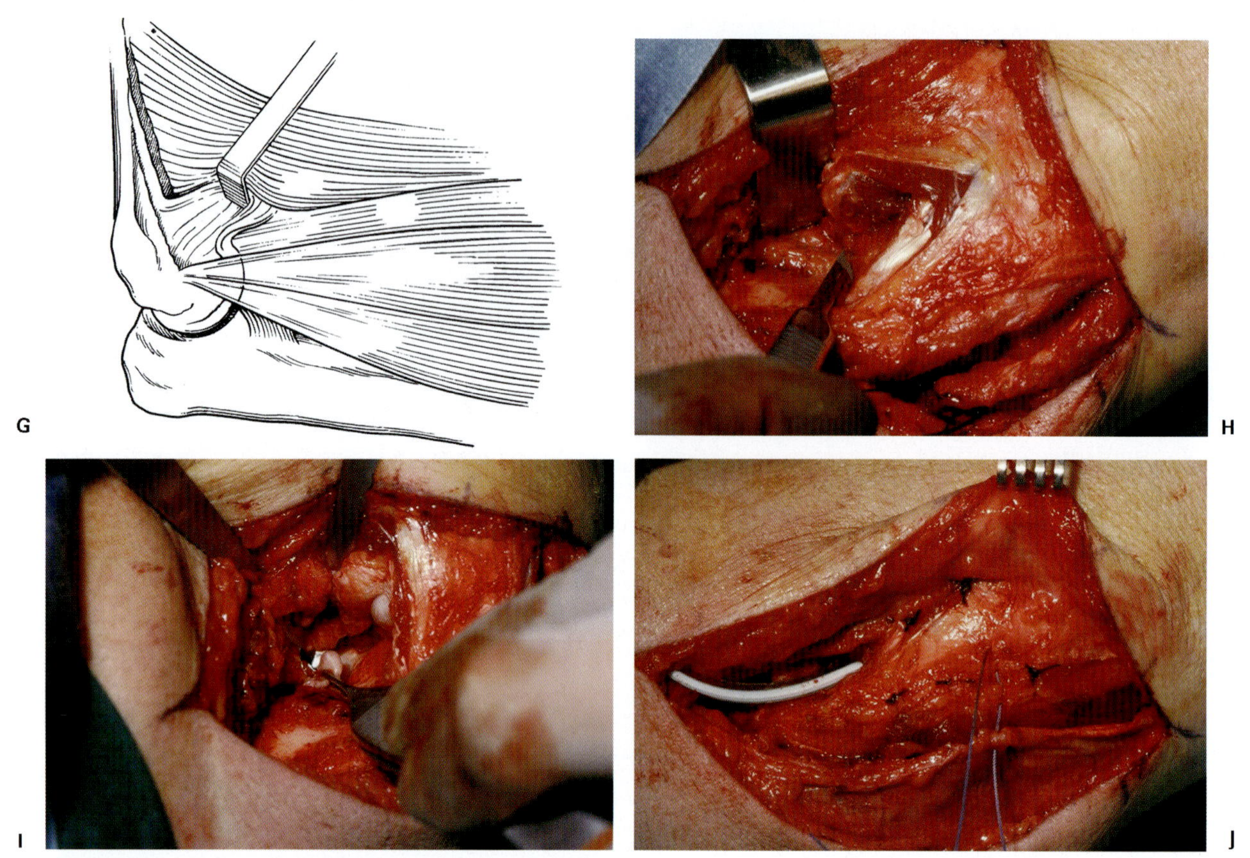

Figure 15–1 (*Continued*) **(G)** An anterior muscle interval is developed between the extensor carpi radialis brevis and the extensor digitorum communis. **(H)** The anterior capsule is exposed and excised. **(I)** The coronoid fossa is cleared and the tip of the coronoid excised as necessary. **(J)** The muscle intervals are closed, followed by skin closure.

capsule, the humerus, and the ulna **(Fig. 15–1D)**. Care is taken to preserve the lateral collateral ligament complex (LCLC) while excising the posterior elbow capsule. The olecranon fossa is cleared out and even burred to deepen it if necessary **(Fig. 15–1E)**. Loose bodies are identified and removed. The tip of the olecranon can also be excised **(Fig. 15–1F)**.

The origin of the extensor carpi radialis and part of the origin if the brachioradialis are released and elevated along with the brachialis off of the anterior humerus and elbow capsule **(Fig. 15–1G,H)**. Distally, an interval is created just anterior to the midportion of the capitellum, roughly corresponding to the split between the extensor carpi radialis brevis and the extensor digitorum communis, although in practice the interval is not precise. Keeping the dissection over the anterior half of the radiocapitellar joint will protect the LCLC. The anterior elbow capsule is excised **(Fig. 15–1I)**. At the medial side of the elbow, the capsulectomy may transition to a capsulotomy for safety depending on visualization. The radial and coronoid fossae can be cleared out and deepened as needed. The tip of the coronoid can be excised. Resection of a deformed radial head may also be helpful in some patients.

Both the anterior and the posterior muscle intervals are sutured **(Fig. 15–1J)**. Drains are used at the discretion of the surgeon. The skin is closed according to surgeon preference.

Medial Elbow Capsulectomy

After skin incision the ulnar nerve is identified on the medial border of the triceps. A complete release of the nerve through the arcade of Struthers, Osborne's ligament, and the flexor-pronator aponeurosis is then performed, along with neurolysis of the ulnar nerve if there is extensive scarring **(Fig. 15–2A)**. Skin flaps can be safely elevated once the ulnar nerve is identified and protected.

The flexor pronator mass is identified and split in half between the interval where the ulnar nerve runs and the anterior margin of the muscle mass. The anterior half of the flexor pronator mass and the brachialis muscle are elevated off of the anterior humerus and elbow capsule **(Fig. 15–2B,C)**. The triceps is elevated off of the distal humerus and the posterior elbow capsule. Capsular excision, fossae deepening, and coronoid and olecranon tip excision are as described for lateral capsulectomy.

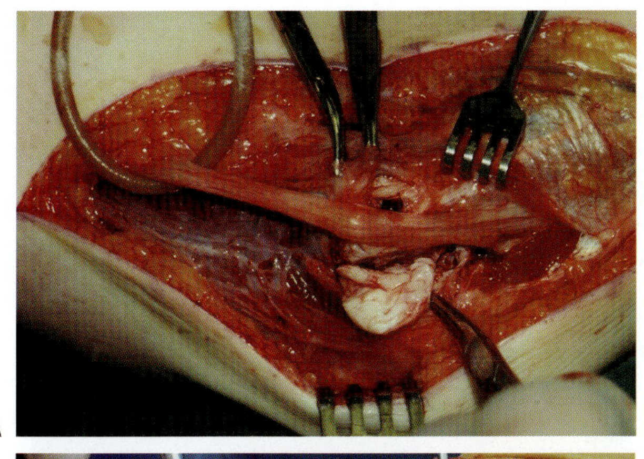

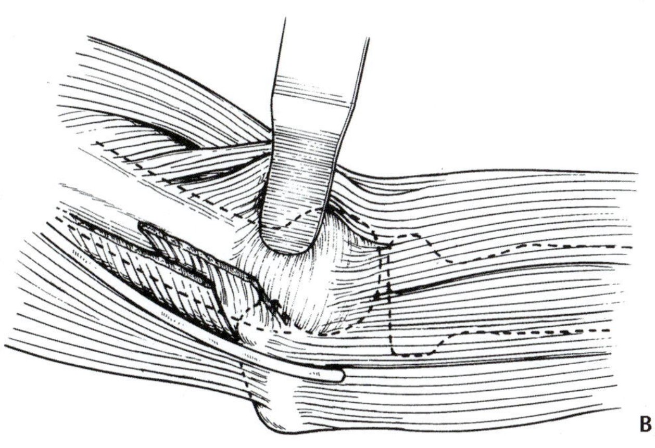

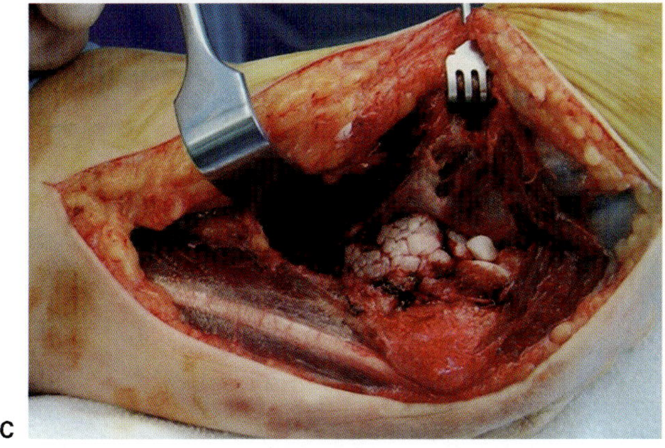

Figure 15–2 Open elbow contracture release through a medial muscle interval. **(A)** A medial or posterior skin incision is used. The ulnar nerve is completely decompressed from the so-called arcade of Struthers through the flexor-pronator aponeurosis distally. External neurolysis is performed as needed. **(B)** The brachialis is elevated off of the anterior surface of the distal humerus and the anterior elbow capsule. **(C)** The flexor-pronator mass is identified and split, and the anterior 50% is retracted anteriorly with the brachialis. In this patient, the anterior elbow capsule has been excised and extensive synovial chondromatosis is apparent.

Heterotopic Bone Excision and Other Factors

Heterotopic bone is excised piecemeal, taking care to identify and protect native bone and articulation. Bleeding bony surfaces are covered with bone wax. Implants are removed after capsulectomy and elbow manipulation to limit the risk of fracture. Malunion and nonunion are addressed as necessary.

Elbow Instability

Lateral Collateral Ligament Reconstruction[1,8]

The instability is confirmed with examination under anesthesia **(Fig. 15–3A,B)**. The interval between the anconeus and the extensor carpi ulnaris is used to expose the lateral elbow joint **(Fig. 15–3C,D)**. The capsular remnant and scar are split in line with the planned reconstruction so that this tissue can be used to reinforce the repair. A single drill hole large enough to pass both limbs of the tendon graft is placed in the lateral epicondyle at the center of rotation – anatomically, this corresponds to the inferior point of a small tubercle on the lateral epicondyle. Two smaller drill holes are made on the anterior and posterior aspect of the lateral epicondyle to be used to pull the tendon grafts up into place.

Two drill holes large enough to pass a single limb of the tendon graft are made at the crista supinatoris on the proximal ulna **(Fig. 15–3D)**. A tendon graft (usually the palmaris longus, but alternatively a foot or hamstring tendon) is obtained. Sutures are applied to each end of the graft in a multiple grasping and locking fashion. The suture/tendon graft is then passed through the ulna holes using a bent 24-gauge wire as a passer. Each end of the graft is then pulled into the lateral epicondyle hole using the sutures passed through the additional holes over the lateral epicondyle. The graft is tensioned appropriately and then the sutures are tied. Any adjacent capsuloligamentous tissue is used to reinforce the repair **(Fig. 15–3E)**.

Posttraumatic Subluxation

A dorsal midline skin incision and ulnar nerve transposition are used. An extended Kocher-type approach is developed,[31] occasionally using a slightly more anterior muscle interval such as that described by Kaplan[32] depending

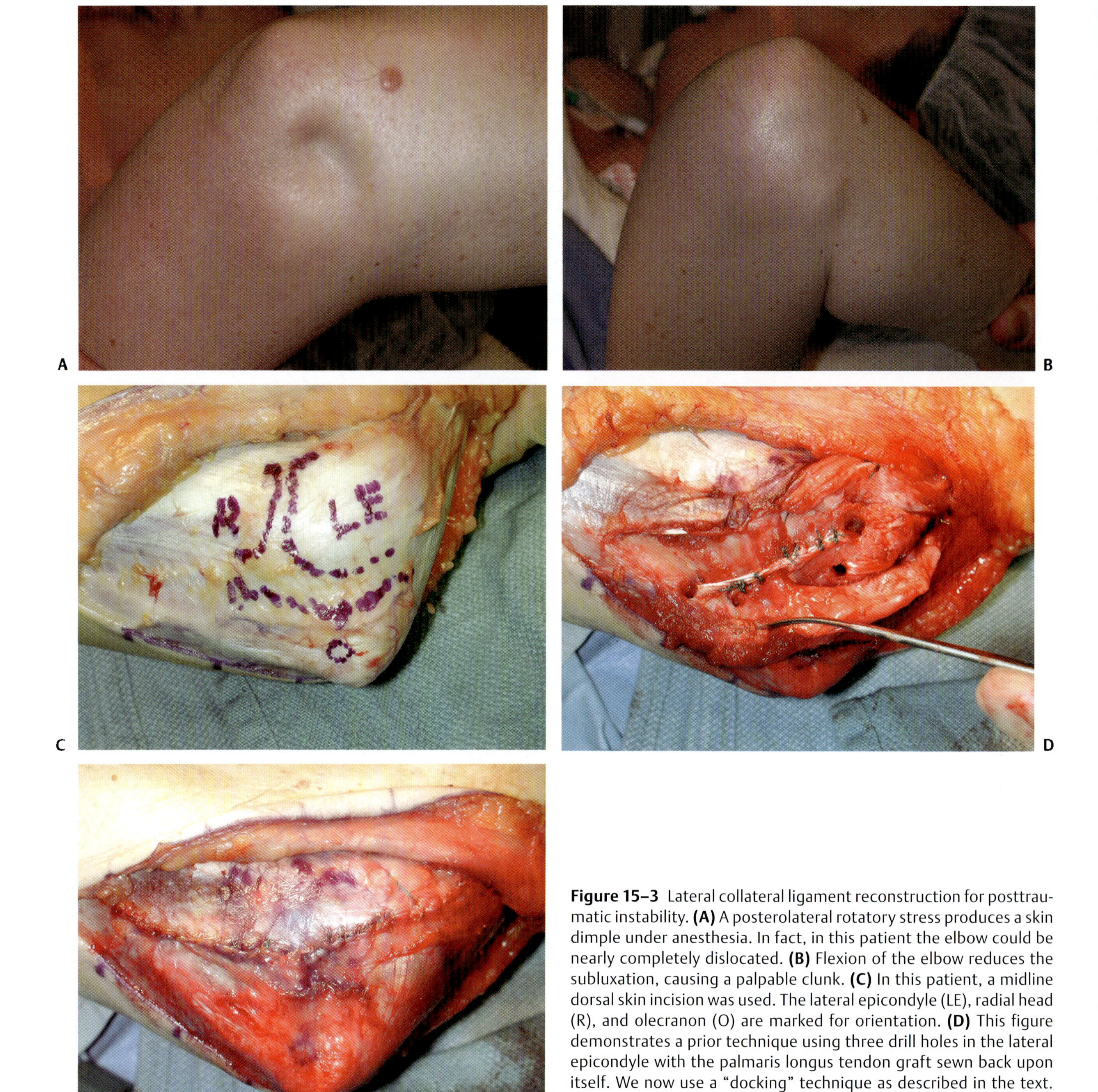

Figure 15–3 Lateral collateral ligament reconstruction for posttraumatic instability. **(A)** A posterolateral rotatory stress produces a skin dimple under anesthesia. In fact, in this patient the elbow could be nearly completely dislocated. **(B)** Flexion of the elbow reduces the subluxation, causing a palpable clunk. **(C)** In this patient, a midline dorsal skin incision was used. The lateral epicondyle (LE), radial head (R), and olecranon (O) are marked for orientation. **(D)** This figure demonstrates a prior technique using three drill holes in the lateral epicondyle with the palmaris longus tendon graft sewn back upon itself. We now use a "docking" technique as described in the text. **(E)** Suture and imbrication of the ligament remnant, and scar, and closure of the muscle interval helps restore stability.

upon what was injured and prior operative exposures. The common extensors and the origin of the LCLC are detached from the lateral epicondyle, recreating the damage that occurred at the original injury. The origin of the extensor carpi radialis longus is detached from the lateral supracondylar ridge and the brachialis is then elevated from the anterior humerus and the anterior elbow capsule. The thickened and contracted anterior elbow capsule is either isolated and excised, or released from the humerus.

The triceps and anconeus are elevated off the posterior surface of the distal humerus and the posterior elbow capsule. The posterior elbow capsule is isolated and excised. Access to the elbow joint is improved by supinating the forearm away from the distal humerus. Fibrous tissue is removed from the joint, and a concentric reduction obtained. Small areas of injury to the articular surface of the trochlea are common and loose cartilage can be débrided. Patients with severe damage will require interpositional arthroplasty or total elbow arthroplasty.

Radiocapitellar contact should be retained or restored. In most patients, this is achieved with a metal radial head prosthesis. In patients with an inadequate coronoid process, a piece of the resected radial head or the tip of the olecranon can be used to reconstruct it. The transferred bone is secured with a screw.

The lateral soft tissue envelope is reattached to the lateral epicondyle with suture anchors or sutures through drill holes through bone. Reconstruction of the collateral ligaments with tendon grafts is rarely necessary. A hinged external elbow fixator is applied for 4 to 8 weeks to protect the healing structures (**Fig. 15–4**).

Subacute or Chronic Dislocation

A dorsal midline incision and ulnar nerve transposition are used. The elbow joint is exposed through both medial and lateral muscle intervals. A complete capsular release is performed and the ulnotrochlear articulation is reduced and a hinged elbow distractor applied. The medial and lateral soft tissue envelope can be sewn closed and reattached to the epicondyle with suture anchors or drill holes.

Complications

Complications include recurrent stiffness (including recurrent heterotopic ossification) and ulnar neuropathy (due to restoration of flexion or to handling of the nerve). Other complications include infection, wound problems, nerve palsy, and complications related to hinged external fixation (broken or infected pins, fractures through pin holes, etc.).

Postoperative Rehabilitation

Patients with LCL reconstruction are immobilized for 1 month in a cast. All other patients begin rehabilitation the morning after surgery. Gravity-assisted and active-assisted range of motion exercises are used to improve elbow motion. Some surgeons like to use continuous passive motion with or without a brachial plexus block, but there are no data to support this. We find it both too costly and too passive (meaning that we prefer that patients realize that their active efforts are critical to recovering motion after trauma) and do not use it. Some hinged external fixators include a worm gear that can be used to mobilize the elbow and provide static progressive stretch. Static progressive or dynamic splints are used in patients that have trouble maintaining motion obtained in surgery. These splints are initiated as soon as the wound is stable.

Results

The majority of published case series reporting the results of open elbow contracture release describe a single technique used to treat patients with a variety of diagnoses. The results of various techniques seem comparable, although very few data are available regarding the use of a medial exposure for posttraumatic contractures.[18,33] In general, ~75% of patients regain at least an 80-degree arc of flexion.[33] Patients with limited flexion – particularly those due to primary osteoarthritis – may be susceptible to ulnar neuropathy after release.[21] The results of excision of subtotal heterotopic ossification may be superior to the results of capsular contracture alone.[34] The results of excision of complete bony ankylosis, although generally rewarding, are less predictable.[7]

We reported on 5 patients with chronic unreduced simple elbow dislocations treated operatively with the techniques described in this chapter.[35] In particular, the use of hinged external fixation for an average of 5 weeks was important. It also seems important that the elbows were widely dislocated, so that the articular surfaces were not damaged by abnormal contact. The results were remarkably good. At an average of 38 months, a stable, concentric reduction had been maintained in all 5 patients, with radiographic signs of mild arthrosis in 4 patients. The average arc of flexion was 123 degrees; all patients had full forearm rotation. The average score on the Mayo Elbow Performance Index[36] was 89 points, with two excellent and three good results. The average scores on the Disabilities of the Arm, Shoulder, and Hand (DASH) and American Shoulder and Elbow Surgeons outcome instruments (13 and 92 points, respectively) reflected mild residual pain and disability.[37] We concluded that the treatment of unreduced elbow dislocations with open reduction and hinged external fixation as much as 30 weeks after the injury can restore a stable, mobile joint without the need for tendon-lengthening or transfer, ligament reconstruction, or deepening of the trochlear notch of the ulna.

We also reviewed our results treating 13 patients with residual subluxation and dislocation after fracture-dislocation of the elbow.[2] All patients had adequate

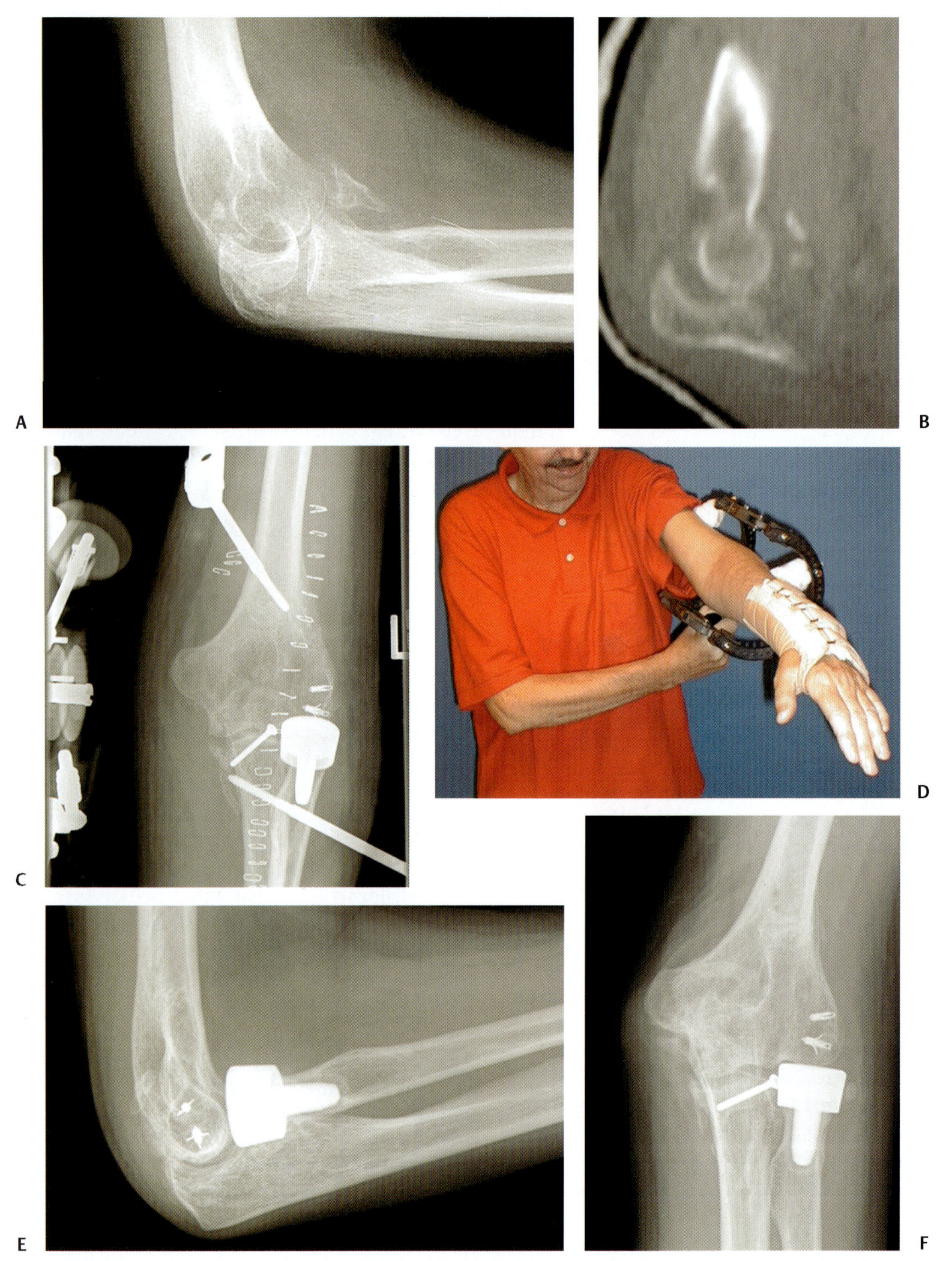

Figure 15–4 A 55-year-old man with subluxation of the elbow 3 months after a terrible triad injury. **(A)** The lateral radiograph shows a coronoid and radial head fracture and problems with alignment, but remains somewhat unclear. **(B)** Computed tomography scans better demonstrate subluxation of the trochlea into the defect created by the coronoid fracture. **(C)** Operative treatment consisted of replacement of the radial head with a metal prosthesis, reconstruction of the coronoid using a fragment of the radial head (secured by the small screw), reattachment of the lateral collateral ligament origin and the lateral soft tissues to the lateral epicondyle, and temporary hinged external fixation. **(D)** This hinged external fixator has a worm-gear that the patient used for static progressive stretch. **(E)** A lateral radiograph 1 year later shows concentric reduction. **(F)** An anteroposterior radiograph also confirms good alignment. Excellent elbow motion was restored.

articular surfaces, and adequate, stable alignment of the olecranon. Treatment included temporary hinged external fixation; preservation or reconstruction of both the coronoid process and radiocapitellar contact; and repair of the LCLC. Seven patients had a terrible triad pattern injury and 6 had a posterior Monteggia pattern injury. All 13 patients had fracture of the radial head and 10 patients had fracture of the coronoid process. At an average follow-up period of 57 months, stability was restored in every patient. The average DASH and Questionnaire Score was 15 and the average Mayo score was 84, with six excellent, four good, and three fair results. The average arc of ulnohumeral motion was 99 degrees. Six patients had radiographic signs of arthrosis including 5 of 6 patients with olecranon fracture-dislocations. We concluded that a stable, functional elbow can be restored in most patients with persistent instability after fracture-dislocation of the elbow using a treatment protocol incorporating hinged external fixation.

Summary

Posttraumatic stiffness without heterotopic bone, malunion/nonunion/articular incongruity, ulnar neuropathy, or errant implants nearly always responds to time, exercises, and static progressive or dynamic elbow splinting. Clearly identified hindrances to elbow motion benefit from operative treatment through either a lateral, medial, or combined approach. Episodic instability in an otherwise functional and well-aligned elbow is uncommon, and well treated by reconstruction of the LCLC. Subacute and chronic subluxation and dislocation are complex problems. The results of operative treatment of subluxation and dislocation depend upon the status of the articular stabilizers of the elbow (the radial head and coronoid in particular), the status of the articular surfaces, and the ability to keep the elbow in a reduced position while the repaired and reconstructed structures heal, for which hinged external fixation is useful.

References

1. O'Driscoll SW, Bell DF, Morrey BF. Posterolateral rotatory instability of the elbow. J Bone Joint Surg Am 1991;73:440–446
2. Ring D, Hannouche D, Jupiter JB. Surgical treatment of persistent dislocation or subluxation of the ulnohumeral joint after fracture-dislocation of the elbow. J Hand Surg [Am] 2004;29:470–480
3. Morrey BF. Post-traumatic contracture of the elbow. Operative treatment, including distraction arthroplasty. J Bone Joint Surg Am 1990;72:601–618
4. Morrey BF, Askew LJ, Chao EY. A biomechanical study of normal functional elbow motion. J Bone Joint Surg Am 1981;63:872–880
5. Doornberg JN, Ring D, Fabian LM, Malhotra L, Zurakowski D, Jupiter JB. Pain dominates measurements of elbow function and health status. J Bone Joint Surg Am 2005;87:1725–1731
6. Viola RW, Hastings H. Treatment of ectopic ossification about the elbow. Clin Orthop Relat Res 2000;370:65–86
7. Ring D, Jupiter J. The operative release of complete ankylosis of the elbow due to heterotopic bone in patients without severe injury of the central nervous system. J Bone Joint Surg Am 2003;85:849–857
8. Nestor BJ, O'Driscoll SW, Morrey BF. Ligamentous reconstruction for posterolateral rotatory instability of the elbow. J Bone Joint Surg Am 1992;74:1235–1241
9. O'Driscoll SW, Jupiter JB, Cohen M, Ring D, McKee MD. Difficult elbow fractures: pearls and pitfalls. Instr Course Lect 2003;52:113–134
10. McKee M, Jupiter JB, Toh CL, Wilson L, Colton C, Karras KK. Reconstruction after malunion and nonunion of intra-articular fractures of the distal humerus. J Bone Joint Surg Br 1994;76:614–621
11. Doornberg JN, Ring D, Jupiter J. Static progressive splinting for post-traumatic elbow stiffness. J Orthop Trauma 2006;20:400–404
12. Jupiter JB, Ring D. Operative treatment of post-traumatic proximal radioulnar synostosis. J Bone Joint Surg Am 1998;80:248–257
13. Viola RW, Hanel DP. Early "simple" release of posttraumatic elbow contracture associated with heterotopic ossification. J Hand Surg [Am] 1999;24:370–380
14. Morrey BF, Adams RA, Bryan RS. Total elbow replacement for post-traumatic arthritis of the elbow. J Bone Joint Surg Br 1991;73:607–612
15. Helfet DL, Kloen P, Anand N, Rosen HS. Open reduction and internal fixation of delayed unions and nonunions of fractures of the distal part of the humerus. J Bone Joint Surg Am 2003;85:33–40
16. Cohen MS, Hastings H. Post-traumatic contracture of the elbow: operative release using a lateral collateral liagment sparing approach. J Bone Joint Surg Br 1998;80:805–812
17. Mansat P, Morrey BF. The column procedure: a limited lateral approach for extrinsic contracture of the elbow. J Bone Joint Surg Am 1998;80:1603–1615
18. Wada T, Isogai S, Ishii S, Yamashita T. Debridement arthroplasty for primary osteoarthritis of the elbow. Surgical technique. J Bone Joint Surg Am 2005;87(Suppl 1 Pt 1):95–105
19. Hotchkiss RN. Elbow contracture. In: Green DP, Hotchkiss RN, Pederson WC, eds. Green's Operative Hand Surgery. Philadelphia, PA: Churchill-Livingstone; 1999:667–682
20. Urbaniak JR, Hansen PE, Beissinger SF, Aitken MS. Correction of post-traumatic flexion contracture of the elbow

by anterior capsulotomy. J Bone Joint Surg Am 1985;67: 1160–1164
21. Antuna SA, Morrey BF, Adams RA, O'Driscoll SW. Ulnohumeral arthroplasty for primary degenerative arthritis of the elbow: long-term outcome and complications. J Bone Joint Surg Am 2002;84:2168–2173
22. Ball CM, Meunier M, Galatz LM, Calfee R, Yamaguchi K. Arthroscopic treatment of post-traumatic elbow contracture. J Shoulder Elbow Surg 2002;11:624–629
23. Haapaniemi T, Berggren M, Adolfsson L. Complete transection of the median and radial nerves during arthroscopic release of post-traumatic elbow contracture. Arthroscopy 1999;15:784–787
24. Jones GS, Savoie FH III. Arthroscopic capsular release of flexion contractures (arthrofibrosis) of the elbow. Arthroscopy 1993;9:277–283
25. Kim SJ, Kim HK, Lee JW. Arthroscopy for limitation of motion of the elbow. Arthroscopy 1995;11:680–683
26. Phillips BB, Strasburger S. Arthroscopic treatment of arthrofibrosis of the elbow joint. Arthroscopy 1998;14: 38–44
27. McKee MD, Bowden SH, King GJ, et al. Management of recurrent, complex instability of the elbow with a hinged external fixator. J Bone Joint Surg Br 1998;80: 1031–1036
28. Dowdy PA, Bain GI, King GJW, Patterson SD. The midline posterior elbow incision. J Bone Joint Surg Br 1995;77: 696–699
29. Patterson SD, Bain GI, Mehta JA. Surgical approaches to the elbow. Clin Orthop Relat Res 2000;370:19–33
30. Ring D, Hotchkiss RN, Guss D, Jupiter JB. Hinged elbow external fixation for severe elbow contracture. J Bone Joint Surg Am 2005;87:1293–1296
31. Kocher T. Textbook of Operative Surgery. 3rd ed. London: Adam and Charles Black; 1911
32. Morrey BF. Surgical exposures of the elbow. In: Morrey BF, ed. The Elbow and Its Disorders. 2nd ed. Philadelphia, PA: WB Saunders; 1993:139–166
33. Ring D, Adey L, Zurakowski D, Jupiter JB. Health status after release of post-traumatic elbow contracture. J Hand Surg [Am] 2006;31:1264–1271
34. Lindenhovius AL, Linzel DS, Doornberg JN, Ring D, Jupiter JB. Comparison of elbow contracture release in elbows with and without heterotopic ossification restricting motion. J Should Elbow Surg 2007;16:621–625
35. Jupiter JB, Ring D. Treatment of unreduced elbow dislocations with hinged external fixation. J Bone Joint Surg Am 2002;84:1630–1635
36. Morrey BF, An KN, Chao EYS. Functional evaluation of the elbow. In: Morrey BF, ed. The Elbow and Its Disorders, 2nd ed. Philadelphia: W.B. Saunders, 1993:86–97
37. Hudak PL, Amadio PC, Bombardier C. Development of an upper extremity outcome measure: the DASH (disabilities of the arm, shoulder and hand) [corrected]. The Upper Extremity Collaborative Group (UECG). Am J Ind Med 1996;29:602–608

16 Nonunions of the Distal Humerus

Peter Kloen and David L. Helfet

Good and excellent results can be expected after anatomic reduction and rigid internal fixation of intraarticular fractures of the distal humerus.[1-3] In a small subgroup of patients, however, complications such as elbow stiffness and periarticular fibrosis, heterotopic ossification, ulnar neuritis, malunions, and delayed unions or nonunions occur.[2] Fortunately, the prevalence of delayed unions and nonunions of the distal humerus is low, ranging between 2 and 10%.[1-4] Although a delayed union or nonunion of the distal humerus can be pain-free and treatable with a brace in a small minority of patients, most patients complain of a frail, painful, and essentially nonfunctional upper extremity. The proximity of the ulnar nerve to the periarticular elbow instability often leads to exacerbation of an existing ulnar neuritis compounding to the patient's disability. Operative intervention of some type is thus often required for these patients. Challenging associated factors that often face the treating surgeon are compromised soft tissues due to previous interventions, poor bone stock, osteopenia, broken hardware, and small fragment size.

Classification

The delayed union and nonunion can be classified according to Mitsunaga[5] and colleagues into supracondylar, transcondylar, T-condylar (or intercondylar), and low transcondylar. The type of nonunion is classified according to Weber and Çech into atrophic, oligotrophic, or hypertrophic.[6] The diagnosis of a synovial pseudarthrosis can only be made intraoperatively and is characterized by a fluid-filled sac with a synovial lining. Infection is diagnosed based on clinical examination (drainage, fistula, etc.) and/or by intraoperatively obtained deep cultures prior to administration of antibiotics.

Patient Asssessment

History

Previous operative reports should be scrutinized for details regarding fracture configuration, position of the ulnar nerve, difficulties (if any) encountered, and comments on bone quality. If hardware is already in place, it should be determined which type so that appropriate instruments are available for removal.

Physical Examination

Preoperative evaluation of the patient's range of elbow motion, neurovascular status, previous scars, and signs of infection is important. A detailed examination of the ulnar nerve is paramount, including its mobility, position, absence or presence of a Tinel's sign, and a detailed sensory and motor function.

Radiographic Assessment

Elbow radiographs in at least two planes will often give sufficient insight into the bony problem **(Fig. 16–1)**. Based on these radiographs, one should be able to classify whether the nonunion is atrophic, oligotrophic, or hypertrophic. The configuration of the nonunion needs to be outlined, especially if it involves the articular surface. Occasionally a computed tomography (CT) scan is needed to identify which portions of the distal humerus are ununited. It can be helpful to evaluate the residual motion at the elbow and/or nonunion site by obtaining two lateral radiographs with the elbow in flexion and extension, respectively. This will often show that most – if not all – motion is at the nonunion site and not at the elbow joint itself.

The goal of all these preoperative evaluations is to understand the exact nonunion configuration, allowing the surgeon to make a line drawing of the various fragments, their reduction, and expected final montage. This preoperative exercise prepares the surgeon in a stepwise fashion for the procedure, its potential problems and pitfalls, and provides both the surgeon and patient with realistic expectations of outcome and potential complications.

Laboratory Studies

Other than routine preoperative laboratory studies no specific blood tests are needed. In case of (suspected) infection, a complete blood count including differential, an erythrocyte sedimentation rate and C-reactive protein can be determined. Aspiration of the nonunion site to

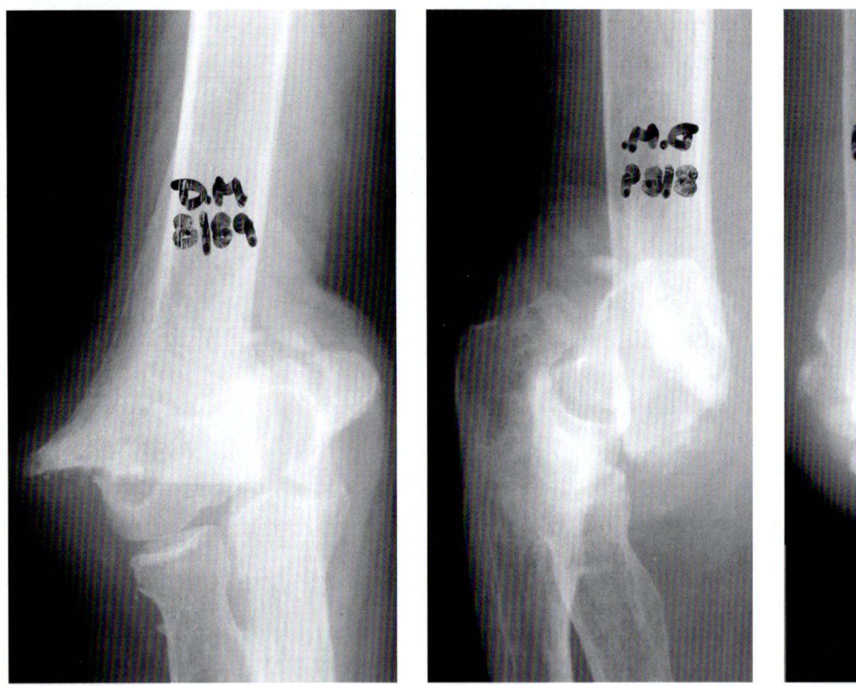

Figure 16–1 (A-C) An 81-year-old man presented 6 months following a right-sided distal humerus fracture with complaints of pain and limited function that was originally treated in a elbow brace. Motion at the nonunion site is obvious radiographically.

determine evidence of infection can be considered, but is seldom done in our practice.

Treatment

Nonsurgical Treatment

Only a very small number of patients will not require surgery and might be considered for brace treatment. In our experience the vast majority of patients with a nonunion of the distal humerus will benefit from operative intervention and are able to undergo the proposed treatment.

Surgical Treatment

Successful operative treatment is based on an extensile release, removal of failed hardware, adequate débridement, and rigid fixation with liberal use of bone graft allowing early motion.

Surgical Reconstructive Procedures

Reconstructive options other than open reduction and internal fixation of distal humerus nonunions are distraction arthroplasty, allograft (cadaveric) replacement, elbow arthrodesis, and total elbow arthroplasty. Better total elbow prosthetic designs as popularized by Morrey and Adams[7] have improved upon the initial relatively poor results of total elbow arthroplasty for distal humeral nonunions. Still, their proponents agree that this should only be used as a salvage procedure, i.e., if stable open reduction and internal fixation are not possible or the articular surface or joint anatomy are not salvageable. Limited data on the use of cadaveric allografts are lacking in long-term results and complications such as instability, resorption, and nonunion may occur.[8] Lastly, the option of distraction arthroplasty for posttraumatic dysfunction as described by Morrey is a technically demanding salvage procedure associated with a high complication rate.[9]

Authors' Recommended Treatment

The operative procedure begins by positioning the patient on a beanbag in the lateral decubitus position. Alternatively the patient can be placed prone with the upper arm resting on a small armrest keeping the elbow at 90 degree's flexion. A sterile tourniquet is inflated and the arm is placed across the chest over a blanket roll if in the lateral position. If an iliac crest bone graft is to be taken, this area is draped out simultaneously. Depending on the surgeon's handedness and preference, the surgeon and first assistant will each be on one side of the arm. Using a sterile marker, all previous incision(s) are marked out. Ideally, old incision(s) are incorporated in a midline posterior approach lowering the risk of ischemic skin necrosis. To facilitate exposure of the ulnar nerve, the procedure is started under tourniquet. The ulnar nerve is best first localized proximally where it emerges beneath the triceps tendon. Any previous surgery around the elbow warrants extra caution, given the possibility of scarring or a change of location of the ulnar nerve. If extensive scarring around the nerve is present, the dissection is more complicated and the surgeon should be prepared for a careful microdissection with the use of surgical loupes. The nerve is followed for at least 7 cm after entering the flexor pronator mass. The first branch of the ulnar nerve (articular branch) is often sacrificed because it tethers the nerve to the joint, preventing adequate release of the nerve. Its next branches should be carefully preserved as they supply the flexor carpi ulnaris. Once the ulnar nerve is dissected free it is tagged with a Penrose drain. Proximally, the distal aspect of the intermuscular septum should be released to increase mobility of the ulnar nerve. If preoperative ulnar neuritis is present, in addition to extensive scarring around the nerve, an external neurolysis should be performed.

In case of an intraarticular nonunion, malunion, or a low transcondylar nonunion, the best exposure of the joint is obtained through a chevron intraarticular olecranon osteotomy (**Fig. 16–2**). However, if the delayed or nonunion is extraarticular (supracondylar), a triceps splitting, triceps preserving/reflecting or dividing approach can be sufficient. A combined medial and lateral approach is, in our experience, insufficient for an intraarticular or low transcondylar nonunion. Only for an isolated medial or lateral condylar delayed union or nonunion can a unilateral approach be considered. In case of a previous olecranon osteotomy that has not yet healed, it is prudent to reutilize this same approach.

Prior to starting an olecranon osteotomy, part of the anconeus and the flexor carpi ulnaris have to be released off the olecranon to identify the exact position of the osteotomy, which is at the thinnest part of the cartilage at the apex of the olecranon fossa. This will generally leave at least 1 cm of intact olecranon proximal to the apex of the osteotomy. Using an oscillating saw under continuous saline cooling to prevent thermal necrosis the osteotomy is started. The osteotomy is completed with an osteotome. The osteotomized olecranon is then reflected superiorly releasing the often adherent triceps from the lower 4 inches of the humerus using finger or periosteal dissection (**Fig. 16–3**). The radial nerve and accompanying vessels should be exposed and tagged if the fracture extends proximally.

After exposure of the nonunion, routine cultures should be obtained (frozen sections to rule out infection are not used in our practice) and routine intravenous antibiotics are given at this stage. If the tourniquet is inflated this should be released prior to infusing antibiotics. All hardware should be removed, although removal of broken screws inside the bone is not warranted if it will lead to additional bone loss. Débridement of intervening scar tissue is next done with a curette or rongeur, while maintaining the soft tissue attachments to avoid devascularization of

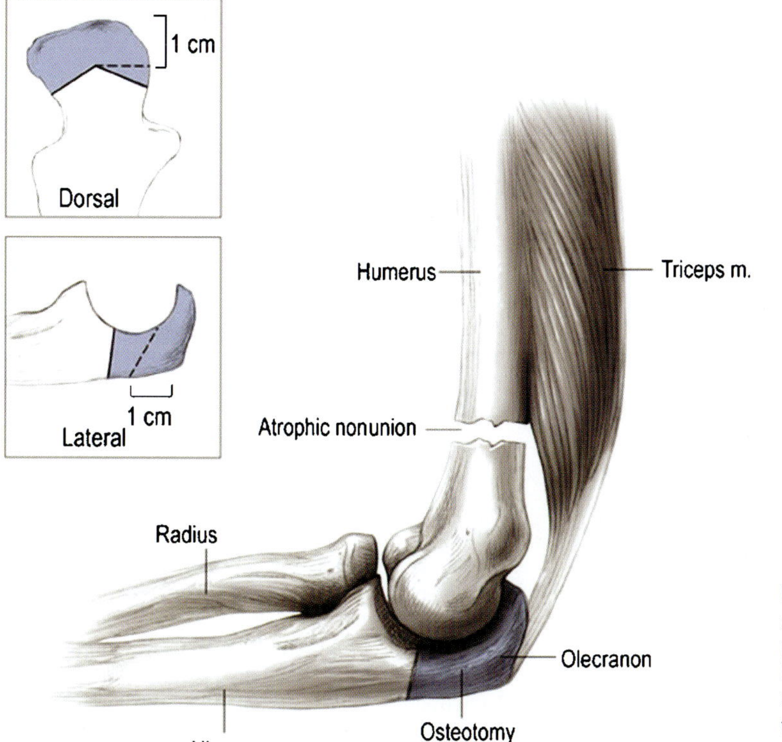

Figure 16–2 The olecranon osteotomy is angulated (as shown in inset), forming an apex to facilitate reduction and providing additional rotational stability for fixation. (From Helfet DL, Kloen P, Anand N, Rosen HS. ORIF of delayed unions and nonunions of distal humerus fractures. Surgical technique. J Bone Joint Surg Am 2004; 86-A(Suppl 1):18-29. Reprinted by permission.)

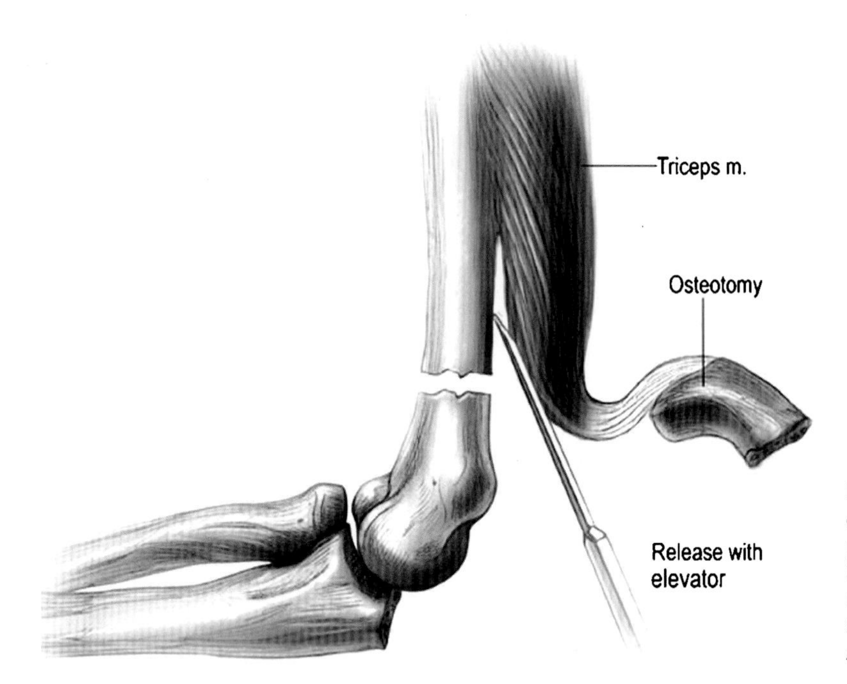

Figure 16–3 After completing the osteotomy, the triceps can be released from the nonunion and the distal part of the shaft by finger or periosteal dissection. (From Helfet DL, Kloen P, Anand N, Rosen HS. ORIF of delayed unions and nonunions of distal humerus fractures. Surgical technique. J Bone Joint Surg Am 2004; 86-A(Suppl 1):18-29. Reprinted by permission.)

the fragments. In case of a synovial pseudoarthrosis, the cavity is opened and excised completely, cleaning the bone ends of all fibrous tissue. Special caution is warranted during this part of the procedure because the anterior neurovascular structures can be adherent to the anterior extent of the pseudarthrosis cavity. The medullary canal of the proximal fragment is often sealed by fibrous nonunion tissue or a sclerotic bony end cap, and needs to be opened with an awl or a 2.5-mm drill to allow migration of osteogenic cells and neovascularization. The appearance of bleeding from these drill holes signifies adequate penetration. If the tourniquet is still inflated at this stage, the absence of bleeding is not an adequate indicator.

Next, the lower fragment is mobilized by freeing the anterior capsule through the nonunion with an elevator or knife (**Fig. 16–4**). The elbow joint is mobilized by freeing the distal fragment anteriorly and posteriorly and by cutting joint adhesions. When extensive periarticular fibrosis

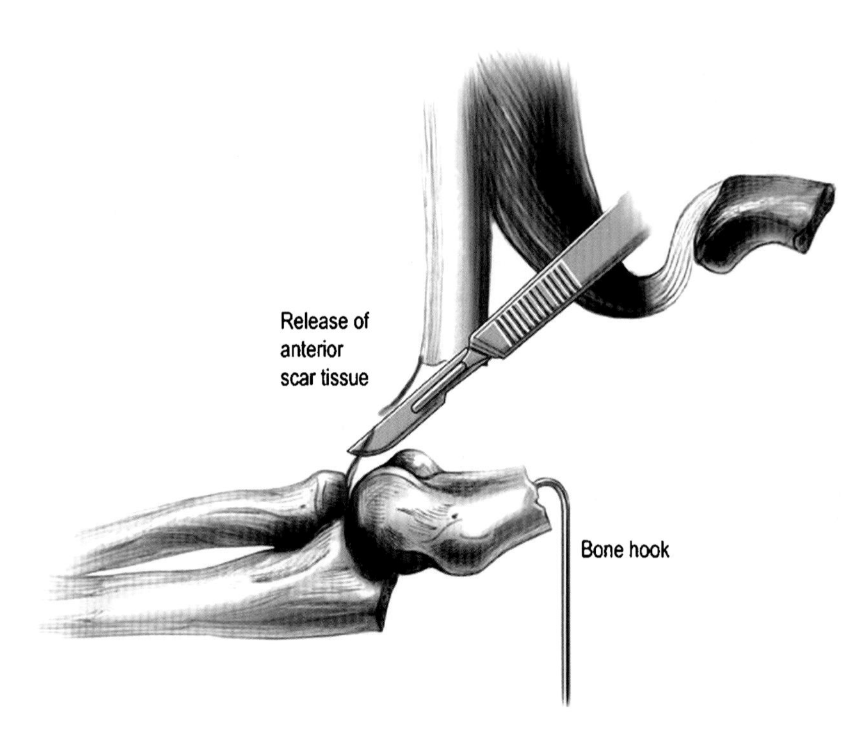

Figure 16–4 Using an elevator or knife the anterior capsule and/or scar tissue can be released throughout the nonunion site from posterior to anterior. (From Helfet DL, Kloen P, Anand N, Rosen HS. ORIF of delayed unions and nonunions of distal humerus fractures. Surgical technique. J Bone Joint Surg Am 2004; 86-A(Suppl 1):18-29. Reprinted by permission.)

is encountered, this scar tissue is sharply dissected to allow for increased mobility. If necessary, an anterior capsulectomy can be performed through the delayed/nonunion. The condylar block can be carefully flexed and extended releasing additional contractures. If full motion of the distal fragment is still not achieved at this point, the lateral collateral ligament and extensor origin from the lateral epicondyle can be incised leaving a small tag of ligament for reattachment. The elbow joint is then opened like a book hinging on the medial collateral ligament, and all remaining adhesions are cut until the joint motion is free. The extensor origin and lateral ligament are sutured back to the lateral epicondyle via the ligamentous tag and/or transosseous drill holes or suture anchors.

The humeral articular surfaces are assessed for nonunion or malunion of the trochlea and capitellum. If these are judged by preoperative tomograms and intraoperative observations of the joint to impede motion or articulate poorly with the proximal ulna and radius, an intraarticular osteotomy is performed and then provisionally stabilized with Kirschner wires (K-wires) replaced by 3.5-mm lag screws **(Fig. 16–5)**. If an articular gap is present, corticocancellous iliac bone can be fashioned to fill the defect, and a fully threaded position screw used to hold the joint surface. Care should be taken to ensure that the reconstructed humeral condyles do not narrow the trochlea, otherwise the trochlea will not fit properly within the trochlear notch. If a nonunion or pseudoarthrosis is a low transcondylar type, then the sealed medullary canal of the distal small osteoporotic fragment is not opened. Instead, it is drilled with multiple 2-mm drill holes.

Using 1.6 or 2.0 K-wires, existing fragments are temporarily reduced and fixed. If an intraarticular component exists, this is reduced first, after which the reconstituted condylar block is reduced to the medial and lateral columns. Depending on the configuration of the delayed union or nonunion, 3.5-mm pelvic reconstruction plates are contoured to fit along the involved columns (Synthes, Paoli, PA). The lateral column plate is contoured around the posterior aspect, whereas the medial column is plated along the medial column **(Fig. 16–6)**. Long screws aiming from the medial or lateral epicondyles through the medial and lateral columns provide additional fixation. Currently, we prefer the use of self-tapping, fully threaded 3.5-mm cortical screws of 60 to 80 mm in length. The recently popularized locked compression plates (locking compression plate [LCP], Synthes) utilize fixed angled screws that might provide superior fixation in osteopenic bone. As they can also be used with only unicortical purchase, there is less risk of joint penetration. In addition, with bicolumnar fixation there is often "crowding" of screws, which is circumvented by using unicortical (short) screws. Until convincing data on the use of these unicortical screws are available, we use at least one long "intramedullary" screw that "crosses over" from the distal medial column into the proximal lateral metaphyseal/diaphyseal junction and similarly from the distal lateral column into the proximal medial metaphyseal/diaphyseal area. These long screws are ideally placed through the plate to improve the stability of the construct **(Fig. 16–7)**. Cross-threading of the screws is often felt during placement and visible on the postoperative radiograph by bending of the screw.

Nonunions in the coronal plane are especially challenging, as these fragments usually are entirely articular and difficult to fix. For capitellar nonunions, we use a

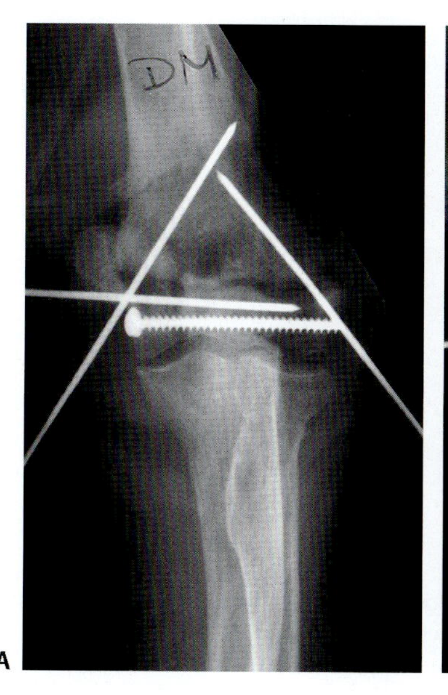

A

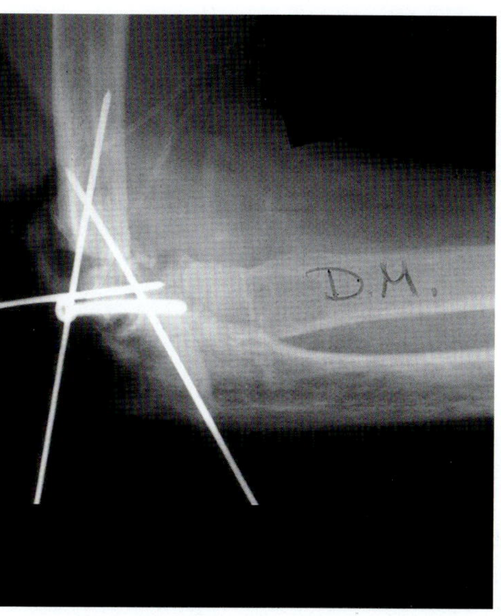

B

Figure 16–5 (A,B) The nonunion/articular surface was provisionally stabilized with insertion of Kirschner wires.

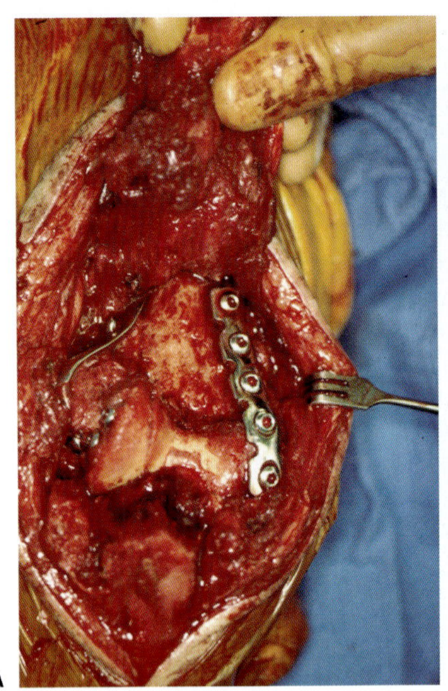

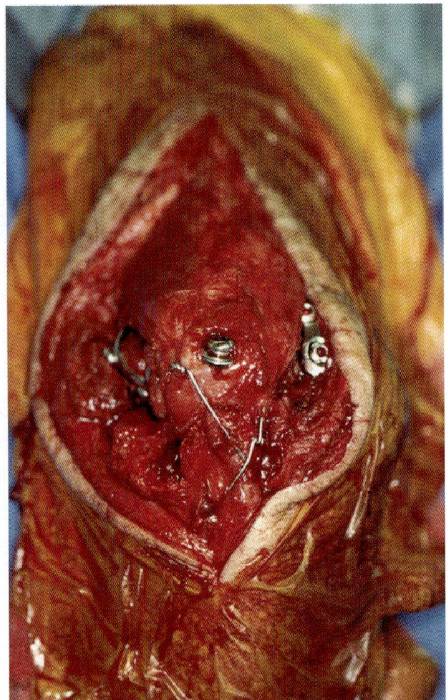

Figure 16–6 The K-wires were then replaced with interfragmentary lag screws. **(A)** Plates and screws were then placed medially and laterally; a seven-hole, one-third tubular plate was contoured and placed on the medial column and a six-hole, 3.5-mm pelvic reconstruction plate was contoured and placed on the posterior aspect for the lateral column. **(B)** The olecranon osteotomy was then repaired using a figure- eight wire tension band construct.

buried minifragment or Herbert screw, and place two screws from opposite directions (anteroposterior and posteroanterior) to enhance fixation.

In the very low transcondylar nonunions, a transcondylar lag screw is placed through the distal hole of one of the contoured plates to gain purchase on the small osteoporotic distal fragment. Occasionally, there is no alternative than to traverse a deformed olecranon notch with screws to obtain adequate distal fixation. These screws rarely impede full extension, but one can resect the tip of the olecranon to prevent this impingement.

To optimize osteogenic and/or osteoconductive potential, some type of bone is often needed. Autogenous bone graft can be harvested from the iliac crest, the olecranon tip, or both. In our series, only 1 patient received a vascularized fibular bone graft in conjunction with iliac crest and olecranon bone graft. Recently, we have used a demineralized bone graft product as it minimizes donor site morbidity (Grafton DBM Crunch; Osteotech Inc., Eatontown, NJ). We have no objective data whether it compares favorably as far as its bone inductive/conductive properties are concerned compared with autogenous bone graft.

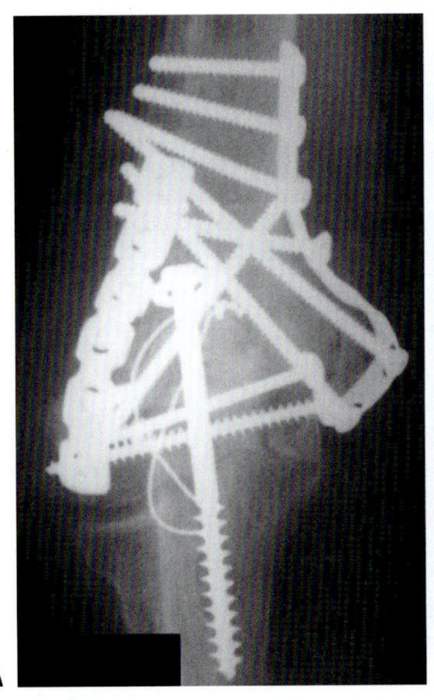

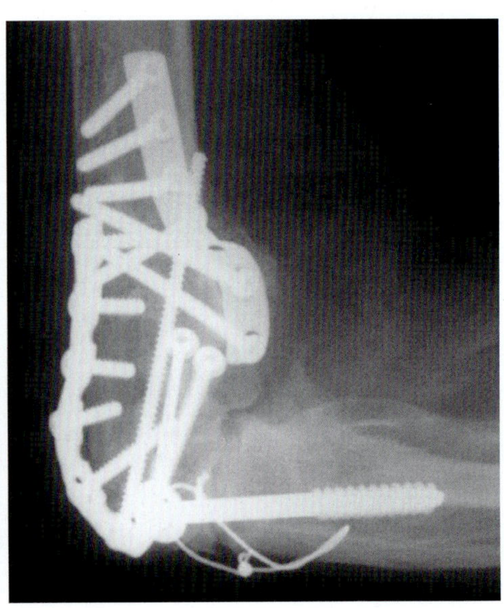

Figure 16–7 **(A)** Anteroposterior and **(B)** lateral views at 3.5 months illustrate a healed distal humerus nonunion.

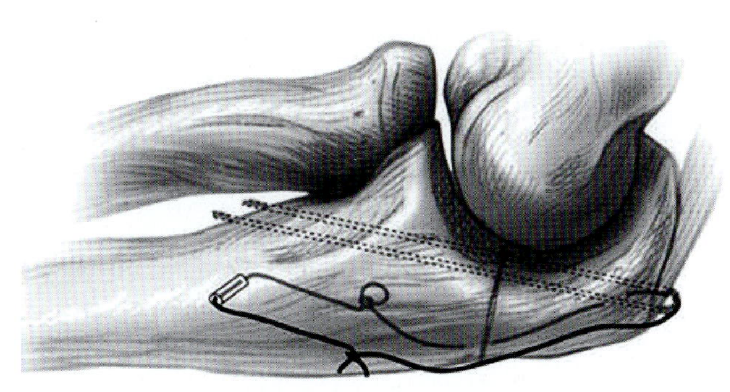

Figure 16–8 Repair of the olecranon osteotomy. (From Helfet DL, Kloen P, Anand N, Rosen HS. ORIF of delayed unions and nonunions of distal humerus fractures. Surgical technique. J Bone Joint Surg Am 2004; 86-A(Suppl 1):18-29. Reprinted by permission.)

After intraoperative radiographs confirm adequate placement of the hardware and reconstitution of the bony anatomy, the elbow is gently taken through a range of motion (ROM). This will test the stability of the repair and guide postoperative rehabilitation goals. If an olecranon osteotomy was performed, this is repaired with two K-wires engaging the anterior cortex **(Fig. 16–8)**, or a screw and a figure-eight wire tension band. To prevent prominence of the hardware, it is important to pass the tension-band wire under the triceps and also to bury the K-wires under the triceps. Prior to closure, the tourniquet is deflated and hemostasis is obtained. We now routinely transpose the ulnar nerve anteriorly into the subcutaneous tissue. It is our experience that this decreases the incidence of iatrogenic ulnar nerve symptoms and facilitates exposure at a later time, if needed. Deep suction drains are placed and the patient's arm is placed in a well-padded posterior splint.

Complications

Ulnar nerve dysfunction is relatively common after operative treatment of distal humerus fractures – even more so after treatment of distal humerus nonunions because the nerve is often already compromised from previous surgery, ongoing instability in the nonunion, and encasement in scar tissue and/or bone. In addition to an external neurolysis, we currently transpose the nerve anteriorly in the subcutaneous tissues.

With the current protocol of early mobilization, formation of heterotopic ossification is relatively uncommon. Risk factors that are associated with its formation are burns or head injuries. We do not routinely use indomethacin and/or postoperative irradiation to prevent recurrence of heterotopic ossification unless there is a previous history of a closed head injury and/or significant ossification. Ongoing nonunion of the distal humerus is rare if adhering to the principles outlined above. A nonunion of the olecranon osteotomy is also rarely seen.

Stiffness after obtaining union – despite an extensile release – was seen in only 4 of our 52 patients.[4] Three of these patients underwent successful manipulation under anesthesia, one underwent a formal release. Hardware-related complications are most often seen after an olecranon osteotomy. Migration or prominence of the K-wires leading to skin irritation or breakdown might warrant removal once the osteotomy is healed.

Postoperative Rehabilitation

After surgery the arm is immobilized in a resting splint overnight. On the first postoperative day, the patient is fitted with a hinged elbow brace, and gentle active and active-assisted ROM exercises are started under supervision of a physical or occupational therapist. We do not utilize continuous passive motion postoperatively. In case of preoperative evidence of heterotopic ossification or head injury, we prescribe oral indomethacin SR (75 mg/day) for 6 weeks started on the first postoperative day. We do not routinely use postoperative radiation for any of these patients. Radiographs are checked at 6 weeks, 12 weeks, and then at 6 months and 12 months until bony healing is confirmed.

Results

In our recently published series of 52 patients, all except 1 patient (98%) obtained bony union following open reduction and internal fixation at an average of 6 months (range: 2 to 24 months).[4,10] The 1 patient that failed to heal his nonunion had severe Parkinsonism and developed a painless nonunion that required no further treatment. All 29 of the olecranon osteotomies healed. The average arc of motion postoperatively was 95 degrees **(Fig. 16–9)**. The preoperative ROM was often hard to assess in these patients because their contracted elbows were painful precluding an adequate clinical evaluation. The measured arc of motion was often through the delayed union or nonunion rather than through the elbow joint. Therefore, the validity of the preoperative ROM testing was questionable.

Fourteen patients (27%) underwent additional surgery after our index procedure. Of these, 13 complained of sufficient pain about the plates and screws warranting removal. In 4 of 13 patients, only the olecranon hardware was removed. During the hardware removal, 2 patients underwent ulnar neurolysis, 3 patients underwent manipulation under anesthesia, and 1 patient underwent arthrotomy and arthrolysis. One of the patients undergoing manipulation under anesthesia sustained a minimally

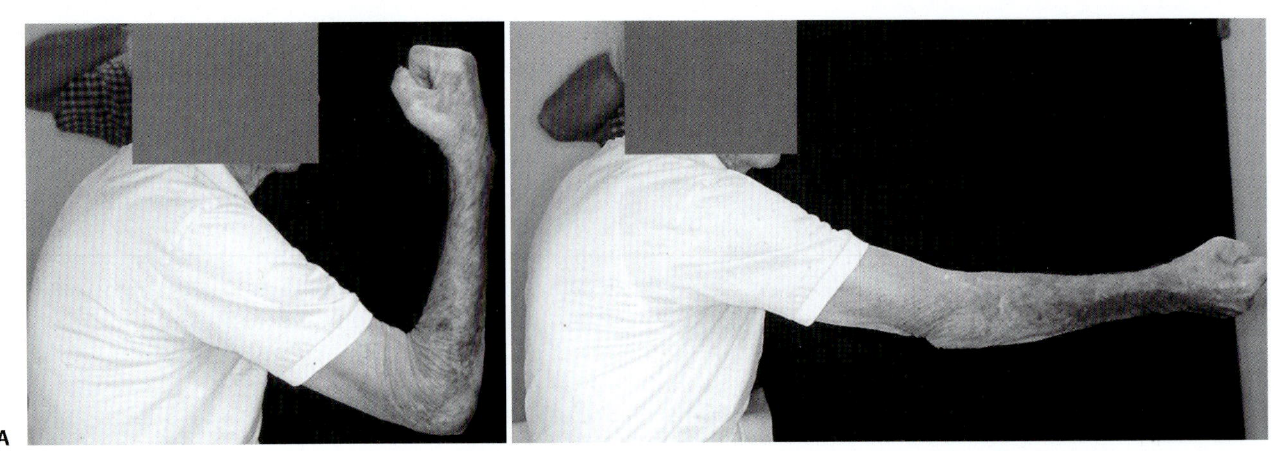

Figure 16–9 (A,B) The patient also has returned to preinjury activity status with a restoration of his elbow function and motion.

displaced fracture of the lateral column that required internal fixation and healed uneventfully.

There were four (8%) postoperative infections, of which two were superficial and resolved with oral antibiotics. The other two were deep infections, requiring irrigation, débridement, and intravenous antibiotics before ultimately leading to resolution. Five patients (14%) developed an ulnar neuropathy after our procedure, in addition to the 15 who had an existing preoperative ulnar neuropathy. One patient was diagnosed with new transient postoperative radial nerve palsy (2%).

Others have reported on the treatment of distal humerus nonunions.[5,11–15] A retrospective, multiple surgeon review of 25 patients published by Mitsunaga et al[5] found healing in 80%, 6 of whom required more than one procedure to obtain union. Postoperative ROM averaged 71 degrees. In contrast to our current series, only 2 patients were judged to have stable enough fixation postoperatively to allow early motion. The authors emphasized the importance of "union first and motion second" which is in contrast to our philosophy of obtaining motion – by extensile release if needed – and union at the same time.

Ackerman and Jupiter reported on 20 patients with a distal humerus nonunion.[11] Their average arc of motion postoperatively was 76 degrees, with union in 95% of patients. They reported improved results after adjusting their surgical tactic combining stable fixation and autogenous bone graft in addition to capsulotomy and ulnar neurolysis.[12–14]

Summary

A delayed union or nonunion of a distal humerus fracture is relatively rare. The largest comparative study to date on their incidence was done by the AO/Association for the Study for Internal Fixation (ASIF) and published in the German literature in 1984.[3] They found a 5.2% incidence of nonunion in 412 patients, which is comparable to other smaller series where the reported nonunion rates ranged from 2 to 10%. Of note is that the nonunion typically involves the supracondylar region, whereas the intercondylar region generally unites.

We believe that to achieve union, surgery must address all contributing factors to the persistence of the nonunion including the complete mobilization of the stiff elbow joint as well as stable fixation with bone grafting of the nonunion. The elbow joint stiffness seen in these lesions is multifactorial. Not only are there intraarticular adhesions and bony incongruence and extraarticular fibrosis, but there are ligamentous and muscular contractures as well. With increasing elbow stiffness, the forces become magnified at the nonunion site, where most of the motion then takes place. The main advantage of releasing the elbow contractures at the time of surgery is the redistribution of normal forces across the elbow joint rather than across the now stabilized delayed union or nonunion site. Such arthrolysis protects the stability of the osteosynthesis. In fact, not mobilizing the elbow joint at the time of nonunion osteosynthesis increases the lever arm and forces on the distal humerus; it probably decreases the chances of union.

Based on our experience, delayed unions and nonunions of the distal humerus are disabling, but fortunately salvageable problems. Careful preoperative planning, adequate exposure and extensive release of contractures and periarticular fibrosis followed by rigid internal fixation with bone grafting and immediate postoperative mobilization can result in a high union rate and an improved arc of elbow motion.

References

1. Jupiter JB, Neff U, Holzach P, Allgöwer M. Intercondylar fractures of the humerus: an operative approach. J Bone Joint Surg Am 1985;67:226–239
2. Ring D, Jupiter JB. Complex fractures of the distal humerus and their complications. J Shoulder Elbow Surg 1999;8:85–97
3. Lob G, Burri C, Feil J. Die operative Behandlung von distalen intraarticularen Humerusfrakturen; Ergebnis von 412 nachkontrollierten Fallen (Ao-Sammelstatistik) [Operative treatment of distal intra-articular humerus fractures; results of 412 follow-up cases (AO-collected statistics)] Langenbecks Arch Chir 1984;364:359–361
4. Helfet DL, Kloen P, Anand N, Rosen HS. Open reduction and internal fixation of delayed and nonunions of fractures of the distal humerus. J Bone Joint Surg Am 2003;85:33–40
5. Mitsunaga MM, Bryan RS, Linscheid RL. Condylar nonunions of the elbow. J Trauma 1982;22:787–791
6. Weber BG, Çech O. Pseudarthrosis; pathophysiology, biomechanics, therapy, results. In: Pseudarthrosis. New York, NY: Grune & Stratton; 1976:14–28
7. Morrey BF, Adams RA. Semiconstrained elbow replacement for distal humeral nonunion. J Bone Joint Surg Br 1995;77:67–72
8. Urbaniak JR, Black KE. Cadaveric elbow allografts: a six-year experience. Clin Orthop Relat Res 1985;197:131–140
9. Morrey BF. Post-traumatic contracture of the elbow: operative treatment, including distraction arthroplasty. J Bone Joint Surg Am 1990;72:601–618
10. Helfet DL, Kloen P, Anand N, Rosen HS. ORIF of delayed unions and nonunions of distal humerus fractures. Surgical technique. J Bone Joint Surg Am 2004;86-A(Suppl 1): 18–29
11. Ackerman G, Jupiter JB. Non-union of fractures of the distal end of the humerus. J Bone Joint Surg Am 1988;70:75–83
12. Jupiter JB, Goodman LJ. The management of complex distal humerus nonunion in the elderly by elbow capsulectomy, triple plating, and ulnar nerve neurolysis. J Shoulder Elbow Surg 1992;1:37–46
13. McKee M, Jupiter J, Toh CL, Wilson L, Colton C, Karras KK. Reconstruction after malunion and nonunion of intra-articular fractures of the distal humerus. Methods and results in 13 adults. J Bone Joint Surg Br 1994;76: 614–621
14. Ring D, Gulotta L, Jupiter JB. Unstable nonunions of the distal part of the humerus. J Bone Joint Surg Am 2003;85: 1040–1046
15. Beredjiklian PK, Hotchkiss RN, Athanasian EA, Ramsey ML, Katz MA. Recalcitrant nonunion of the distal humerus. Treatment with free vascularized bone grafting. Clin Orthop Relat Res 2005;435:134–139

17 Nonunions and Malunions of Monteggia Fracture Dislocations

Peter Kloen and David C. Ring

Monteggia originally described a fracture of the ulna with dislocation of the proximal radioulnar joint.[1] His name is now applied to a variety of injuries that fit this definition. Bado placed numbers on the variations that had long been recognized: apex anterior fracture of the ulna with anterior dislocation of the radial head (type I), apex posterior fracture of the ulna with posterior dislocation of the radial head (type II), apex lateral fracture of the ulna with lateral dislocation of the radial head (type III), and diaphyseal fractures of both the radius and the ulna with proximal radioulnar dislocation (type IV).[1] Bado also introduced many "Monteggia variants," which are not very useful because they are not truly forearm fracture dislocations as the Monteggia originally defined them.[1]

The posterior Monteggia lesion has been the focus of some dispute in this regard because the fractures that are close to the ulnohumeral joint are associated with relatively limited displacement of the proximal radioulnar joint.[3] Jupiter and colleagues have emphasized that posterior Monteggia lesions occur on a spectrum from the diaphysis to intraarticular fractures.[4] Although the more proximal fractures have less obvious proximal radioulnar dislocation, the injuries have so many factors in common that it is useful to consider them together. This holds true for the consideration of malunion and nonunion as well.[5]

Patient Assessment

Malunions and nonunions of Monteggia injuries in adults (often older women) occur mainly with posterior (Bado type II) Monteggia lesions that have inadequate plate fixation leading to collapse of the fracture and either malunion or nonunion.[5]

In many cases, a plate has been applied to the medial or lateral surface of the ulna and only two or three screws have been placed in the proximal metaphyseal fragment (**Fig. 17–1A**).[5,6] Many of the patients are older women with osteoporosis. The proximal screws loosen resulting in recurrence of the apex posterior fracture deformity and posterior dislocation of the radial head from the radiocapitellar and proximal radioulnar joints (**Fig. 17–1B**). Patients often complain of pain and lack of supination. Associated factors that can challenge the treating physician are compromised soft tissues, osteopenia, failed hardware, and an already compromised ulnar nerve.

Physical Examination

The preoperative examination and documentation should include a detailed neurovascular examination, location of previous incision(s), and range of motion. The elbow should be scrutinized for signs of infection.

Radiographic Assessment

Standard radiographs in two planes provide generally enough data for preoperative planning. In cases of associated instability and/or suspicion of a coronoid fracture, a preoperative computed tomography (CT) scan is helpful (despite often-present hardware). The type of nonunion should be noted, whether oligotrophic, atrophic, or hypertrophic.

Laboratory Studies

Other than routine preoperative laboratory studies, no specific blood tests are needed. In case of (suspected) infection, a complete blood count including differential, an erythrocyte sedimentation rate and C-reactive protein can be determined. Aspiration of the nonunion site to determine evidence of infection can be considered, but is seldom done in our practice.

Treatment

Nonsurgical Treatment

Anterior Malunions

It is always reasonable to consider no treatment. Patients with anterior malunions often have good elbow mobility and limited pain, particularly children. Adults with anterior malunions often present after decades of good elbow function and it is sometimes unclear what finally brings them in. If they desire greater elbow flexion, this can often be accomplished with radial head resection.

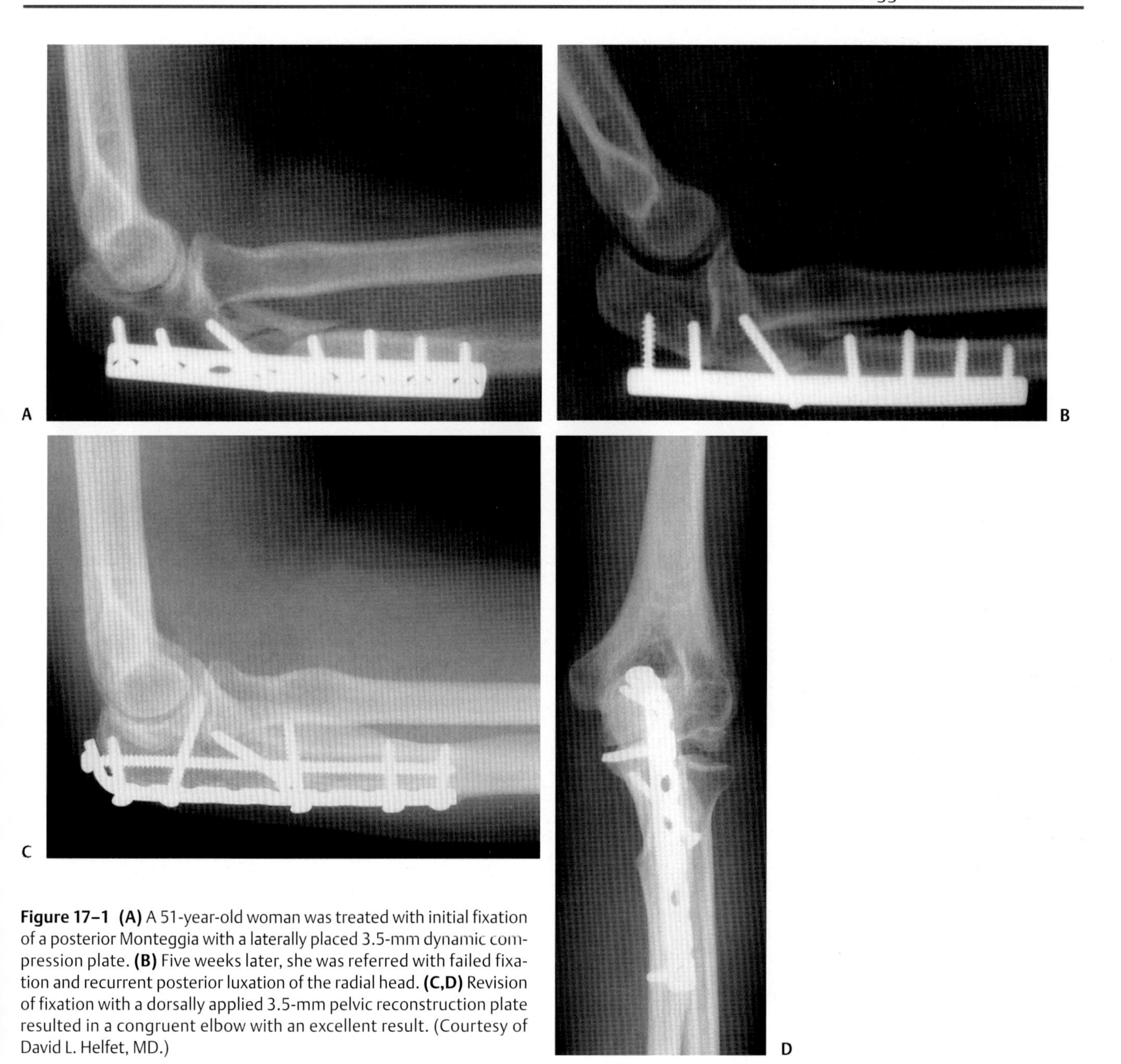

Figure 17–1 **(A)** A 51-year-old woman was treated with initial fixation of a posterior Monteggia with a laterally placed 3.5-mm dynamic compression plate. **(B)** Five weeks later, she was referred with failed fixation and recurrent posterior luxation of the radial head. **(C,D)** Revision of fixation with a dorsally applied 3.5-mm pelvic reconstruction plate resulted in a congruent elbow with an excellent result. (Courtesy of David L. Helfet, MD.)

Surgeries for pain or deformity are less satisfying and not recommended.

Posterior Malunion or Nonunion without Instability

Patients that are functioning well despite malunion can be managed nonoperatively. Pain and limitation of motion lead to operative intervention in most patients.[5] The ulna is either osteotomized or the nonunion débrided, a posterior contoured plate applied, bone graft used as needed, and the radial head is addressed as needed **(Fig. 17–1C,D)**.

Posterior Malunion or Nonunion with Instability

If there is subluxation or dislocation of the elbow concomitant with malunion or nonunion the situation is far more complex.[5,7] There may be a coronoid fracture of coronoid deficiency that needs to be addressed **(Fig. 17–2A)**. If inadequate fixation is obtained, instability will develop with subsequent failure of hardware **(Fig. 17–2B)**. The radial head must be repaired or replaced and the ligaments must be repaired. When treated at a subacute or chronic stage, these repairs will usually need to be protected with hinged external fixation.

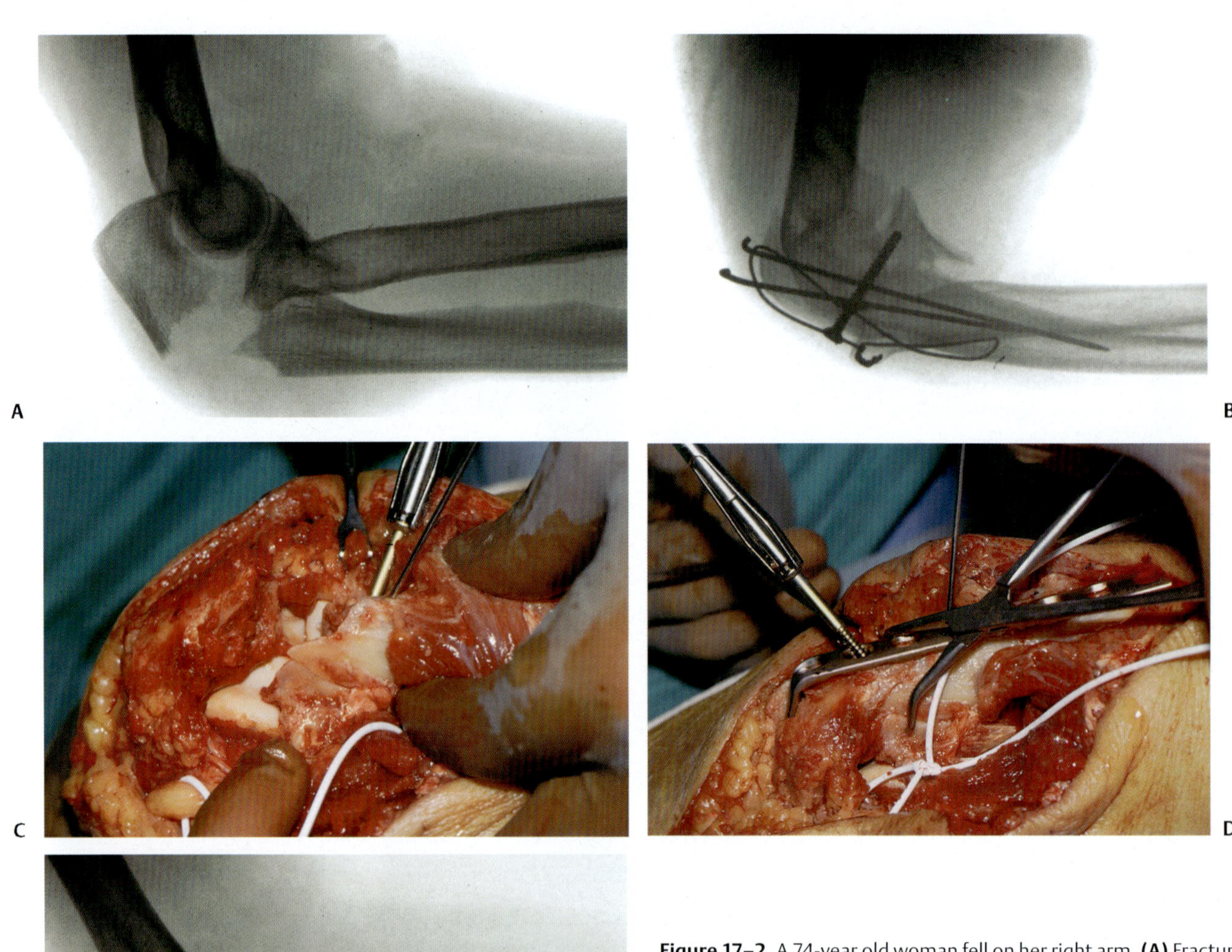

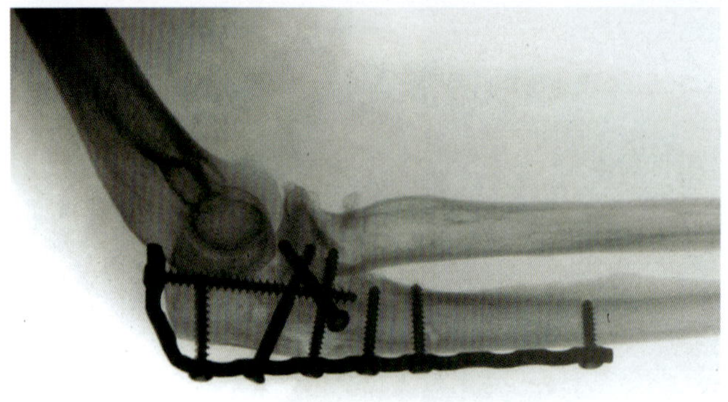

Figure 17–2 A 74-year old woman fell on her right arm. **(A)** Fractures of the radial, olecranon, and coronoid were seen. **(B)** Initial fixation was done with Kirschner wires and tension band and one lag screw into the coronoid fragment was insufficient. Two weeks after the initial surgery, a revision was done. **(C)** Via a posterior approach the shaft of the ulna was reduced to the large coronoid fragment and a lag screw was placed. **(D)** A contoured 3.5-mm dynamic compression plate was then contoured to curve around the olecranon tip. **(E)** The fracture healed with good alignment with a stable ulnohumeral articulation. A good functional result was obtained. (Courtesy of Jesse B. Jupiter, MD.)

Surgical Treatment

Posterior Malunion or Nonunion without Instability

If the ulnohumeral joint is concentrically reduced and stable, the situation is straightforward. In most patients the problem is identified prior to solid fracture healing. With the patient supine or in the lateral position, the arm is prepped and draped. We generally use a sterile tourniquet to increase the operative field. The iliac crest is prepped and draped as well if autogenous bone graft is needed. The prior incision is opened and extended proximally. Previous surgery around the elbow warrants a careful dissection to find the ulnar nerve first. The ulnar nerve is identified proximally and followed distally through Osborne's fascia. If ulnar nerve symptoms are present before the index procedure, an external neurolysis can be considered followed by an anterior subcutaneous or submuscular transposition. Prior loose internal fixation is then removed and the fracture site identified and mobilized either via osteotomy or by débriding the nonunion site of callus and fibrous tissue. Cultures are obtained after which time intravenous antibiotics are given (if the tourniquet is inflated at that time we generally give antibiotics immediately prior to releasing the tourniquet). After thorough débridement using drills, curettes, and rongeurs a temporary stabilization of the ulna is obtained with smooth Kirschner wires (K-wires). Next, a lateral interval between the anconeus and extensor carpi ulnaris, or more anteriorly between the extensor carpi radialis brevis and the extensor digitorum communis, is developed. The radiocapitellar proximal radioulnar joint is cleared to accept the relocated radial head. If the radial head is fractured and not salvageable, it should be excised. Consideration is given to replacing the radial head if there is any possibility of ulnohumeral instability.

The ulna is stabilized with a 3.5-mm limited contact dynamic compression (LCDC) plate or 3.5-mm locking compression (LC) plate applied to the dorsal surface of the proximal ulna and contoured to wrap around the olecranon process **(Fig. 17–2C)**. Recently, precontoured plates for the olecranon have become commercially available (Accumed, Beaverton, OR). The proximal contour increases the number of screws in the proximal fragment. In addition, the most proximal screws are orthogonal to the more distal screws, creating an interlocking construct. Distally the plate lies on the apex of the ulnar diaphysis and the interval between the extensor and flexor carpi ulnaris muscles is incised just enough to get the plate touching periosteum. If the fracture site had delayed healing, autogenous cancellous bone graft from the iliac crest or the tip of the olecranon is applied **(Fig. 17–2D,E)**.

Posterior Malunion or Nonunion with Instability

When instability is present, the coronoid, radial head, and collateral ligaments must be addressed. In subacute cases the coronoid can often be identified and repaired. The later one intervenes, the less likely this will be possible. Consideration can be given to reconstructing the coronoid with a fragment of the radial head of olecranon. Radiocapitellar contact should be preserved or restored. In most patients, this requires a metal radial head prosthesis. The lateral collateral ligament is reattached to the lateral epicondyle using suture anchors. The entire construct is protected with a hinged external fixator.

Complications

Posterior malunions and nonunions have been associated with loss of fixation, nonunion, continued instability, and arthrosis. Temporary ulnar neuropathy is often seen despite external neurolysis and/or anterior transposition.

Postoperative Rehabilitation

Patients are encouraged to do active-assisted exercises and use the arm for light daily activities within a few days of surgery. If the elbow is slow to mobilize, static progressive and dynamic splints may be used to assist with restoration of elbow mobility. Strengthening exercises are delayed until healing is established. Hinged external fixation is removed between 4 and 8 weeks after surgery.

Results

Nonunion/Malunion without Instability

We recently reviewed 17 patients with malalignment after surgical treatment of a posterior Monteggia fracture (Bado type II). Of these, 9 patients initially had a coronoid fracture. A radial head fracture was seen in 16 of 17 patients (seven Mason type II, nine Mason type III) including all of the 9 patients with a coronoid fracture. There was instability with either subluxation (9 patients) or dislocation (2 patients) of the ulnohumeral joint. All patients were treated according to the protocol as outlined above. Index surgery was performed at an average of 7 weeks (range: 1 to 16 weeks) after the injury. Posterior plating of the ulna was performed in all 17 patients. Bone graft was added in 5 patients. Treatment of the radial head evolved over time with the development of improved radial head prostheses and increased appreciation of its role in elbow stability. Because of ulnohumeral instability, 5 patients were treated with an external hinged fixator (Compass Hinge; Richards, Memphis, TN) as part of the reconstructive procedure. At the final follow up at 59 months (24 to 130 months) all ulnar fractures had united in good alignment with a stable ulnohumeral joint. Average ROM was 108 degrees (range: 75 to 135 degrees) with average flexion of 130 degrees (range: 100 to 150 degrees) and a flexion contracture of 22 degrees (range: 0 to 55 degrees). Pronation and supination averaged 70 degrees (range: 20 to 80 degrees) and 64 degrees (range: 10 to 80 degrees), respectively. Results were rated as excellent in 5, good for 9, fair for 2, and poor for 1 patient according to the system of Broberg and Morrey.[2]

Complications that were seen after the index procedure were failure of coronoid fixation (1 patient), recurrent radioulnar synostosis (1 patient), elbow dislocation necessitating adjustment of the hinged external fixator (1 patient), nonunion of the olecranon (1 patient) necessitating revision osteosynthesis and bone grafting, wound infection (1 patient, self-inflicted), and persistent ulnar nerve symptoms that needed submuscular nerve transposition (1 patient). Only 1 patient requested hardware removal of the ulnar plate.

Summary

Patients with malunited and nonunited Monteggia fractures often have restriction of forearm rotation, ulnohumeral instability, and incongruity of the elbow joint leading to arthrosis. Salvage of these malaligned Monteggia lesions can often be obtained by realignment of the ulna with a dorsally applied plate contouring around the tip of the olecranon. Patients with instability are more challenging and the result is determined by the status of the joint and other associated problems.

References

1. Bado JL. The Monteggia lesion. Clin Orthop Relat Res 1967;50:71–76
2. Broberg MA, Morrey BF. Results of delayed excision of the radial head after fracture. Bone Joint Surg Am 1986;68:669–674
3. Bruce HE, Harvey JP, Wilson JC. Monteggia fractures. J Bone Joint Surg Am 1974;56:1563–1576
4. Jupiter JB, Leibovic SJ, Ribbans W, Wilk RM. The posterior Monteggia lesion. J Orthop Trauma 1991; 5:395–402
5. Ring D, Kloen P, Tavakolian J, Helfet DL, Jupiter JB. Loss of alignment after operative treatment of posterior Monteggia fractures: salvage with dorsal contoured plating. J Hand Surg [Am] 2004;29:694–702
6. Ring D, Jupiter JB, Simpson NS. Monteggia fractures in adults. J Bone Joint Surg Am 1998;80:1733–1744
7. Ring D, Hannouche D, Jupiter JB. Surgical treatment of persistent dislocation or subluxation of the ulnohumeral joint after fracture-dislocation of the elbow. J Hand Surg [Am] 2004;29:470–480

18 Nonunions, Malunions, and Synostosis of Forearm Fractures

Diego L. Fernandez and Ladislav Nagy

The forearm should be considered as a joint consisting of two long bones and three ligamentous restraints: the annular ligament complex, the interosseous membrane (IOM), and the triangular fibrocartilage complex (TFCC). There are two articular components as well: the proximal (PRUJs) and distal radioulnar joints (DRUJs), which permit rotation of the radius on a relatively fixed ulnar axis.

If the forearm is now looked upon as a joint, diaphyseal fractures should be considered intraarticular and therefore deserve – as in any other fracture that disrupts an articular surface – accurate anatomic reduction to guarantee full restoration of function. This same principle should be taken into consideration for the surgical reconstruction of nonunited and malunited forearm fractures.

Although open reduction and compression plate fixation of forearm fractures invariably restores anatomy and function with a relatively low rate of complications,[1–5] surgical reconstruction of forearm nonunions and malunions represents a more difficult challenge in which despite achieving bony union, correcting deformity, and relieving pain, complete and symmetrical restoration of forearm rotation is difficult to obtain, but may be certainly improved to a reasonable functional arc of pronation and supination.

This is due to the frequent concomitant derangement of the PRUJS and DRUJs as well as the IOM commonly associated with the bony deformity of the nonunited or malunited forearm bones. In both scenarios, symmetric shortening of both bones may not alter the congruity of the PRUJ or the DRUJ, provided there is no significant associated angular deformity. Conversely, shortening of a single forearm bone with or without angular deformity will automatically affect the articular anatomic relationships of either the PRUJ or DRUJ. Loss of the physiological bow of the radius is responsible for limited pronation, whereas reduction of the interosseous space associated with angular or ad latus (translation) deformity leads to secondary contracture of the IOM and decreases forearm rotation.

Posttraumatic radioulnar synostosis is a less frequent complication, but its management, although currently well standardized, does not exclude recurrence in patients with special risk factors.

In this chapter, we describe the current principles of management of both simple and complex diaphyseal forearm nonunions and malunions in adults, and present treatment recommendations for both primary and recurrent radioulnar synostosis.

Diaphyseal Forearm Nonunion

Because cast treatment of displaced forearm fractures in adults is practically "past history," we are commonly confronted with nonunions following insufficient surgical stabilization with implants associated with extensive devascularization, infection, or extensive bone loss after high-energy injuries and open comminuted fractures. Occasionally, a well-vascularized nonunion may develop after a conservative trial of a minimally displaced forearm bone. These are treated with minimal decortication of the callus to provide a flat surface for the compression plate, and successful outcome is to be expected, provided that the construct is biomechanically sound.

Classification

The types of presentation of a forearm nonunion include the following combinations:

1. Radius or ulna alone without radioulnar joint disruption
2. Radius or ulna alone with associated radioulnar joint disruption
3. Nonunion of one forearm bone with malunion of the other
4. Both bone nonunions

Each of these may be further subgrouped according to Weber and Çech's classification[6] into

1. Vital or well-vascularized
   a. hypertrophic
   b. oligotrophic
2. Nonvital or avascular
   c. necrotic fragment
   d. comminuted necrotic area
   e. large defect
   f. atrophic

Finally, any of the above can be aggravated by infection, soft tissue defects, soft tissue contracture, neurovascular deficit, and stiffness of the neighboring joints (elbow and wrist).

Treatment

The goals of treatment must extend beyond obtaining bony union to ensure anatomic restoration of skeletal alignment and both congruity and stability of the PRUJs and DRUJs. Preoperative assessment should include a careful clinical examination of the whole upper extremity to document the residual forearm function and that of the neighboring joints, the soft tissue condition, and the neurovascular status. Laboratory studies including an electromyogram for nerve lesions or aspiration and cultures in infected cases are routinely performed. For the radiographic assessment, comparative x-rays of both forearms including the elbow and wrist joints are considered essential for the preoperative planning and correction of deformity or shortening associated with the nonunion. Most of the simple, straightforward cases do not need additional imaging. Computed tomography (CT) may be helpful to rule out the presence of sequestrae in infected cases, and assess rotatory deformity and congruity of the DRUJ. Magnetic resonance imaging is reserved to evaluate additional soft tissue lesions such as the TFCC, the IOM, and muscle defects. Arteriograms are useful to document the patency of the vascular axes in nonunions following severe high-energy trauma, particularly when planning microvascular reconstruction of large bony defects.

Surgical Treatment

General Principles

Disregarding the localization of the forearm nonunion, hypertrophic well-vascularized nonunions are managed with decortication of the callus and stable plate fixation, whereas atrophic nonunions need rigid fixation and autologous bone grafting. These principles of nonunion management advocated by Müller[7] and Weber and Çech[6] over 40 years ago have stood the test of time and are associated with a high success rate.

Small diaphyseal defects may be bridged with a structural corticocancellous iliac graft, fixed to the plate. In larger diaphyseal bone defects up to 10 cm, in which a circumferential well-vascularized soft tissue bed is present, long bridging plates and morcellized iliac bone grafts are the procedure of choice because diaphyseal stability and skeletal continuity, length, and alignment are readily achieved along with rapid functional recovery.[8]

Vascularized bone grafts are reserved for those situations of large defects in which conventional bone grafting procedures have failed and in those cases with poor vascularized bed and massive scarring as in chronically infected cases or in situations with composite soft tissue and skeletal defects following mutilating injuries.[9,10]

Creation of a one-bone forearm for the treatment of large diaphyseal defects (most commonly in the ulna) is a valid alternative,[11–13] but skeletal continuity is restored at the expense of loss of forearm rotation. For this reason this modality remains, in our view, the ultimate salvage procedure. Other valid alternatives of nonunion management such as electrical stimulation,[14,15] the use of bone morphogenic protein,[16,17] or the use of the Ilizarov technique[18] will not be discussed because we do not routinely use these options.

Tactics

Approaches

Our preferred surgical exposure for the radius is the extensile approach described by Henry,[19] in which the whole bone from the radial head to the wrist joint can be exposed medially to the brachioradialis on the volar aspect of the forearm. In the proximal third the major advantage is that both the deep and superficial branches of the radial nerve can be protected as the supinator muscle is detached from the proximal shaft. Extension of the incision proximally to the elbow flexion crease further permits exposure of the anterior capsule of the elbow joint, particularly the lateral compartment and the PRUJ. In the midshaft area the insertion of the pronator teres is well visualized, and the insertion of the central part of the IOM can be exposed at this level. In the distal point the radius may be widely exposed partially elevating the insertion of the flexor pollicis longus muscle and further distally the pronator quadratus.

The whole of the ulna is exposed with a longitudinal incision over its subcutaneous border between the extensor and flexor carpi ulnaris (FCU) muscles. If exposure of the DRUJ is needed, the incision may be extended distally by swinging it dorsally over the ulnar head at the neck level ending at the junction of the fourth and fifth carpometacarpal joints. In this manner the superficial branch of the ulnar nerve remains safely in the medial subcutaneous flap. The PRUJ is exposed through a posterolateral approach between the anconeus and extensor carpi ulnaris. (ECU) If scars of previous surgery are present, usually these are utilized to avoid additional soft tissue disruption and iatrogenic devascularization.

Preparation, Reduction, Fixation, and Bone Grafting

Hypertrophic nonunions require minimal exposure of the nonunion site to preserve the well-vascularized a callus on both fragments. Limited decortication at the surface of plate application is all that is needed. Because these nonunions are generally elastic, the associated deformity is usually corrected by carefully molding the plate to the normal anatomy of the shaft segment. The plate is securely fixed to the proximal fragment and deformity correction is gradually obtained with strategic use of the compression device and bone clamps applied to the distal fragment. This works very nicely when the plate comes to lie on the convexity of the angulation, acting as a tension band implant. If the convexity of the angulation faces the opposite bone reducing the interosseous space, associated IOM release is mandatory. The prebent plate is then fixed in a bridging mode to which one screw is inserted in the most proximal and one in the most distal plate hole. Thereafter using Verbrugge bone clamps the ununited bone ends are approximated to the plate, thus recreating the interosseous space.[6] Following reduction, axial compression can be achieved with eccentric introduction of screws of a dynamic compression (DC) plate. Molding of the plate with the appropriate curvature is particularly important in the midshaft area of the radius, whereas less plate bending is needed in the proximal and distal thirds. For the ulna, being practically a straight long bone, a slight bend at the nonunion site is helpful to obtain compression at the opposite cortex as in acute fracture fixation.

Atrophic nonunions require a more careful preparation of the site including resection of necrotic areas to bleeding bone, as well as devitalized intermediate fragments. The obliterated medullary canal on both ends is routinely opened with an awl or a drill bit that accommodates to its diameter. Although relatively small defects created after débridement of a bone forearm nonunion may be stabilized with plates creating a symmetric skeletal shortening, whenever possible we prefer to maintain length using bridging plates and interpositional bone grafting. This is particularly important in the treatment of large defects of one bone, while the opposite bone is intact.

If the radius presents with a pseudoarthrotic defect, there is severe radial deviation and shortening of the distal fragment, as well as disruption of the DRUJ with a positive ulnar variance, which equals the amount of radial shortening (**Fig. 18–1**). A pronatory rotational deformity is frequently present as well as palmar displacement of the distal fragment.

Because these chronic nonunions are invariably associated with soft tissue contracture, restoration of length and realignment of the DRUJ can be obtained with a combination of soft tissue release and intraoperative temporary distraction. Soft tissue release includes resection of

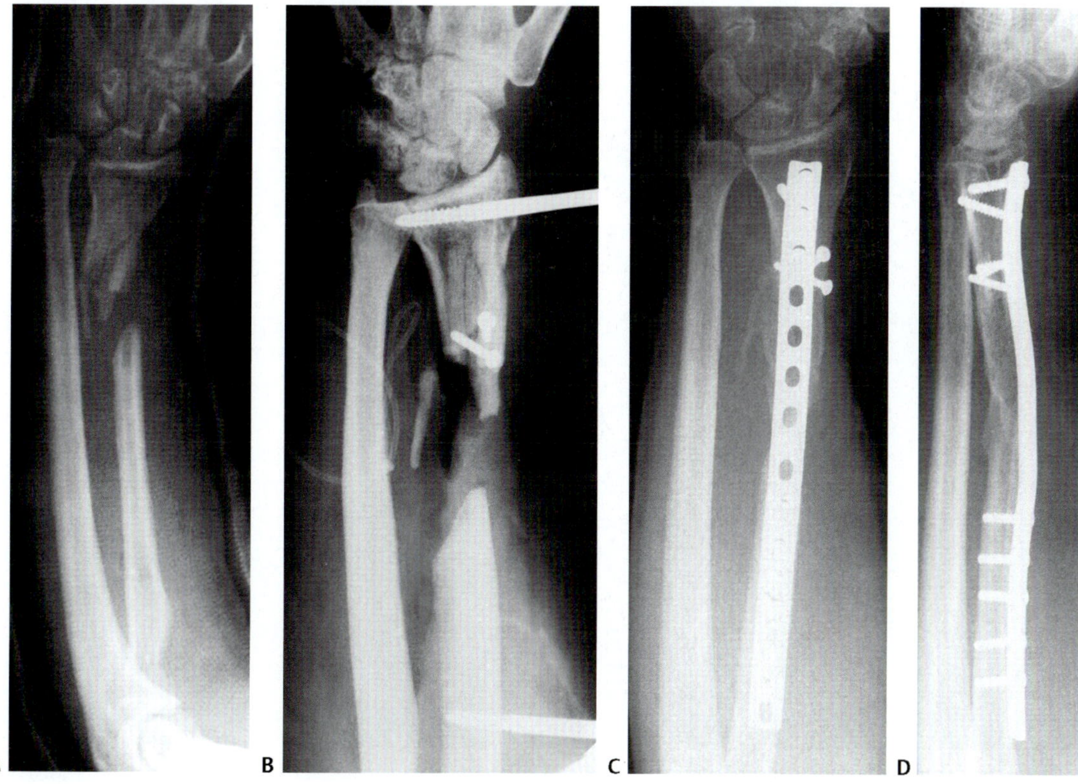

Figure 18–1 (A,B) Large defect nonunion of the distal third of the radius. Notice distal radioulnar joint disruptions, severe shortening, and radial deviation of the distal fragment. Middle: Intraoperative roentgenograms with the distractor in place. Notice realignment of the distal radioulnar joint. **(C,D)** Radiographs at 12 months following volar bridge plating and autologous morcellized iliac crest cancellous bone grafting. Notice cortical remodeling of the interposed graft.

scarred nonviable tissue surrounding the nonunion area, detachment and partial resection of the contracted IOM, and subperiosteal detachment of the brachioradialis tendon from the distal radius. If severe contracture of the DRUJ is present, release of the pronator quadratus and resection of the volar DRUJ capsule are recommended.

Intraoperative progressive distraction of the nonunion is achieved with the use of the AO femoral distractor,[20] placing one 4.5-mm Schanz pin into each radial fragment. Distraction should be performed slowly over a period of 30 minutes **(Fig. 18–1)**. Visual control of the median nerve to avoid excessive sudden tension is important, although one stage restoration of posttraumatic skeletal shortening up to 2.5 to 3 cm is usually not associated with neurapraxia. However, this may occur if the peripheral nerve is tethered and adherent to scarred tissue. Therefore, inspection of the nerve and neurolysis should be performed accordingly. Realignment of the DRUJ is assessed with fluoroscopy, and passive forearm rotation is controlled at this point. If reduction of the DRUJ is not obtained despite distraction, a shortening osteotomy of the ulna may be performed simultaneously or delayed to a later date. If severe incongruity of the joint is present with secondary degenerative changes, prosthetic replacement is advocated. We no longer perform distal ulna resections because loss of the ulnar head invariably leads to radioulnar convergence and painful instability of the ulnar stump.[21]

While the distractor maintains alignment, the premolded plate is applied in a bridging fashion. Although most forearm nonunions are stabilized with 3.5 limited-contact dynamic compression (LCDC) plates with a minimum of 6 to 8 cortices for screw fixation on each fragment, the 4.5 narrow DC plate may be recommended as a stronger implant to bridge large defects. Locking plates with angular stability may be also used, especially in osteoporotic bone. Augmentation of screw holding power with bone cement is still a valid alternative to increase stability of plate fixation in such situations.

The defect is then grafted with morcellized autologous bone grafts, taking care not to place them close to the IOM. If a soft tissue defect is present in this area, Gelfoam (Pfizer, New York, NY) is applied as a barrier to obliterate the dead space to reduce the danger of radioulnar synostosis. For smaller defects up to 3 cm, a corticocancellous strut graft may be interposed and fixed with screws to the plate **(Fig. 18–2)**. The cortical border of the graft is placed

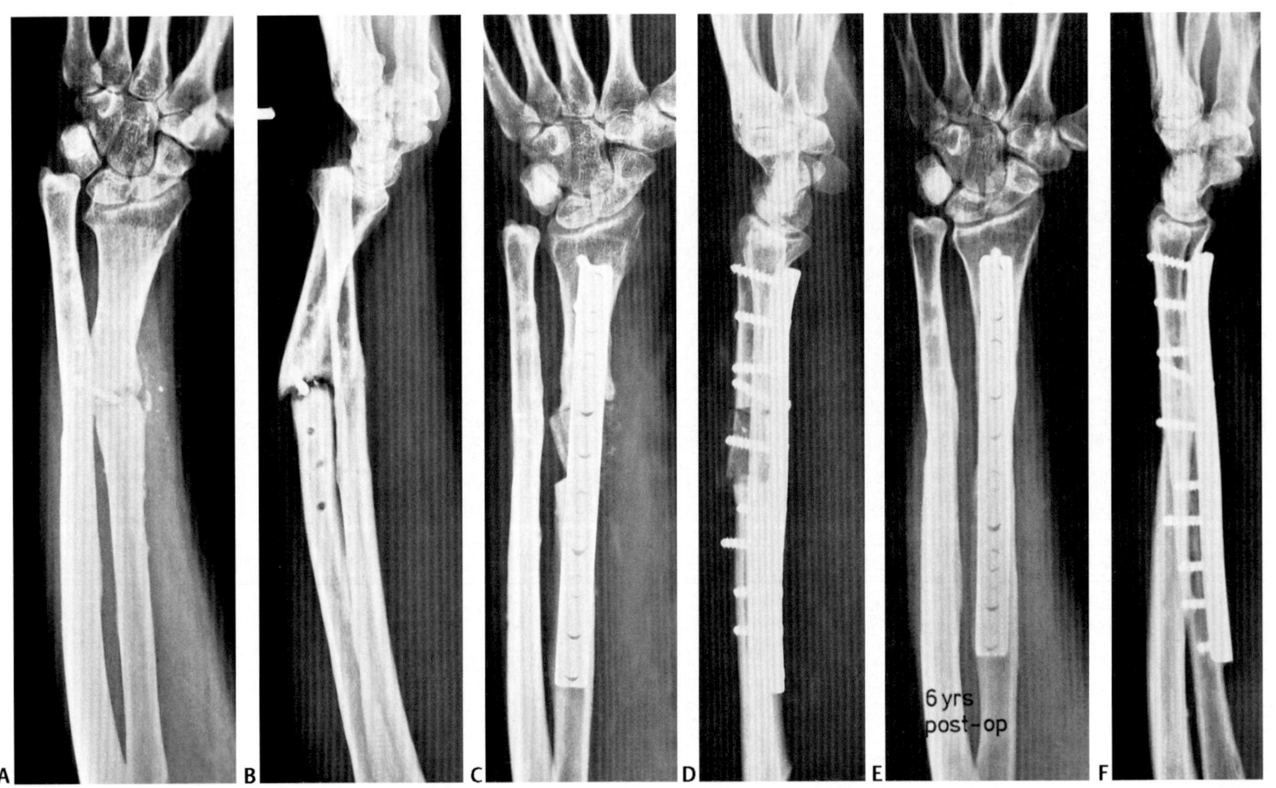

Figure 18–2 **(A,B)** Oligotrophic nonunion of the radial shaft following insufficient internal fixation of an Galeazzi fracture and early removal of the plate. Notice severe palmar angulation, shortening, and complete disruption of the distal radioulnar joint. **(C,D)** Following débridement of the necrotic bone ends, the nonunion was realigned and stabilized with a 3.5 dynamic compression plate; the 3-cm defect was filled with a corticocancellous structural iliac graft fixed to the plate with one screw. **(E,F)** Radiographs 6 years after the operation. Notice full remodeling of the graft and restoration of the interosseous space. The patient regained full pronation and supination of her left forearm.

opposite to the plate surface while the cancellous surface lies on the plate.[22] Morcellized cancellous grafts are additionally placed in the proximal and distal junctions of the construct.

Restoration of length in smaller defects is achieved by fixing the plate with screws to the distal fragment and applying the articulating tension device in distraction mode on the proximal end of the plate. This device permits a maximal excursion of 40 mm. Alternatively, for shorter distances and absence of soft tissue contractures a laminar spreader applied between the plate and a separate cortical screw can be used.[23,24]

A less common scenario is the nonunited ulna with a large defect and an intact radius. According to the shortening and angulation, a concomitant dislocation of the radial head may be present. Similar tactical steps as described for the radius are recommended. In longstanding cases, an open reduction of the radial head and annular ligament reconstruction may become necessary. If degenerative cartilage changes are present, prosthetic replacement of the radial head is preferred to resection, to obviate late proximal radius migration and secondary disruption of the DRUJ.

Infected Nonunions

If the nonunion presents with a draining sinus and active infection, an aggressive débridement; removal of implants, external fixation, temporary irrigation-suction; and a prolonged course of parenteral antibiotics are performed as the first stage of the treatment. Sequential débridements and repeat cultures may become necessary in cases where the inflammatory signs persist. Definitive reconstruction as described for the atrophic nonunion with large defects is indicated as soon as both the clinical and laboratory parameters of active infection have normalized. It must be kept in mind, that revascularization of free morcellized cancellous graft is directly dependent on the vascularity of the soft tissue envelope. If the soft tissues surrounding a chronic infected nonunion reveal massive scarring, are devitalized, or are associated with loss of muscle substance microvascular free tissue transfer is advisable **(Fig. 18–3)**. The most commonly used graft is an osteocutaneous fibular graft pedicled on the peroneal vessels.[25,26] The composite graft is placed into the defect having the peroneal vessels in an appropriate position for an optimal anastomosis to the radial or ulnar recipient vessels according to the particular scenario. To minimize instability and prevent delayed union, the graft junctions are stabilized to the recipient bone ends with plate or screw fixation or a combination of both. The cutaneous portion of the graft is sutured into the overlying soft tissue defect.

Postoperative Rehabilitation

Except in those cases where maximal implant stability cannot be achieved such as in patients with severe osteoporosis or in the free fibular grafts in which additional initial cast or removable splints are indicated, functional after-treatment with early range of motion (ROM) exercises of the forearm and neighboring joints are permitted. Forceful passive physiotherapy measures or dynamic splints to restore pronation and supination should be used with caution in the first 3 months following surgery. Thereafter, strengthening exercises and progressive loading is allowed as soon as radiographic signs of bony healing and incorporation of the grafts are present.

Results and Complications

The results reported in recent articles in which the above-mentioned techniques were used are highly satisfactory. Barbieri et al[22] obtained union in 10 out of 12 cases treated with structural corticocancellous grafts in an average of 4 months. Ring and coworkers[8] obtained complete union in 35 patients with an average defect of 2.2 cm (range: 1 to 6 cm) in an average time of 6 months. Jupiter et al[27] reported the use of vascularized fibular grafts for segmental defects of the radius averaging 7.9 cm. Eight out of 9 patients treated (6 of whom had chronic osseous infection) presented radiographic union at both the proximal and distal junctions of the graft. The functional results were satisfactory and 6 out of 9 patients had returned to their preinjury occupation. Safoury[28] recently reported 18 infected nonunions and segmental defects of the forearm treated with vascularized fibular grafts. In this series, all nonunions healed with resolution of infection in an average time of 4 months.

Although the overall reported rate of complications in the articles reviewed is relatively low, the most common problems requiring subsequent surgery were the DRUJ (Darrach resections), failure to obtain union, persistence or reactivation of infection, and very seldom creation of an "iatrogenic" radioulnar synostosis. The functional outcome is undoubtedly multifactorial. Better results with a balanced arc of functional forearm rotation are usually observed in those patients with anatomic realignment of the forearm bones and radioulnar congruity. If the soft tissue and muscle envelope is contracted and scarred or suffered segmental loss as in sequelae of high-energy trauma or chronic infection, function will be limited despite restoration of skeletal stability. Affectation of the neighboring joints with residual stiffness will also influence the functional outcome. Revascularization of autologous cancellous or corticocancellous bone grafts require a well-vascularized soft tissue envelope along with environmental stability provided by

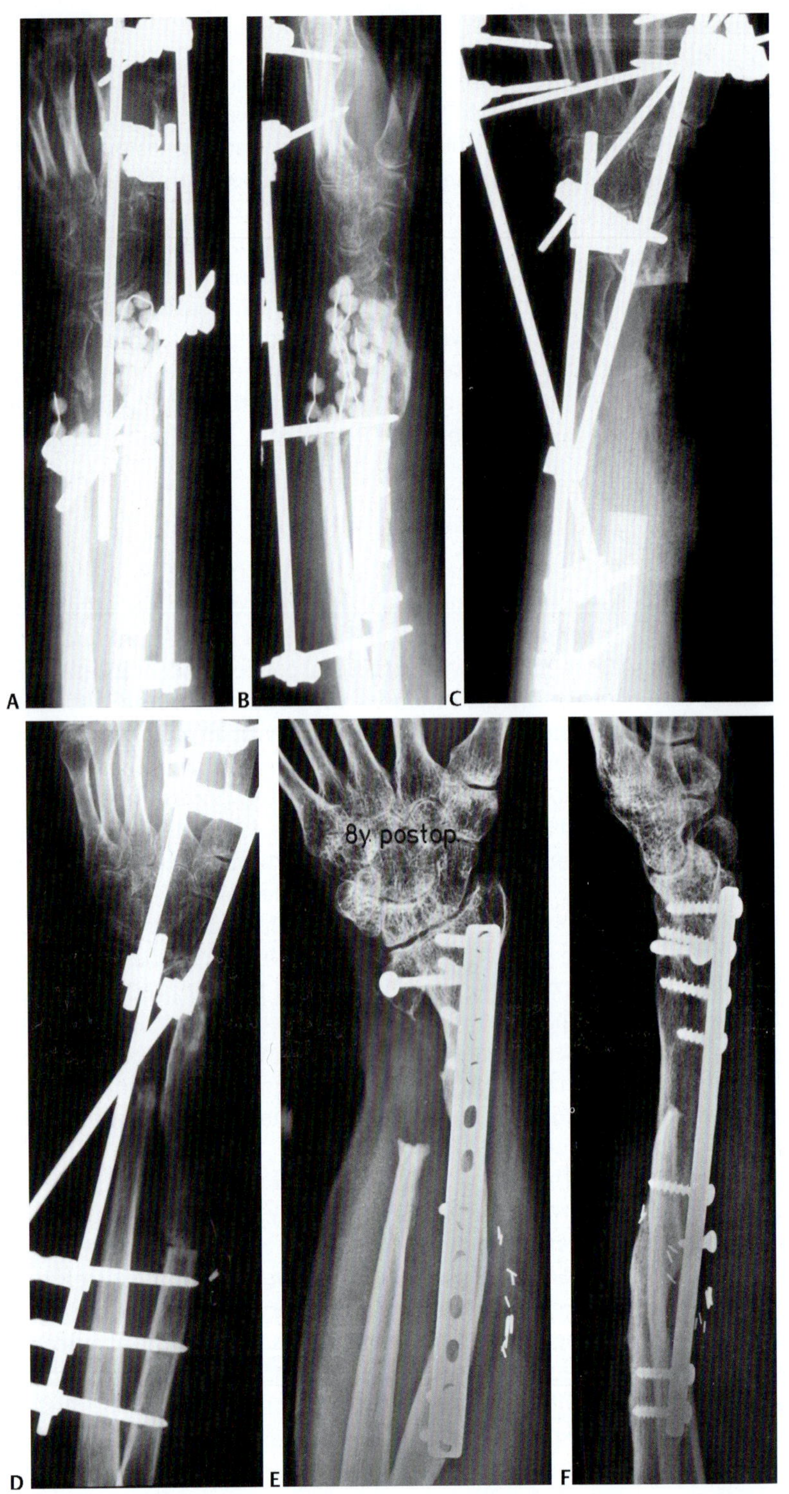

Figure 18–3 (A,B) Radiographs of an infected nonunion of the distal third of the radius following an open complex comminuted fracture. The radiographs demonstrate the presence of PMMA gentamicin beads and a diaphyseal radius plate after repeated débridements for a period of 10 months. Notice massive disuse atrophy of the carpus. **(C,D)** Following radical débridement and partial diaphysectomy, the defect was bridged with an iliac crest vascularized bone graft pedicled on the deep iliac circumflex artery and veins. Definite volar plate fixation through a Henry approach and a Sauvé–Kapandji procedure (undertaken because of the segmental loss of the distal third of the ulna) were performed 4 weeks after the microvascular reconstruction. At the same time the external fixator was removed. **(E,F)** Radiographs 8 years following reconstruction reveal a solid remodeling of the interposed vascularized graft. The patient regained a functional but limited arc of forearm rotation, adequate strength. There was no recurrence of the infection.

rigid plate fixation. Although revascularization and incorporation of morcellized grafts is faster, remodeling into a "cortical-like" structure takes a longer time. However, successful long-term results have been recently reported using this technique for atrophic nonunions of the femur[29,30] and humerus.[31] The advantage of the use of "pressure resistant corticocancellous bone blocks," as suggested by Weber and Çech,[6] is the immediate reconstruction of the loading capacity of the cortical part of the graft opposite to the plate. If corticocancellous blocks are used, screw fixation to the plate is mandatory to reduce micromotion to a minimum and enhance undisturbed revascularization. His recommendation for this grafting modality was, however, for defects of not more than 3 cm.

Union and incorporation of the grafts are directly dependent on the length of the defect, the vascularity of the recipient ends, the local perfusion of the soft tissues, the mechanical stability, and the absence of infection. These prerequisites should be carefully assessed to decide whether or not to use a vascularized bone graft.

Malunion of the Forearm Bones

Diaphyseal malunion in adults results after insufficient reduction following conservative or operative treatment, or may present as an iatrogenic deformity after attempted osteotomies. The deformity may include one or both bones of the forearm. Treatment goals in the care of forearm fractures are bone healing and restoration of function. Bone union of the forearm shaft in a nonanatomic position impairs motion of the wrist, especially the rotation of the forearm. This may present as restriction of motion, clicking, pain, and giving-way during forearm rotation (instability), or as a cosmetic problem. All of these complications can be avoided by correcting all components of the deformity: discrepancies in length, angulation, and rotation. Complex three-dimensional (3D) features of the bony architecture such as the bowing of the radius are equally important, thus its reconstruction must be considered as well. This is easily accomplished during initial fracture treatment, but once the bone has healed in malalignment, the chances for spontaneous correction are only realistic in early childhood. In children older than 10 years and adults, only a corrective osteotomy can reestablish normal bony architecture of the forearm bones. This together with the appropriate soft tissue release will reduce restriction of forearm rotation; with congruency of the radioulnar joints the stability will be restored as well. For the planning of the surgical correction the opposite healthy forearm is used, as there are no generally valid normative values. Additionally, 3D templates may be utilized. Our clinical experience with this preoperative assessment has been positive.

Potential for Spontaneous Correction during Growth

The immature skeleton has a considerable potential to spontaneously correct residual deformities, that is, angulations after fractures.[32–35] The amount of correction is defined by multiple factors as, for example, the distance between fracture and physis/growth plate, residual growth time until maturity, and, of course, the amount of angulation.[32,36,37] Deformities in the vicinity of highly active growth plates have a better prognosis, as their growth arrest will arrive substantially later in comparison to less-active physical plates.[38–42] Consequently, the lowest corrective potential is in the diaphysis.

Several authors[43–45] have observed residual deformity following diaphyseal fractures in children. After the age of 10, a complete correction of diaphyseal malunions during growth could not be observed either in boys or in girls.[43] It was concluded that only an angulation of up to 10 degrees, ad latus deformity of 100%, and rotational malalignment up to 45 degrees should be accepted.[44,45] A separate entity is the plastic deformation of the forearm.[46,47] It usually occurs in the intact forearm bone associated with a fracture of the other.

To avoid symptomatic malunion, unnecessary manipulations, as well as operative interventions, it is extremely important to be aware of the evident, but limited potential for spontaneous correction during growth.[48]

Pathomechanics and Clinical Correlation of Posttraumatic Forearm Deformity

Kinematics of Forearm Rotation in Forearm Malunions

The forearm bones with the PRUJs and the DRUJs and the rotational axis connecting the centers of these two have been looked upon as one single bicondylar joint.[48] The impact of the malalignment of the forearm bones on rotation of the forearm has been demonstrated by multiple experimental osteotomies on cadaver forearms.[49–53] A correlation between the amount of angulation and the restriction of prosupination was found. Deformities in the distal third of the forearm had more impact on pronation than in the middle and proximal thirds.[49] Angulations in the middle third of one or both forearm bones up to 10 degrees do not interfere with prosupination. Deformities of 20 degrees restricted forearm rotation by at least 30%.[51] However, a malalignment of more than 20 degrees resulted in a severe deformity,[51] or was impossible to create due to excessive tension in the intact IOM.[49] The same held true for the creation of ulnar deviation of the ulna more than 10 degrees. Rotational deformities shift and decrease the prosupination sector[54]; hence, supination deformity of the radius was associated with a more significant reduction of prosupination than a pronational deformity, especially when exceeding 50 degrees or in the presence of combined rotatory malalignment of both bones.[55]

Associated Derangement of the Radioulnar Joints

Diaphyseal Deformity and Instability of the Distal Radioulnar Joint

Multiple experimental investigations have demonstrated that the stability of the DRUJ is maintained by the 3D anatomy of the forearm bones, the joint capsule,[56] musculotendinous structures,[57,58] and ligaments,[59] including the IOM.[60] Instability can occur following malunion – angulation, rotation, and length discrepancy of one or both forearm bones.[61–63] Thus, it remains unclear whether the ligamentous stabilizers are affected by the same insult and do not heal, or if left intact, undergo gradual stretching and deterioration over time because of undue continuous tension. In fresh lesions of the TFCC, anatomical fracture reduction and stable fixation will generally avoid later instability of the DRUJ, suggesting spontaneous healing of the ligamentous structures, that is of the TFCC. If however fracture healing occurs in nonanatomical shape with subsequent deformity, instability, subluxation, or frank dislocation with incompetence of the TFCC can occur.[64] Angular rotatory malunion may cause recurrent subluxation and dislocation; length discrepancy following shortening of the radius will result in ulnocarpal impaction syndrome.[64]

Palmar subluxation of the distal ulna is associated with dorsally angulated diaphyseal malunions. Conversely, malreduced Galeazzi fractures with persistent palmar angulation and pronatory rotational malalignment will present with a chronically dorsally displaced distal ulna and complete loss of active supination. If the ligaments withstand the initial trauma as well as the following micro-trauma and stretch, a limitation of ROM without instability will result.

Affectation of the Proximal Radioulnar Joint

Chronic dislocation of the radial head can be the result of old unreduced Monteggia fractures with persistent angulation of the ulna or because of malunions with length discrepancy between the radius and the ulna. Angulated metaphyseal malunions of the proximal radius lead to significant incongruity of the radial head in the sigmoid notch and result in severe limitation of pronation. Usually, there is valgus malalignment of the proximal radius that results in lateral subluxation of the radial head creating a substantial incongruity of both the PRUJ and the radiocapitellar joint. The diaphyseal fragment proximal to the insertion of the pronator teres is usually supinated by the biceps and supinator muscles; therefore, a supination rotatory malalignment also contributes to the pronatory loss.

Finally, more complex proximal forearm fracture patterns with associated articular disruption of the radial head as in high-energy multifragmentary fractures may develop massive rotatory forearm contracture due to posttraumatic degenerative changes in the PRUJ and severe soft tissue contracture including the IOM (**Fig. 18–4**).

Interosseous Membrane

The IOM and especially its strongest/stiffest part, the central band, contributes to the longitudinal stability of the forearm,[65,66] the dorsal oblique bundle stabilizes the PRUJ, and the distal membranous part is an adjunct stabilizer of the distal radial joint,[67] but clearly it is less important than the radioulnar ligaments.[68,69]

In experimental malunions, the intact IOM prevented the creation of extreme deformities[18] and its increasing tension limited the rotational motion.[51,70] With regard to physiologic tension, the experimental data are confusing. The interbone distance appeared longest in neutral position and shortest in maximal pronation.[70] Tension was indeed found to be highest in a neutral position, but decreased with rotation to both sides.[71] Other authors[65,66] have shown that the longitudinal stiffness of the IOM was highest in supination and lowest in pronation.

On the other hand, the IOM can become contracted. In paralytic conditions apparently this contracture can result in limited forearm rotation. According to Zancolli,[72] supination contractures due to contracture of the IOM occur secondarily and develop progressively, following lesions of the brachial plexus, poliomyelitis, or tetraplegia. In these cases, surgical sectioning of the IOM did not entail instability of the forearm or the DRUJ, as long as the method was applied to patients with an intact and stable PRUJ. There is clinical evidence that contracture of the IOM occurs in posttraumatic conditions as well; therefore, release of the IOM has been applied in the treatment of limited forearm rotation in posttraumatic cases or malunion along with corrective osteotomy.

Corrective Osteotomy of the Forearm Bones

Our literature review has shown that, to date, only Trousdale and Linscheid[53] have reported on the results of corrective osteotomies for malunited shaft fractures of the forearm. There were 27 patients, 20 had diminished forearm rotation, 6 patients had instability of the DRUJ, and 1 had a purely cosmetic problem. In the first group, 9 patients treated within 12 months after the initial injury

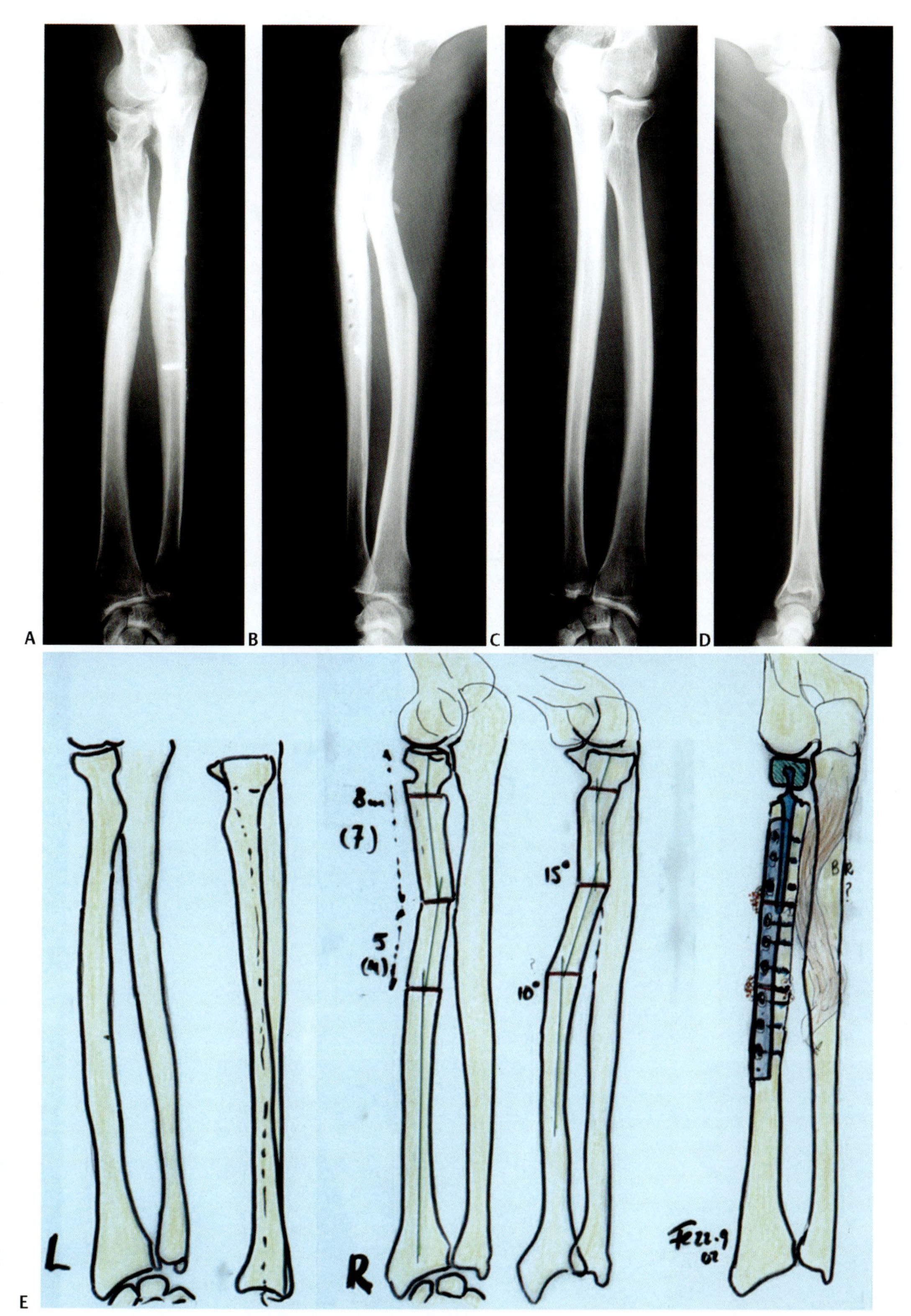

Figure 18–4 **(A,B)** Complex "double angled" proximal diaphyseal malunion of the radius associated with an intraarticular fracture of the radial head and post traumatic incongruity. Notice substantial narrowing of the interosseous space. Forearm rotation was blocked in 10 degrees of pronation, and the patient had lateral elbow pain due to the posttraumatic arthritic changes of the radiocapitellar joint. **(C,D)** Comparative x-rays of the left forearm for preoperative planning. **(E)** Physician's sketch. Restoration of the radial anatomy has been planned with a double radial osteotomy bridged with a long narrow dynamic compression plate associated with prosthetic replacement of the radial head. The operation was performed through the proximal part of the Henry approach with anterior exposure of the radiocapitellar joint through the same incision.

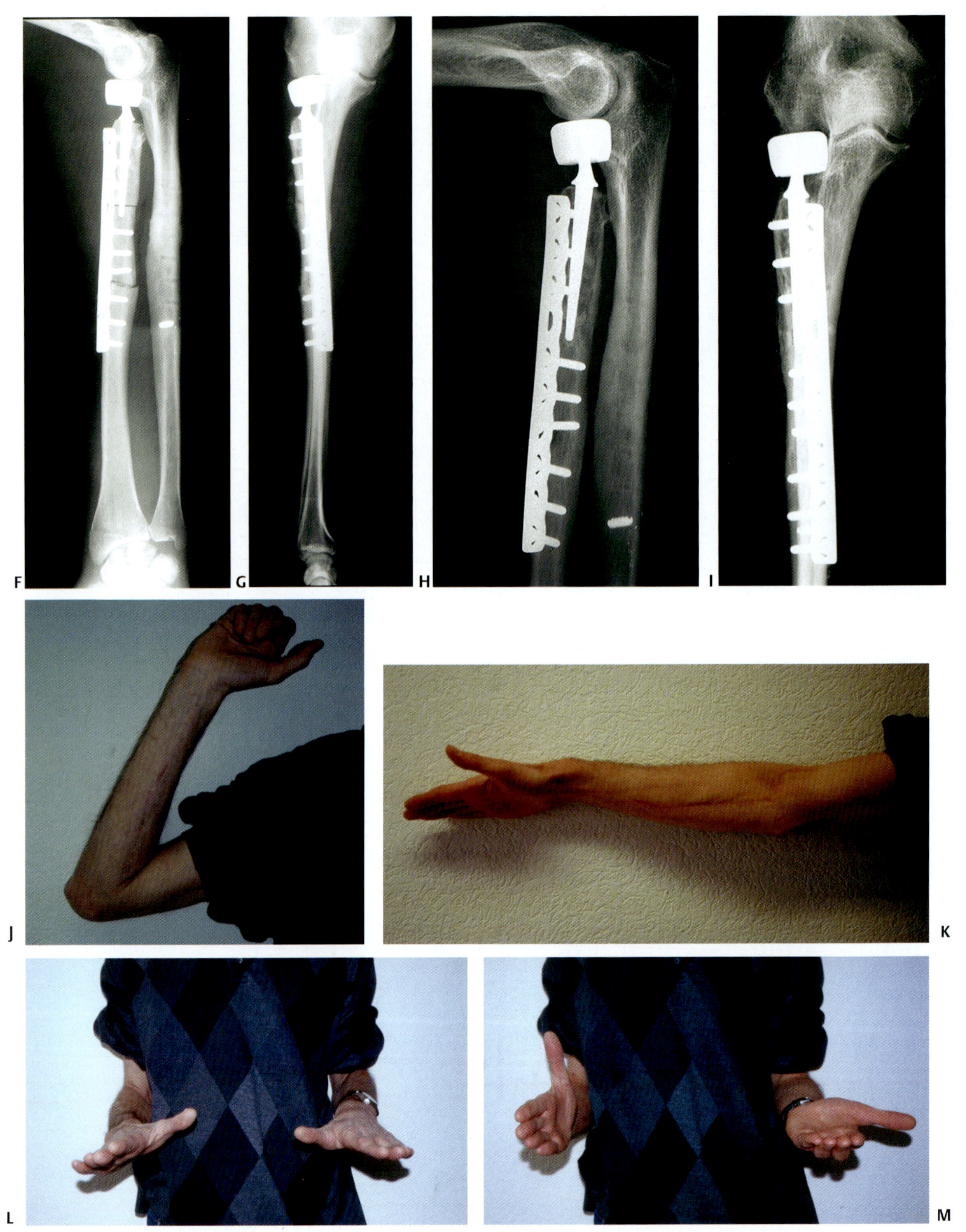

Figure 18–4 *(Continued)* **(F,G)** Immediate postoperative x-rays show adequate realignment of the proximal radial shaft and a well-aligned cemented Judet bipolar prosthesis. **(H,I)** Uneventful healing of both osteotomies and a stable radial head prosthesis 3 years after surgery. **(J–M)** The functional result showed an adequate restoration of elbow motion. Pronation was improved from 10 to 60 degrees while supination was only improved 10 degrees.

gained 79 degrees of rotation on average after the osteotomy, whereas 11 patients treated with a delay longer than 12 months gained only 30 degrees on average. Out of the 6 patients who were operated on for an unstable DRUJ, 3 patients obtained a pain-free, stable wrist, but lost 7 degrees of rotation on average. The patient who was managed for a deformity alone lost 10 degrees of rotation.

In our own retrospective cohort study, 17 patients were divided into three groups according to the clinical problem and presentation of the deformity: limitation of pronation, limitation of supination, and patients with DRUJ instability. These patients underwent 28 corrective osteotomies (mostly radius and ulna). The goal of the osteotomies was to reproduce exactly the geometry of the opposite healthy forearm bones. In 9 patients, the IOM was released. The healing was uneventful in all cases, no complications, infections, fractures, or synostoses occurred. Sixteen out of 17 patients reported subjective improvement, the last patient needed a repeat osteotomy for residual symptomatic deformity and improved finally as well. Patients with restricted supination gained more motion and improved better than those with limited pronation. DRUJ instability was eliminated in all respective cases. IOM release did not result in loss of strength or stability. These results have been confirmed furthering an additional 10 cases.

Osteotomy Types

For simple shortening osteotomies or derotation a transverse osteotomy is preferred. Shortening of the proximal radius is indicated in cases with ulnar shortening and chronic dislocation of the radial head. Both the radial shortening and open reduction of the radial head can be performed through the Henry approach extending the exposure to the anterior aspect of the elbow capsule. Ulnar shortening is useful for DRUJ impaction syndrome secondary to radial shortening. Occasionally, a short oblique osteotomy is useful to regain length of maximally 5 to 10 mm. For complex angular deformities, multiplanar osteotomies are recommended. These include closing wedge osteotomies with one plane of the cut perpendicular to the long axis to permit derotation. Opening wedge osteotomies require additional bone grafting, except in children, in which rapid periosteal bone healing fills the bony defect. Severe deformity with massive soft tissue contracture is better addressed with distraction/osteogenesis techniques.

Authors' Recommended Treatment

The preoperative planning relies upon the opposite healthy side, as the correctional osteotomy intends to reproduce the osseous geometry of the normal side as it were a template. Therefore, conventional radiographs of both forearms including the neighboring joints in full length are taken, with special attention to obtain exact anteroposterior (AP) and exact lateral projection of either the radius or the ulna. This may be difficult, especially when the limitation of forearm rotation does not allow neutral rotation. In these cases, the correct position for exposure must be determined under the image intensifier. Moreover, it may be necessary to produce individual exposures for the radius and the ulna in both AP and lateral projection – four films for one forearm. For exact orientation of the radius the distal epiphysis is considered, whereas for the ulna the humeroulnar joint is used.

The contours of the healthy and deformed bones in both projections are drawn on separate sheets of tracing paper. By simple superposition of the respective drawings the location of maximal deformity can be determined as well as the angular deformity in both planes ($\partial - x$ and $\partial - y$) can be measured. Deriving from these projected angles, the true angle of deformity (∂)[73] is determined using the appropriate table. By analogy the orientation of the deformity in space (β)[73] can be found. If in correct AP and lateral radiographs the profiles of the bicipital tuberosity and the ulnar styloid present differently, relevant axial rotatory malalignment must suspected (**Figs. 18–5** and **18–6**). The exact amount of radial and ulnar torsion can be measured using comparative CT scans of both forearms.[74] After systematic assessment of alternative landmarks, the bicipital tuberosity and the square section of the radius at the level of the Lister's tubercle for the ulna the trochlea humeri and the styloid were most reliable (**Fig. 18–7**).[75,76] Considerable intraindividual side to side differences were found, however.[76] Thus, only a relevant difference, corresponding to the rotatory component (π) of the malunion, can be calculated and included into the preoperative planning.

When deciding whether an opening or a closing wedge osteotomy is suitable, the ulnar variance of the malunited and the healthy side need to be compared. Generally, a closing wedge osteotomy will result in further shortening. Therefore, it is appropriate in the presence of a relative overlength of the malunited bone or when both forearm bones are corrected. In this case, their individual length can be adjusted upon the neighbor bone. In the planning of any closing wedge osteotomy, the height of the base of the wedge (including the true angle of deformity ∂) should be measured at the determined osteotomy site. In an opening wedge osteotomy, a variable amount of lengthening can be achieved using an interpositional bone graft, preferably a compression-resistant, corticocancellous graft from the iliac crest. Moreover, this graft, with its triangular or trapezoidal shape, again includes the true angle of deformity ∂.

The surgical approach is predetermined in incomplete closing and opening wedge osteotomies only, as the cortex

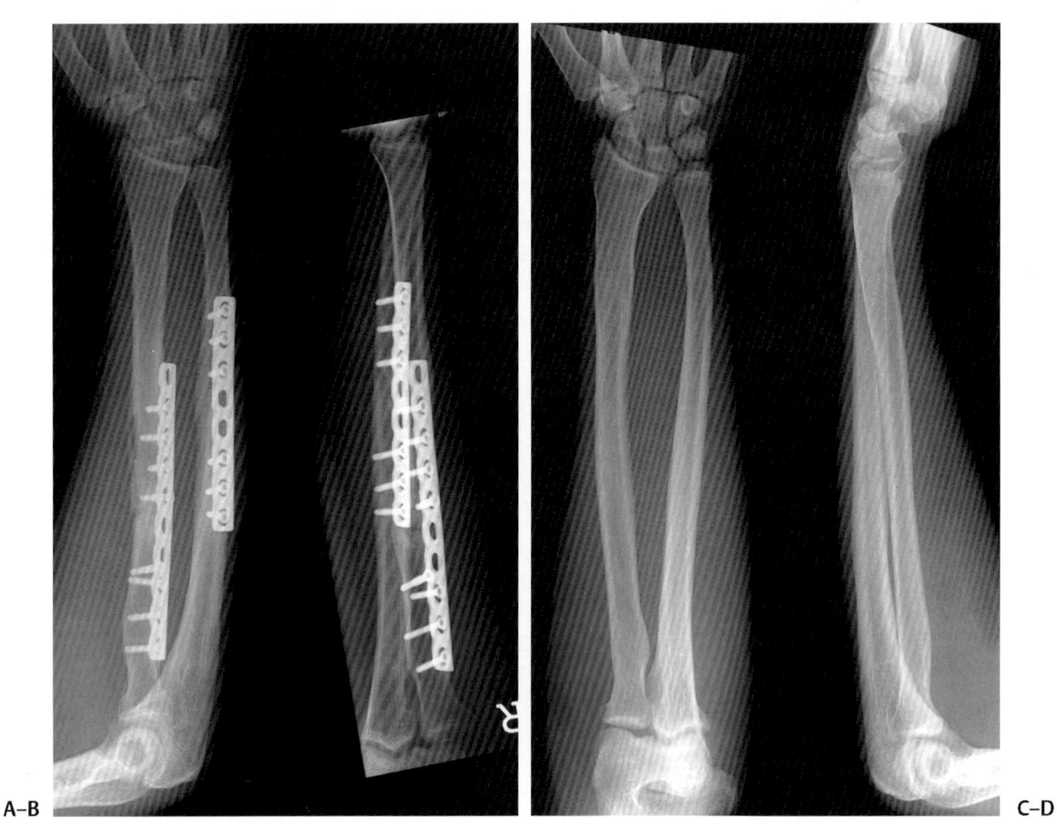

Figure 18–5 (A,B) A 20-year-old man who sustained a closed forearm fracture, treated with open reduction and internal fixation 1 year ago. Malunion and complete loss of supination after failed internal fixation of the radius. **(C,D)** Contralateral x-rays. The contralateral side was asymptomatic despite a distal radius malunion. Comparison of different projections of the bicipital tuberosities suggests rotational malalignment.

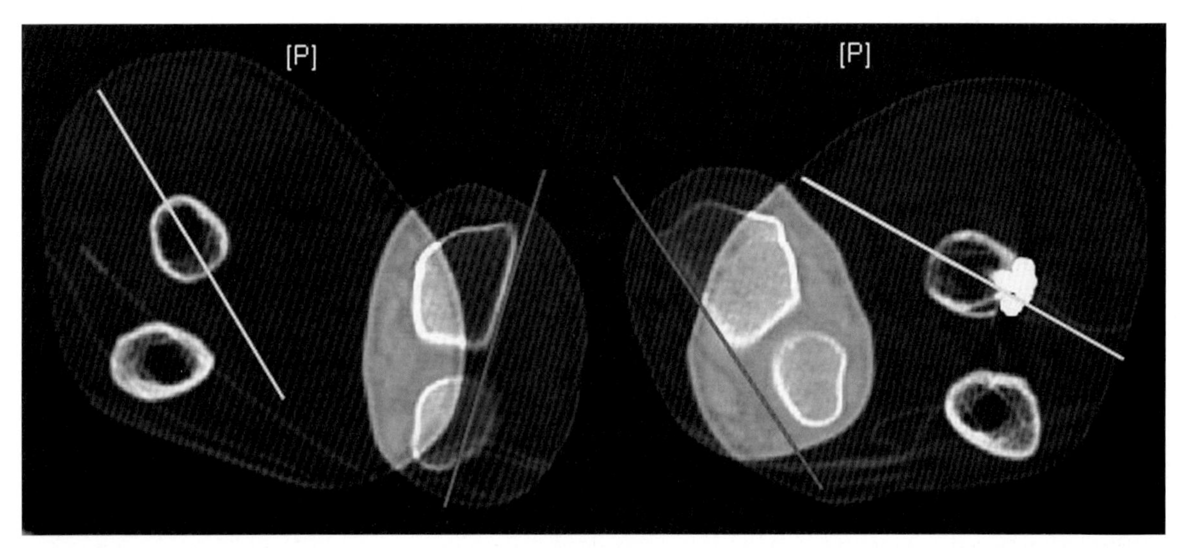

Figure 18–6 Determination of torsion profiles of the radius with comparative computed tomography scans. Lines were drawn through the bicipital tuberosities and tangential to the distal radius body. The subtended angles represent the difference in torsion of each radius. The difference between left and right is the amount of malrotation: angle π.

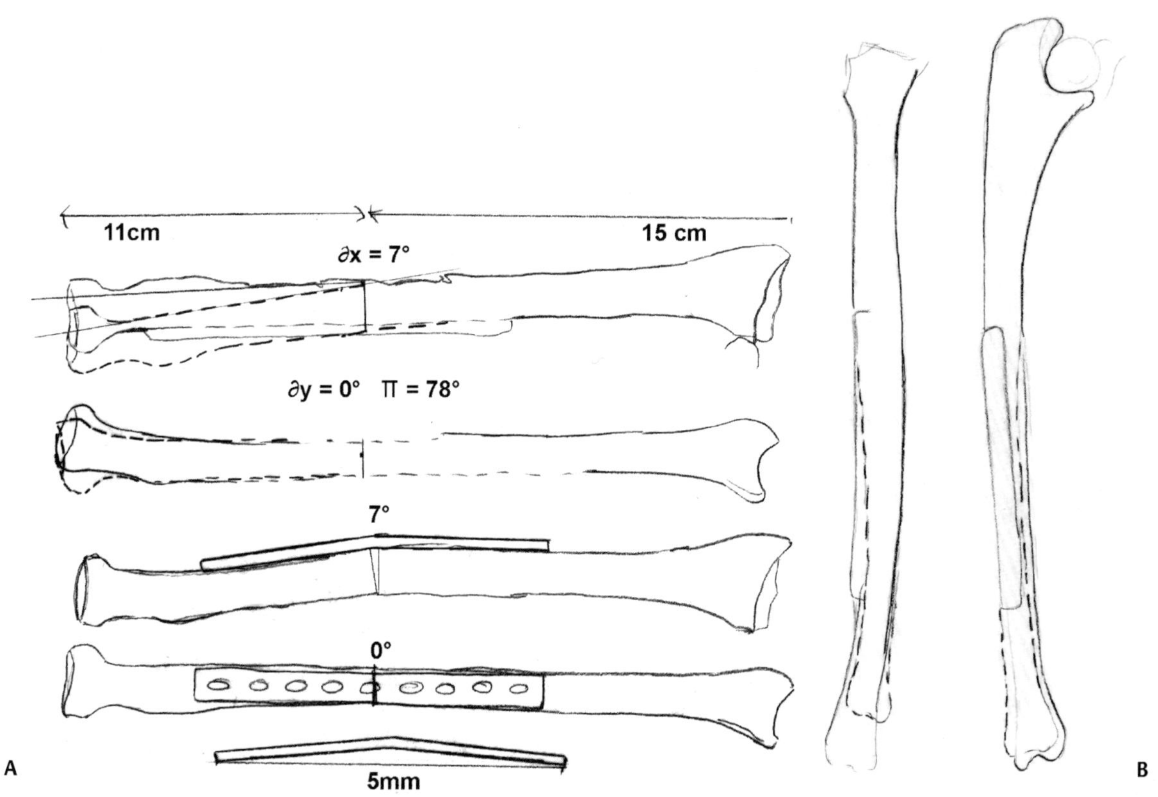

Figure 18–7 **(A)** The contours of the malunited and the contralateral (*dotted line*) radius have been superimposed. Correct shape distally. This allows detection of the site of the maximal deformity (osteotomy) and the projected angles of deformity in the two planes: ∂x, ∂y. Physician's sketch after osteotomy: The planned angle of correction has been placed between the proximal and distal fragment. The length can be compared with the ulna to decide whether an opening or closing wedge osteotomy is needed. The wedge subtends the angle of deformity ∂. The implant can be drawn at the osteotomy site and its shape can be predetermined (expressed in bow in mm). This increases the safety and ease of correction. **(B)** The contours of both ulna have been superimposed (cave: different magnification). Apparently the shape is almost identical; therefore, no correction is needed.

opposite to the hinge has to be exposed and also the plate is best placed here. In complete (all rotational and larger interpositional) osteotomies the approach depends on the surgeon's preference. Whenever possible, as for nonunions, we prefer the Henry approach for the whole radius and the interval between the FCU and ECU muscles for the ulna.

The planned level of the osteotomy is determined by measuring the distance from the distal and the proximal end of the bone. Before cutting, orientation Kirschner wires marking the exact AP or lateral plane must be inserted on both sides of the osteotomy. Often the plate (mostly a 6- or 8-hole 3.5-mm LCDC plate) can be temporarily fixed to one of the future fragments and contoured according the intended correction. It is then removed, but will later help to reduce the osteotomy and also to control the amount of correction.

Then the height of the planned wedge is drawn on the bone. From these marks converging saw cuts (incorporating the true angle of deformity = ∂) are made to remove an incomplete bone wedge in the proper orientation (in the plane of the true deformity = β). This allows for closing the osteotomy around an intact hinge. The plate is then reapplied and fixed to the other fragment mostly in the compression mode. In cases with documented rotatory malalignment (π) exceeding 30 degrees, rotational correction at the side of the osteotomy must be included **(Fig. 18–8)**. Intraoperatively, the accuracy of angular correction is routinely checked by standard biplanar radiographs. If the correct reconstruction of the true anatomical shape of the forearm bones does not result in free motion, the IOM is exposed mostly at the level of the osteotomy and sectioned in both directions until rotation is free. In some cases, the contracted IOM may impede the reduction of the osteotomy and needs to be split to permit reduction and ease of forearm rotation.

The incision is closed over a suction tube and a protective cock-up splint is worn until the pain subsides. On the second day, active- and passive-assisted motion therapy are begun. If passive motion does not reach 60% of the opposite side at 4 weeks, dynamic splinting in pronation or/and supination is begun. Strengthening is started in

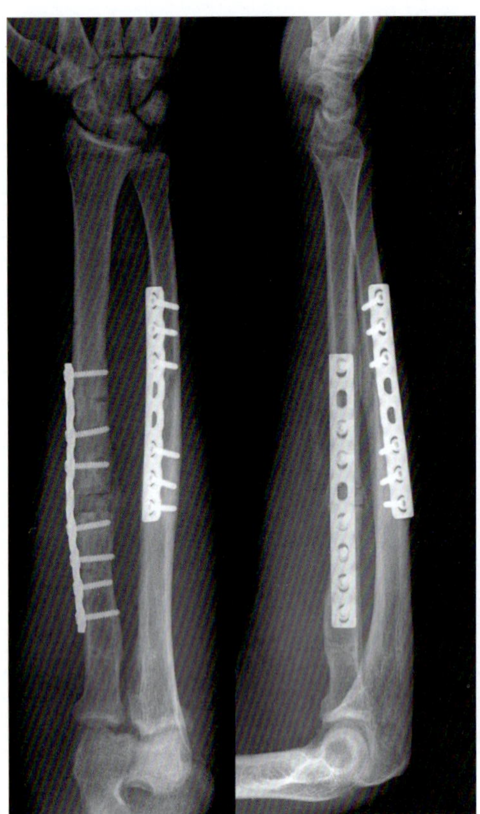

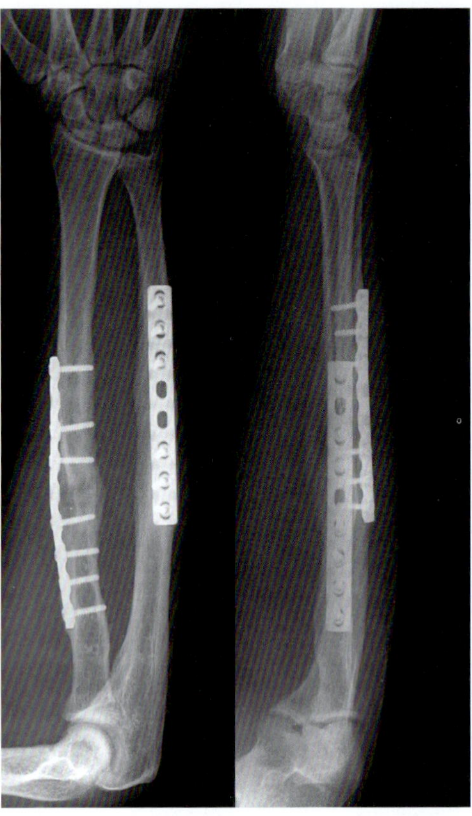

Figure 18–8 (A,B) Radiographs immediately after corrective osteotomy of the radius with interposition of a corticocancellous graft. The height of the graft was adjusted to the size of the defect after resection of fibrotic, hypovascular bone. Notice widening of the interosseous space. The ulna was left alone. **(C,D)** Radiographic appearance of the osteotomy 6 months after surgery showing complete incorporation of the interposed graft.

week 6 to 8 with full weight bearing and sports after documentation of bone consolidation **(Fig. 18–9)**.

Results

The clinical scenario of patients with forearm malunion may present as restriction of rotational movement or instability of the DRUJ. Both can be reliably treated by corrective osteotomy and release of the IOM contracture. Furthermore, malunited proximal ulna fractures have associated radial head dislocation, whereas malunited proximal radius fractures result in incongruity and subluxation of the PRUJ. Additional open reduction of the radial head and creation of an annular ligament is required in the first clinical setting together with the corrective osteotomy.

Patients with limited supination appear to have more functional improvement from osteotomy than those with limited pronation. In general, following skeletal realignment DRUJ instability disappears without adjunct ligament reconstruction and without loss of mobility. The release of the contracted IOM in cases with correct 3D anatomy of the forearm bones and stable radioulnar joints does not result in any impairment, especially with regard to strength or stability.

The methods for assessment of deformity, especially the rotational component, are (despite the increase in sophistication) only of relative usefulness, as they are based on anatomical structures with variable morphology.

The definition of deformity, leading to the diagnosis and ultimately the basis for the preoperative planning, is based upon the assumption of symmetrical 3D anatomy. Despite considerable contralateral variations in healthy subjects, based on plain radiographs, the healthy contralateral side allows for a quite simple geometrical analysis of deformity, careful preoperative planning, and successful correction.

Corrective osteotomies of diaphyseal forearm malunions reliably improve forearm rotation and restore cosmesis and function of the radioulnar joints, provided they are meticulously planned and rigidly fixed. Restoration of the radial bow, angular and rotational malalignment, release of soft tissue contracture (capsular, IOM), and reconstruction of the RUJs are all equally important additional surgical measures to guarantee a good result.

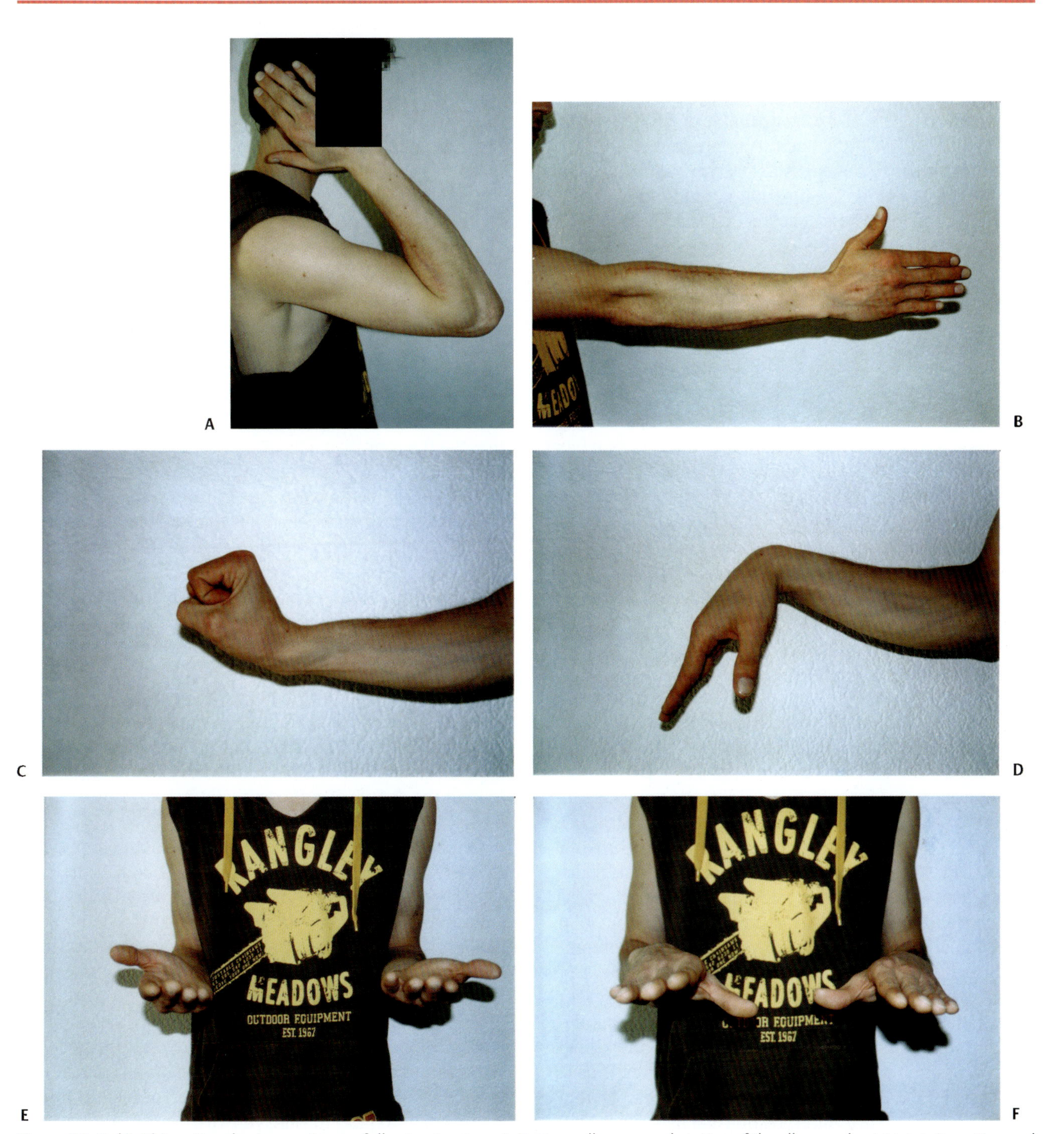

Figure 18–9 (A–F) Functional outcome 2 years following treatment. Notice well-preserved motion of the elbow and wrist joint. Pronation and supination were almost symmetrical and the patient was free of symptoms.

Posttraumatic Radioulnar Synostosis

Synostosis of the forearm bone following fractures is relatively uncommon. In Anderson and coworkers'[2] series of 112 fractures treated with plate fixation, only 3 had a complete synostosis. In Ring and Jupiter's series, three synostoses were observed out of 48 Monteggia fractures, most commonly in Bado type II patterns with posteriorly dislocated radial heads.[77] Vince and Miller[78] reported an overall 2% incidence of synostosis in their series. Patients in whom a synostosis develops frequently have a history of high-energy trauma, head injury, or have a displaced comminuted fracture at the same level. Other etiologic factors are the use of excessive bone graft at the IOM level, malreduction of the fracture, or presence of too long implants contacting the opposite forearm bone. Vince and Miller[78] developed a classification system based on the anatomic location of the synostosis. Type I involves the distal forearm and was the least common in their series. Type II is localized in the midshaft area and was the most common in their study. Type III involves the proximal third and is overall the most common localization because of the close proximity of the radius and ulna over a long distance, the presence of metaphyseal cancellous bone, as well as the higher incidence of complex combined comminuted fracture dislocation and associated soft tissue injuries at this level. Jupiter and Ring further subclassified proximal radioulnar synostoses into three types: A, synostosis at or distal to the bicipital tuberosity; B, synostosis involving the radial head and the PRUJ; and C, synostosis contiguous with bone extending across the elbow to the distal aspect of the humerus.[79]

Treatment

If a synostosis develops and the forearm rotation is blocked in a relatively functional position (usually 20 to 40 degrees of pronation) nonoperative treatment may be considered if the patient is asymptomatic.

Surgical procedures that do not resect the synostosis include the rotational osteotomy to place the forearm in a functional position[80] or the creation of a pseudarthrosis of the radius distal to a proximal synostosis.[81] The first modality does not restore forearm rotation; the second aims at reestablishing a functional arc of pronation and supination. Resection of the synostosis is, however, the most common and direct treatment indicated for this condition. Because of the concern of recurrence after simple resection, several authors have reported the use of biologic or foreign interposition material. Following excision of the bony bridge, the interposition material theoretically would create a biologic barrier between the raw bony surfaces, thereby preventing recurrence. Interposition barriers have been composed of free fat,[79–82] local muscle, and silicone rubber sheets.[84–89] The reported number of patients treated in all these studies are small and nonrandomized, therefore not statistically significant. Furthermore, because nonvascularized tissue is eventually replaced with scar tissue, these interposition materials do not completely control the risk of recurrence, nor do they guarantee functional improvement in either congenital or posttraumatic forearm synostosis.[84,90] Coadjuvant radiation therapy has also been proposed to reduce the risk of recurrence.[91–94] Adding up the patients treated in the four studies referenced, no recurrences were observed in a total of 14 patients treated with early excision and single-dose radiation with doses of 5 to 10 gray (500 to 1,000 rad). Pre- and postoperative low-dose prophylactic radiation is now a routine adjuvant treatment modality in patients with high risk of recurrence.

Conversely, Jupiter and Ring[79] reported highly satisfactory results in 16 out of 17 patients, in whom no adjuvant radiotherapy or nonsteroidal antiinflammatory medication was used following wide resection of the bony bridge. Free fat interposition was used in 8 out of 17 patients in their series. The only recurrence of synostosis was in a patient with a closed head trauma. The authors found that the ultimate ROM was not affected by any of the variables generally cited as contributing factors: size and location of the synostosis, severity of initial trauma, use of a free nonvascularized fat interposition, and especially time between injury and excision. Excision between 6 and 12 months after initial injury did not increase the risk of recurrence; they also found that patients with earlier resections had better motion than those treated at a later date.

The timing of resection is dictated by the presence of distinct margins and linear trabecular orientation of the synostosis in plain radiographs. Cessation of osteogenic activity and maturity of the bony bridge are usually complete by 6 months following injury.[95] Bone scans or assessment of alkaline phosphatase in serum to determine the maturity of heterotopic ossification are no longer necessary. Early resection is preferable because of its potential ability to limit the degree of soft tissue contracture, as well as the overall period of severe disability.

Our current treatment recommendations are to perform an early and wide resection of types II and III primary synostoses followed by immediate active mobilization. Low-dose radiotherapy or indomethacin are not likely needed, except if recurrence risk factors are present. These include severe initial soft tissue injury, head trauma, prior recurrence, and skeletal immaturity.[78,84,96]

The management of distal forearm synostosis (type I) is slightly different. Either a resection interposition arthroplasty of the DRUJ with resection of the cross-union may be selected, or a pseudarthrotic gap of the distal ulna is created proximal to the synostosis to restore forearm rotation. In the first treatment modality, a wide resection of the bony bridge between the distal radius and ulna is performed along with a remodeling of the distal ulna as described by Watson and colleagues in their matched distal ulnar resection technique.[97] The space left after resection is filled with viable muscle utilizing the pronator quadratus and/or an "anchovy" of a proximally based musculotendinous segment of the ECU muscle.[98] Alternatively, following wide resection of the distal ulna and the bony bridge, an ulnar head prosthesis with long neck can

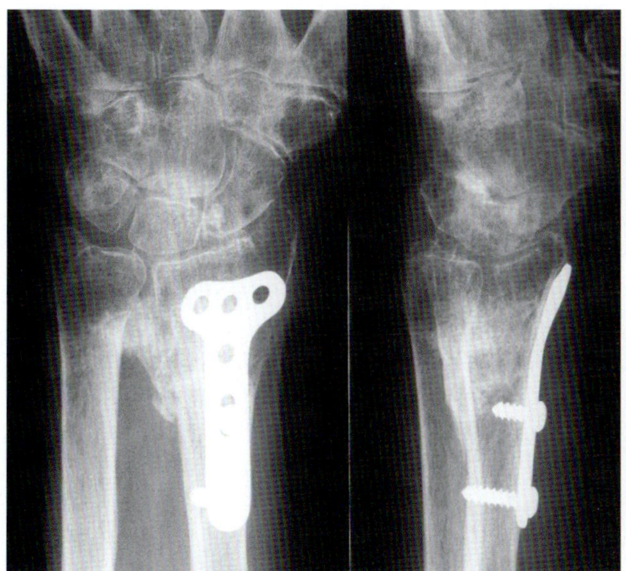

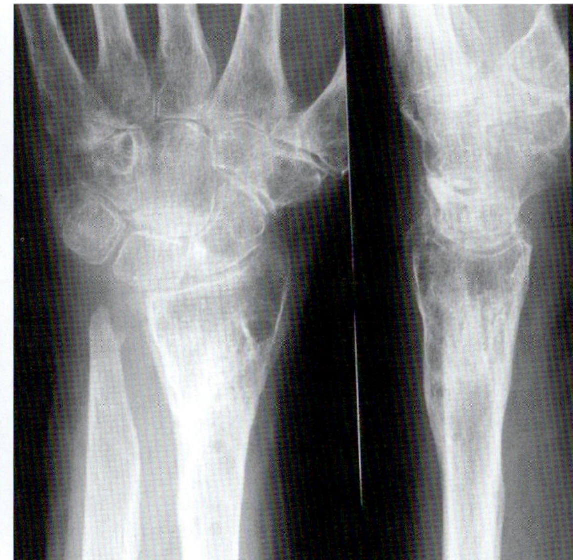

Figure 18–10 (A,B) Radiographs before and **(C,D)** after management of a distal radioulnar synostosis with resection of the bony bridge and a distal radioulnar joint resection interposition arthroplasty. The distal ulna was shaped as in a Watson procedure and a combined muscle interposition with pronator quadratus and an anchovy with a 6-cm long strip of half of the extensor carpi ulnaris muscle was performed.

be inserted to reconstruct the DRUJ (**Fig. 18–10**). The second option is to maintain the distal synostosis (provided that the DRUJ is congruous and no length discrepancy of the radius and ulna is present) and create an 8- to 10-mm pseudarthrosis gap proximal to the synostosis as in a Sauvé–Kapandji procedure.[99,100]

Recurrent Forearm Synostosis

Although recurrence rates following primary resection of posttraumatic radioulnar synostosis with[83,91] or without[79] coadjuvant radiation therapy have been significantly reduced, management of the recurrence after primary excision continues to represent a difficult challenge because rerecurrence is not uncommon. This is especially true in children and in patients for whom the use of adjuvant low-dose radiation therapy is contraindicated.

For proximal (type III) synostosis, the average overall recurrence rate following excision of a primary synostosis is 32% (60% in Vince and Miller's,[78,97] 33% in Failla et al's,[84] and 5% in Jupiter and Ring's series[79]). In children, the recurrence rates are significantly higher, with a 66% recurrence in type III lesions and 33% in type II lesions. Periosteal-increased osteogenic potential in the immature skeleton is believed to be responsible for the higher incidence of recurrence in children. Due to the unpredictability of the use of foreign materials or nonvascular tissue to control recurrence in primary radioulnar synostosis, the use of the vascularized muscle[101] and vascularized fat flaps[102] as interposition material was subsequently reported. Kanaya and Ibaraki successfully used a free vascularized fasciocutaneous graft for the treatment of congenital radioulnar synostosis in 7 patients with good functional outcomes.[103] Following the same reasoning, we have interposed vascularized muscle tissue in a wrap-around fashion in 5 patients with recurrent posttraumatic synostosis. Our objective was to obliterate the space left following wide resection with viable muscle tissue that would maintain its contractility, prevent rerecurrence, and restore a functional arc of forearm rotation. The first author (DLF) reported the management of three proximal and two midshaft recurrent radioulnar synostoses with a wrap-around vascularized muscle interposition after excision of the heterotopic bone. A proximally pedicled brachioradialis flap was used for the proximal forearm and elbow synostoses, and the FCU muscle was used for the midshaft area (**Fig. 18–11**).[104]

The only contraindication for the use of the brachioradialis flap is a nonfunctioning or damaged biceps brachii. The biceps must be available to compensate for the loss of supination force when the supinator is damaged or partly ossified at the level of the synostosis. This proximally pedicled flap is elevated through a Henry approach, protecting its main vascular pedicle arising from the recurrent radial artery. The synostosis is resected through a second incision between the anconeus and ECU muscle. Exposure of the synostosis requires elevation of the supinator. Careful protection of the posterior interosseous nerve during resection of the synostosis is mandatory. The brachioradialis muscle flap is now passed around the proximal radius with a strong stay-suture in the distal

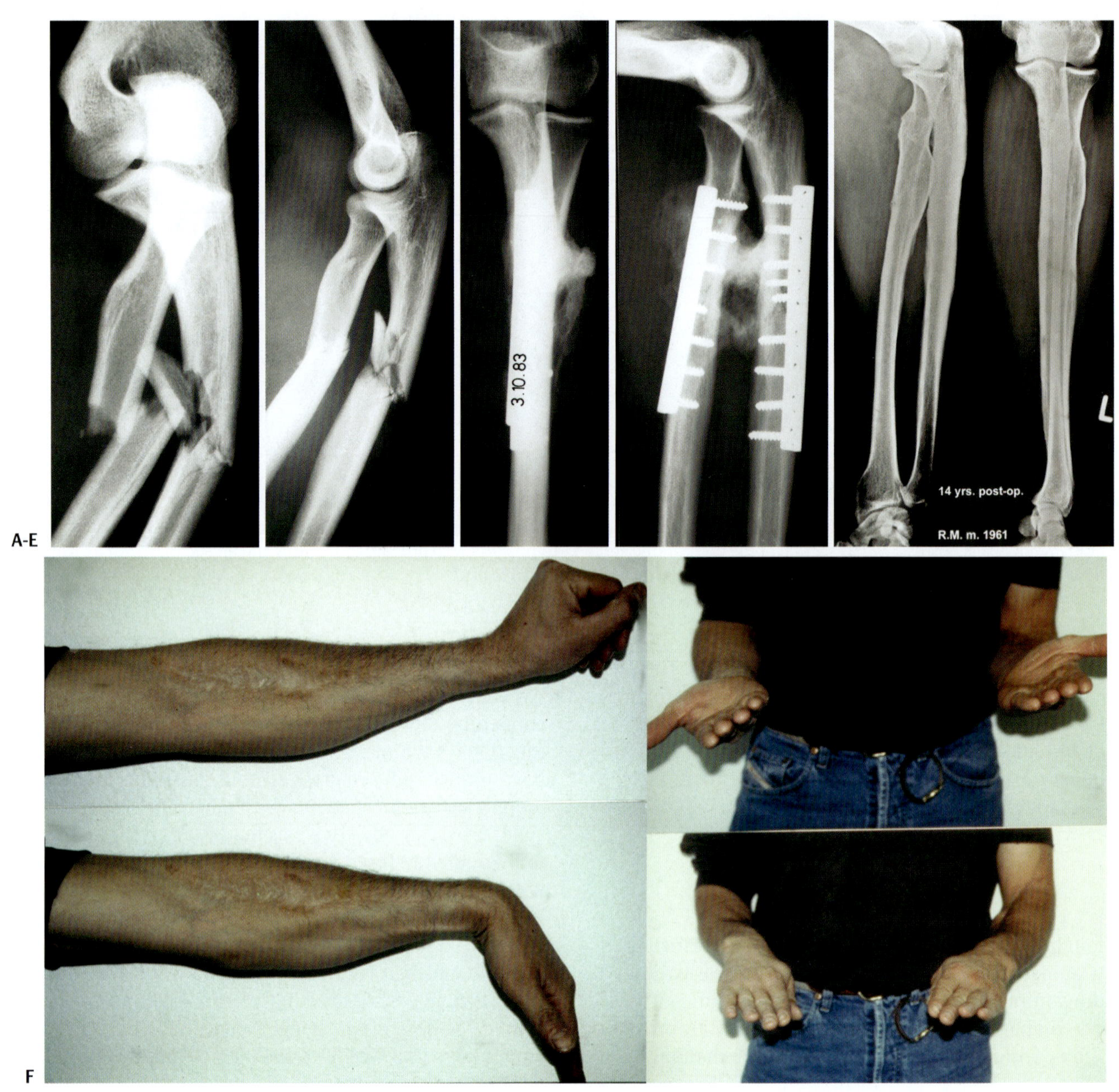

Figure 18–11 (A–D) Recurrent radioulnar synostosis following internal fixation of a comminuted proximal forearm fracture. The patient had already had a prior resection with free fat interposition. **(E)** Radiographic and **(F,G)** clinical result 14 years after resection of the synostosis and wrap around interposition with a flexor carpi ulnaris muscle flap. The patient regained a functional forearm rotation arc of 80 degrees.

tendon and brought out through the posterior incision. Passive forearm rotation is then tested. Secondary contractures of the IOM that may contribute to limitation of prosupination should be released at this point of the procedure. Thereafter, the muscle flap is sutured to itself to envelop the proximal radius and cover the site of the resected bony bridge. For diaphyseal (type II) recurrent synostosis, we have used the FCU muscle because of its anatomic proximity to the ulna and its length. A single longitudinal incision along the ulnar border of the forearm is usually sufficient to expose both the synostosis and the FCU muscle. The synostosis is exposed by retracting the ECU muscle dorsally and the origin of the flexor digitorum profundus on the volar side. Extreme caution not to damage the innervation of these muscles must be taken throughout the whole procedure. Following excision of the synostosis and additional IOM release, the FCU muscle is then detached from its distal insertion and is carefully dissected proximally, stopping at a point 7 to 10 cm distal to the medial epicondyle. During distal elevation of the muscle flap, the superficial branch of the ulnar nerve is visualized and protected. The distal tendinous portion of the muscle is tagged with a large suture and passed with a right angle clamp around the middle third of the ulna from the anterior into the posterior compartment. The muscle is then sutured to itself to envelop the middle third of the ulna in a wrap-around fashion and cover the site of the resected bony bridge.

Postoperatively, in both the brachioradialis and the FCU muscle flaps, the wounds are closed over drains and a splint is applied with the elbow in 90 degrees of flexion. Immobilization is used only for edema control. After 5 to 7 days, once the swelling has decreased, rehabilitation is begun with an emphasis on active ROM.

Our patients were followed up for an average of 8 years (range: 3 to 14 years). There were no recurrences. The functional outcome regarding forearm rotation, elbow motion, and working capacity was highly satisfactory in all 5 patients. These results were very rewarding when compared to the outcomes of two studies[78,84] which addressed this issue of recurrent synostosis – nearly two thirds of the patients had a rerecurrence.

The interposition of viable muscle tissue not only obliterates the critical interosseous space, but also acts as a biologic barrier to prevent another synostosis. We believe that vascularized muscle with intact innervation will retain its contractility, maintain its volume, and therefore function as a dynamic spacer during active use of the forearm. Our current indication for the wrap-around technique is reserved for patients with recalcitrant, recurrent radioulnar synostosis that has failed prior surgical intervention in children or in patients whose risk factors preclude the use of adjuvant radiation therapy.

References

1. Chapman MW, Gordon JE, Zissimos AG. Compression-plate fixation of acute fractures of the diaphysis of the radius and ulna. J Bone Joint Surg Am 1989;71:159–169
2. Anderson LD, Sisk D, Tooms RE, Pard WI III. Compression-plate fixation in acute diaphyseal fracture of the radius and ulna. J Bone Joint Surg Am 1975;57:287–297
3. Wei SY, Born CT, Abene A, Ong A, Hayda R, DeLong WG Jr. Diaphyseal forearm fractures treated with and without bone graft. J Trauma 1999;46:1045–1048
4. Stern PJ, Drury WJ. Complications of plate fixation of forearm fractures. Clin Orthop Relat Res 1983;175:25–29
5. Schemitsch EH, Richards RR. The effect of malunion on fuctional outcome after plate fixation of fractures of both bones of the forearm in adults. J Bone Joint Surg Am 1992;74:1068–1078
6. Weber BG, Cech O. Pseudarthrosis. Bern: Hans Huber Publishers; 1976:85–94
7. Müller ME. Treatment of nonunion by compression. Clin Orthop Relat Res 1965;43:83–91
8. Ring D, Allende C, Jafarnia K, Allende BT, Jupiter JB. Ununited diaphyseal forearm fractures with segmental defects: plate fixation and autogenous cancellous bone-grafting. J Bone Joint Surg Am 2004;86:2440–2445
9. Weiland AJ, Kleiner HE, Kutz J, Danie RK. Free vascularized bone grafts in surgery of the upper extremity. J Hand Surg Am 1979;4:129–144
10. Wood MB. Upper extremity reconstruction by vascularized bone transfer: results and complications. J Hand Surg Am1987;12:422–427
11. Castle ME. One-bone forearm. J Bone Joint Surg Am 1974; 56:1223–1227
12. Haddad RJ, Drez D. Salvage procedures for defects of the forearm bones. Clin Orthop Relat Res 1974;104:183–190
13. Reid RL, Baker GI. The single-bone forearm: a reconstructive technique. Hand 1973;5:214–219
14. Paterson D. Treatment of nonunion with a constant direct current: a totally implantable system. Orthop Clin North Am 1984;15:47–59
15. Scott G, King JB. A prospective, double-blind trial of electrical capacitive coupling in the treatment of non-union of long bones. J Bone Joint Surg Am 1994;76:820–826
16. Johnson EE, Urist MR, Finerman GA. Resistant nonunions and partial or complete segmental defects of long bones: treatment with implants of a composite of human bone morphogenetic protein (BMP) and autolyzed, antigen-extracted, allogeneic (AAA) bone. Clin Orthop Relat Res 1992;277:229–237
17. Kawamura M, Urist MR. Induction of callus formation by implants of bone morphogenetic protein and associated bone matrix noncollagenous proteins. Clin Orthop Relat Res 1988;236:240–248
18. Catagni MA, Guerreschi F, Holman JA, Cattaneo R. Distraction osteogenesis in the treatment of stiff hypertrophic nonunions using the Ilizarov apparatus. Clin Orthop Relat Res 1994;301:159–163
19. Henry AK. Extensile Exposure. 2nd ed. Baltimore, MD: Williams & Wilkins; 1957
20. Jupiter JB, Ruedi T. Intraoperative distraction in the treatment of complex nonunions of the radius. J Hand Surg 1992;17:416–422
21. van Schoonhoven J, Fernandez DL, Bowers WH, Herbert TJ. Salvage of failed resection arthroplasties of the distal radioulnar joint using a new ulnar head endoprosthesis. J Hand Surg Am 2000;25:438–446
22. Barbieri CH, Mazzer N, Aranda CA, Pinto MM. Use of a bone block graft from the iliac crest with rigid fixation to correct diaphyseal defects of the radius and ulna. J Hand Surg Br 1997;22:395–401
23. Mast J, Jakob R, Ganz R. Planning and Reduction Techniques in Fracture Surgery. New York, NY: Springer; 1989:3–5

24. Mast JW, Teitge RA, Gowda M. Preoperative planning for the treatment of nonunions and the correction of malunions of long bones. Orthop Clin North Am 1990;21:693–714
25. Dell PC, Sheppard JE. Vascularized bone grafts in the treatment of infected forearm nonunions. J Hand Surg Am 1984;9:653–658
26. Hurst LC, Mirza MA, Spellman W. Vascular fibular graft for infected loss of the ulna: case report. J Hand Surg Am 1982;7:498–501
27. Jupiter JB, Gerhard HJ, Guerrero J, Nunley JA, Levin LS. Treatment of segmental defects of the radius with use of the vascularized osteoseptocutaneous fibular autogenous graft. J Bone Joint Surg Am 1997;79:542–550
28. Safoury Y. Free vascularized fibula for the treatment of traumatic bone defects and nonunion of the forearm bones. J Hand Surg Br 2005;30:67–72
29. Brunner CF, Weber BG. Special Techniques in Internal Fixation. Telger TC, translator. New York, NY: Springer; 1982
30. Blatter G, Weber BG. Wave plate osteosynthesis as a salvage procedure. Arch Orthop Trauma Surg 1990;109:330–333
31. Ring D, Jupiter JB, Quintero J, Sander RA, Marti RK. Atrophic ununited fractures of the humerus with a bony defect: treatment by wave-plate osteosynthesis. J Bone Joint Surg Br 2000;82:867–871
32. Blount WP. Forearm fractures in children. Clin Orthop Relat Res 1940;51:93–107
33. Davis DR, Green DP. Forearm fractures in children: pitfalls and complications. Clin Orthop Relat Res 1976;120:172–183
34. Friberg KS. Remodelling after distal forearm fractures in children. III. Correction of residual angulation in fractures of the radius. Acta Orthop Scand 1979;50:741–749
35. Perona PG, Light TR. Remodeling of the skeletally immature distal radius. J Orthop Trauma 1990;4:356–361
36. Blount WP. Fractures in Children. Baltimore, MD: Williams & Wilkins; 1955:2–7
37. Gandhi RK, Wilson P, Mason Brown JJ, Macleod W. Spontaneous correction of deformity following fractures of the forearm in children. Br J Surg 1962;50:5–10
38. Slongo T, Jakob RP. Surgical correction following shaft fractures in childhood and adolescence: indications. Z Unfallchir Versicherungsmed 1990;83:91–103
39. Friberg KS. Remodeling after distal forearm fractures in children. I. The effect of residual angulation on the spatial orientation of the epiphyseal plates. Acta Orthop Scand 1979;50:537–546
40. Friberg KS. Remodeling after distal forearm fractures in children. II. The final orientation of the distal and proximal epiphyseal plates of the radius. Acta Orthop Scand 1979;50:731–739
41. Karaharju EO, Alho A, Nieminen J. The results of operative and non-operative management of tibial fractures. Injury 1975;7:47–52
42. Larsen E, Vittas D, Torp-Pedersen S. Remodeling of angulated distal forearm fractures in children. Clin Orthop Relat Res 1988;237:190–195
43. Fuller DJ, McCullough CJ. Malunited fractures of the forearm in children. J Bone Joint Surg Br 1982;64:364–367
44. Price CT, Scott DS, Kurzner ME, Flynn JC. Malunited forearm fractures in children. J Pediatr Orthop 1990;10:705–712
45. Daruwalla JS. A study of radioulnar movements following fractures of the forearm in children. Clin Orthop Relat Res 1979;139:114–120
46. Borden S IV. Traumatic bowing of the forearm in children. J Bone Joint Surg Am 1974;56:611–616
47. Borden S IV. Roentgen recognition of acute plastic bowing of the forearm in children. Am J Roentgenol Radium Ther Nucl Med 1975;125:524–530
48. Prommersberger KJ, Lanz U. Malunited fractures of the forearm during the growth period with special reference to the forearm longitudinal axis. Case reports. Handchir Mikrochir Plast Chir 2000;32:250–259
49. Sarmiento A, Ebramzadeh E, Brys D, Tarr R. Angular deformities and forearm function. J Orthop Res 1992;10:121–133
50. Graham TJ, Fischer TJ, Hotchkiss RN, Kleinmann WB. Disorders of the forearm axis. Hand Clin 1998;14:305–316
51. Matthews LS, Kaufer H, Garver DF, Sonstegard DA. The effect on supination-pronation of angular malalignment of fractures of both bones of the forearm. J Bone Joint Surg Am 1982;64:14–17
52. Tynan MC, Fornalski S, McMahon PJ, Utkan A, Green SA, Lee TQ. The effects of ulnar axial malalignment on supination and pronation. J Bone Joint Surg Am 2000;82:1726–1731
53. Trousdale RT, Linscheid RL. Operative treatment of malunited fractures of the forearm. J Bone Joint Surg Am 1995;77:894–902
54. Tarr RR, Garfinkel AI, Sarmiento A. The effects of angular and rotational deformities of both bones of the forearm. An in vitro study. J Bone Joint Surg Am 1984;66:65–70
55. Dumont CE, Thalmann R, Macy JC. The effect of rotational malunion of the radius and the ulna on supination and pronation. J Bone Joint Surg Br 2002;84:1070–1074
56. Kleinman WB, Graham TJ. The distal radioulnar joint capsule: clinical anatomy and role in posttraumatic limitation of forearm rotation. J Hand Surg Am 1998;23:588–599
57. Spinner M, Kaplan EB. Extensor carpi ulnaris. Its relationship to the stability of the distal radio-ulnar joint. Clin Orthop Relat Res 1970;68:124–129
58. Lengsfeld M, Strauss JM, Koebke J. Functional importance of the m. extensor carpi ulnaris for distal radioulnar articulation. Handchir Mikrochir Plast Chir 1988;20:275–278
59. Kihara H, Short WH, Werner FW, Fortino MD, Palmer AK. The stabilizing mechanism of the distal radioulnar joint during pronation and supination. J Hand Surg Am 1995;20:930–936
60. Palmer AK, Werner FW. Biomechanics of the distal radioulnar joint. Clin Orthop Relat Res 1984;187:26–35
61. Darrach W. Forward dislocation of the inferior radioulnar joint, with fracture of the lower third of the shaft oh the radius. Ann Surg 1912;56:801–802
62. Essex-Lopresti P. Fractures of the radial head with distal radioulnar dislocation: report of two cases. J Bone Joint Surg Br 1951;33:244–247
63. Hughston JC. Fracture of the distal radial shaft; mistakes in management. J Bone Joint Surg Am 1957;39:249–264

64. Bowers WH. The distal radioulnar joint. In: Green, ed. Operative and Surgery, Vol. 1. 3rd ed. New York, NY: Churchill Livingstone; 1999
65. Hotchkiss RN, An KN, Sowa DT, Basta S, Weiland AJ. An anatomic and mechanical study of the interosseous membrane of the forearm: pathomechanics of proximal migration of the radius. J Hand Surg Am 1989;14: 256–261
66. Ofuchi S, Takahashi K, Yamagata M, Rokkaku T, Moriya H, Hara T. Pressure distribution in the humeroradial joint and force transmission to the capitellum during rotation of the forearm: effects of the Sauvé-Kapandji procedure and incision of the interosseous membrane. J Orthop Sci 2001;6:33–38
67. Poitevin LA. Anatomy and biomechanics of the interosseous membrane: its importance in the longitudinal stability of the forearm. Hand Clin 2001;17:97–110
68. Ward LD, Ambrose CG, Masson MV, Levaro F. The role of the distal radioulnar ligaments, interosseous membrane, and joint capsule in distal radioulnar joint stability. J Hand Surg Am 2000;25:341–351
69. Gofton WT, Gordon KD, Dunning CE, Johnson JA, King GJ. Soft-tissue stabilizers of the distal radioulnar joint: an in vitro kinematic study. J Hand Surg Am 2004;29: 423–431
70. Christensen JB, Adams JP, Cho KO, Miller L. A study of the interosseous distance between the radius and ulna during rotation of the forearm. Anat Rec 1968;160:261–271
71. Skahen JR III, Palmer AK, Werner FW, Fortino MD. The interosseous membrane of the forearm: anatomy and function. J Hand Surg Am 1997;22:981–985
72. Zancolli EA. Paralytic supination contracture of the forearm. J Bone Joint Surg Am 1967;49:1275–1284
73. Nagy L. Malunion of the distal end of the radius. In: Fernandez DL, Jupiter JB, eds. Fractures of the Distal Radius, a Practical Approach to Management. 2nd ed. New York, NY: Springer; 2002: 289–344
74. Bindra RR, Cole RJ, Yamaguchi K, et al. Quantification of the radial torsion angle with computerized tomography in cadaver specimens. J Bone Joint Surg Am 1997;79: 833–837
75. Dumont C, Nagy L, Ziegler D, Pfirrmann C. Assessment of the radial and the ulnar torsion profiles with fluoroscopy coupled with goniometry and with MR cross-sectional imaging in volunteers. J Bone Joint Surg Am 2006
76. Dumont C, Nagy L, Ziegler D, Pfirrmann C. Assessment of the radial and the ulnar diaphyseal axial torsions with magnetic resonance imaging in volunteers. J Hand Surg Am 2006
77. Ring D, Jupiter RB, Simpson NS. Monteggia fractures in adults. J Bone Joint Surg Am 1998;80:1733–1744
78. Vince KG, Miller JE. Cross-union complicating fracture of the forearm. Part I: Adults. J Bone Joint Surg Am 1987;69: 640–653
79. Jupiter JB, Ring D. Operative treatment of post-traumatic proximal radiounlar synostosis. J Bone Joint Surg Am 1998;80:248–257
80. Canale ST. Campbell's Operative Orthopaedics, Vol. 3. 10th ed. Philadelphia, PA: Mosby; 2003:3103–3105
81. Kamineni S, Maritz NG, Morrey BV. Proximal radial resection for posttraumatic radioulnar synostosis: a new technique to improve forearm rotation. J Bone Joint Surg Am 2002;84-A:745–751
82. Yong-Hing K, Tschang SPK. Traumatic radioulnar synostosis treated by excision and a free fat transplant: a report of two cases. J Bone Joint Surg Br 1983;65:433–435
83. Yong-Hing K, Tchang SP. Post-traumatic radio-ulnar synostosis treated by excision and free fat transplant: a report of two cases. J Bone Joint Surg Br 1983;65:433–435
84. Failla JM, Amadio PC, Morrey BV. Post-traumatic proximal radio-ulnar synostosis: results of surgical treatment. J Bone Joint Surg Am 1989;71:1208–1213
85. Carstam N, Eiken O. The use of silastic sheet in hand surgery. Scand J Plast Reconstr Surg Hand Surg 1971;5: 57–61
86. Corless IR. Post-traumatic radioulnar synostosis. J Bone Joint Surg Br 1977;59:510
87. Watson FM, Eaton RG. Post-traumatic radioulnar synostosis. J Trauma 1978;18:467–468
88. Poilvache G. Correction de synostose radio-cubitale post-trauamtique par interposition d'une lame de silastic. Acta Orthop Belg 1977;43:206–211
89. Garland DE, Dowling V. Forearm fractures in the head-injured adult. Clin Orthop Relat Res 1983;176:190–196
90. Dal Monte A, Andrisano A, Mignani G, et al. A critical review of the surgical treatment of congenital proximal radio-ulnar synostosis. Ital J Orthop Traumatol 1987;13: 181–186
91. Cullen JP, Pellegrini VD, Miller RJ, Jones JA. Treatment of traumatic radioulnar synostosis by excision and postoperative low-dose irradiation. J Hand Surg Am 1994;19: 394–401
92. Abrams RA, Simmons BP, Brown RA, Botte MJ. Treatment of post-traumatic radioulnar synostosis with excision and low-dose radiation. J Hand Surg Am 1993;18: 704–707
93. Thurston AJ, Spry NA. Post-traumatic radioulnar synostosis treated by surgical excision and adjunctive radiotherapy. Aust N Z J Surg 1993;63:976–980
94. Beingessner DM, Patterson SD, King GJ. Early excision of heterotopic ossification at the elbow following long-term coma. J Hand Surg Am 2000;25:483–488
95. Hastings H, Graham TJ. The classification and treatment of heterotopic ossification about the elbow and forearm. Hand Clin 1994;10:417–437
96. Vince KG, Miller JE. Cross-union complicating fracture of the forearm. Part II: Children. J Bone Joint Surg Am 1987;69:654–661
97. Watson HK, Ryu JY, Burgess RC. Matched distal ulnar resection. J Hand Surg Am 1986;11:812–817
98. Fernandez DL. Radial osteotomy and Bowers arthroplasty for malunited fractures of the distal end of the radius. J Bone Joint Surg Am 1988;70:1538–1551
99. Sauvé L, Kapandji M. Nouvelle technique de traitement chirurgical des luxations récidivantes isolées de l'extrémité inférieure du cubitus. J Chir (Paris) 1936;47:589–594
100. Lamey DM, Fernandez DL. Results of modified Sauvé-Kapandji procedure in the treatment of chronic post-

traumatic derangement of the distal radioulnar joint. J Bone Joint Surg Am 1998;80:1758–1769
101. Bell SN, Benger D. Management of radioulnar synostosis with mobilization, anconaeus interposition, and a forearm rotation assist splint. J Shoulder Elbow Surg 1999;8: 621–624
102. Sugimoto M, Masada K, Ohno H, et al. Treatment of traumatic radioulnar synostosis by excision, with interposition of a posterior interosseous island forearm flap. J Hand Surg Br 1996;21:393–395
103. Kanaya F, Ibaraki K. Mobilization of a congential proximal radioulnar synostosis with use of a free vascularized fascio-fat graft. J Bone Joint Surg Am 1998;80:1186–1192
104. Fernandez DL, Joneschild E. 'Wrap around' pedicled muscle flaps for the treatment of recurrent forearm synostosis. Tech Hand Up Extrem Surg 2004;8:102–109

Index

Note: Page numbers followed by *f* indicate figures.

E

F

G

R

S

T

U